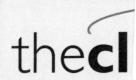 

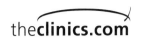

theclinics.com

CLINICS IN
GERIATRIC MEDICINE

Rheumatic Diseases in the Elderly

GUEST EDITOR
Arthur Kavanaugh, MD

August 2005 • Volume 21 • Number 3

SAUNDERS

An Imprint of Elsevier, Inc
PHILADELPHIA   LONDON   TORONTO   MONTREAL   SYDNEY   TOKYO

W.B. SAUNDERS COMPANY
A Division of Elsevier Inc.

Elsevier, Inc. • 1600 John F. Kennedy Blvd., Suite 1800 • Philadelphia, PA 19103-2899

http://www.theclinics.com

CLINICS IN GERIATRIC MEDICINE
August 2005
Editor: Maria Lorusso

Volume 21, Number 3
ISSN 0749-0690
ISBN 1-4160-2648-7

Reprints. For copies of 100 or more, of articles in this publication, please contact the Commercial Reprints Department, Elsevier Inc., 360 Park Avenue South, New York, New York 10010-1710. Tel. (212) 633-3813; Fax: (212) 462-1935; e-mail: reprints@elsevier.com.

The ideas and opinions expressed in the *Clinics in Geriatric Medicine* do not necessarily reflect those of the Publisher. The Publisher does not assume any responsibility for any injury and/or damage to persons or property arising out of or related to any use of the material contained in this periodical. The reader is advised to check the appropriate medical literature and the product information currently provided by the manufacturer of each drug to be administered to verify the dosage, the method and duration of administration, or contraindications. It is the responsibility of the treating physician or other health care professional, relying on independent experience and knowledge of the patient, to determine drug dosages and the best treatment for the patient. Mention of any product in this issue should not be construed as endorsement by the contributors, editors, or the Publisher of the product or manufacturers' claims.

Clinics in Geriatric Medicine (ISSN 0749-0690) is published quarterly by W.B. Saunders Company. Corporate and editorial offices: Elsevier, Inc. 1600 John F. Kennedy Blvd., Suite 1800, Philadelphia, PA 19103-2899. Accounting and circulation offices: 6277 Sea Harbor Drive, Orlando, FL 32887-4800. Periodicals postage paid at Orlando, FL 32862, and additional mailing offices. Subscription price is $160.00 per year (US individuals), $260.00 per year (US institutions), $205.00 per year (Canadian individuals), $320.00 per year (Canadian institutions), $210.00 per year (foreign individuals), and $320.00 per year (foreign institutions). Foreign air speed delivery is included in all *Clinics* subscription prices. All prices are subject to change without notice. POSTMASTER: Send address changes to *Clinics in Geriatric Medicine* W.B. Saunders Company, Periodicals Fulfillment, Orlando, FL 32887-4800. **Customer Service: 1-800-654-2452 (US). From outside of the US, call 1-407-345-4000. E-mail:hhspcs@harcourt.com.**

Clinics in Geriatric Medicine is covered in *Index Medicus, EMBASE/Excerpta Medica, Current Contents/Clinical Medicine (CC/CM), and the Cumulative Index to Nursing & Allied Health Literature.*

Printed in the United States of America.

GUEST EDITOR

ARTHUR KAVANAUGH, MD, Professor of Medicine, Director, Center for Innovative Therapy, Division of Rheumatology, Allergy and Immunology, University of California, San Diego, La Jolla, California

CONTRIBUTORS

DIANA S. BARKIN, AA, Editorial Associate, American Journal of Therapeutics, Lake Bluff, Illinois

STACY J. BARKIN, MA, MED, PSYD CANDIDATE, NBCC, CSAC, Department of Behavioral Health, Saint Luke's Behavioral Health Hospital, Scottsdale, Arizona

ROBERT L. BARKIN, PharmD, MBA, DAAPM, FCP, NHA, Associate Professor, Department of Anesthesiology, Family Medicine, Pharmacology, and Psychiatry, Rush Medical College, Rush University Medical Center, Chicago; Rush Pain Center, North Shore Pain Center, Rush North Shore Medical Center, Skokie, Illinois

LAUREN A. BEAUPRE, PhD, Orthopaedic Research Director, Division of Orthopaedics, Department of Surgery, Capital Health, Edmonton, Alberta, Canada

SUSAN L. CHARETTE, MD, Assistant Clinical Professor, Division of Geriatrics, University of California, Los Angeles, Los Angeles, California

JOHN J. CUSH, MD, Chief, Rheumatology & Clinical Immunology, Presbyterian Hospital of Dallas, Dallas, Texas

BRUCE A. FERRELL, MD, Associate Professor, Division of Geriatrics, University of California, Los Angeles, Los Angeles, California

DANIEL E. FURST, MD, Carl M. Pearson Professor of Rheumatology, Division of Rheumatology, Department of Medicine, David Geffen School of Medicine at UCLA, Los Angeles; VA Greater Los Angeles Healthcare System, Los Angeles, California

D.W.C. JOHNSTON, MD, FRCS(C), Orthopaedic Surgeon, Division of Orthopaedics, Department of Surgery, Capital Health, Edmonton, Alberta, Canada

C. ALLYSON JONES, PhD, Assistant Professor, Department of Physical Therapy, Faculty of Rehabilitation Medicine, University of Alberta, Edmonton, Alberta; Department of Public Health Sciences, Faculty of Medicine and Dentistry, University of Alberta, Edmonton, Alberta; and Institute of Health Economics, Edmonton, Alberta, Canada

KENNETH C. KALUNIAN, MD, Professor of Medicine, Center of Innovative Therapies at the University of San Diego at California, La Jolla, California

ARTHUR KAVANAUGH, MD, Professor of Medicine, Director, Center for Innovative Therapy, Division of Rheumatology, Allergy and Immunology, University of California, San Diego, La Jolla, California

CAROL A. LANGFORD, MD, MHS, Director, Center for Vasculitis Care and Research, Department of Rheumatic and Immunologic Diseases, The Cleveland Clinic Foundation, Cleveland, Ohio

BILL H. MCCARBERG, MD, Founder, Chronic Pain Management Program, Kaiser Permanente, San Diego; Assistant Clinical Professor (voluntary), University of California School of Medicine, San Diego, California

G. ANDRES QUICENO, MD, Assistant Medical Director, Rheumatology & Clinical Immunology, Presbyterian Hospital of Dallas, Dallas, Texas

VEENA K. RANGANATH, MD, Professor of Rheumatology, Division of Rheumatology, Department of Medicine, David Geffen School of Medicine at UCLA, Los Angeles, California

LEE S. SIMON, MD, Associate Clinical Professor of Medicine, Division of Rheumatology and Metabolic Bone Disease, Beth Israel Deaconess Medical Center, Harvard Medical School, Boston, Massachusetts

MARIA E. SUAREZ-ALMAZOR, MD, PhD, Professor, Baylor College of Medicine, Houston, Texas

ZUHRE TUTUNCU, MD, Assistant Professor of Medicine, Division of Rheumatology, Allergy and Immunology, University of California, San Diego, La Jolla, California

CHRISTOPHER M. WISE, MD, W. Robert Irby Professor, Internal Medicine, Division of Rheumatology, Allergy, and Immunology, Medical College of Virginia, Virginia Commonwealth University Health System, Richmond, Virginia

CHRISTOPHER W. WU, MD, Fellow, Center of Innovative Therapies at the University of San Diego at California, La Jolla, California

CONTENTS

Twenty to 50% of community elderly suffer from pain. Up to 80% of the institutionalized elderly report at least one pain problem. Multiple pain etiologies that occur in elderly patients may be the occurrence of multiple chronic diseases: osteoarthritis, RA, cancer, DJD, bone/joint disorders, osteoporosis, surgical pain, trauma, neuropathic pain, and nociceptive pain. The incidence of unrelieved pain inhibits respiration, decreases mobility, and decreases their functional status, which may lead to iatrogenic events, which include pneumonia, constipation and deep vein thrombosis. Prolonged inpatient stays and extended care facilities or nursing homes may decrease the elderly patient's expectations of quality of life and initiate social isolation. There exists some roadblocks or barriers to the detection of pain in the elderly client. These include social, emotional, cognitive, and subjective issues with the patient.

Since the original descriptions of the involvement of crystals in arthritis, our understanding of the clinical syndromes of gout and pseudogout, and the role of basic calcium crystals in arthritis has increased. Gout is usually considered an affliction confined to middle-aged men, but has an increasing prevalence in older populations, with unique and often atypical features. Calcium pyrophosphate dihydrate crystal deposition disease is common in elderly patients. The diagnosis of both of these common forms of arthritis and the need to individualize therapy in patients with other medical problems remain important clinical challenges to the practicing physician.

Rheumatic Disease in the Elderly: Rheumatoid Arthritis

Zuhre Tutuncu and Arthur Kavanaugh

This review summarizes the different aspects of rheumatoid arthritis and the spectrum of diseases that can present as rheumatoid arthritis-like arthritis in the elderly population. With the aging of Western population, different forms of inflammatory arthritis' prevalence and incidence are increasing in the elderly persons. Difficulties in establishing the diagnosis and introducing new treatment modalities in this patient group poses a great challenge for the clinicians. The management of inflammatory arthritis in the elderly requires special consideration in regard to the comorbidities and increased frequency of adverse events. There is definitely a substantial need for improving different aspects of diagnostic and therapeutic interventions that will reduce the impact of inflammatory arthritis in the growing elderly population.

Total Joint Arthroplasties: Current Concepts of Patient Outcomes after Surgery

C. Allyson Jones, Lauren A. Beaupre, D.W.C. Johnston, and Maria E. Suarez-Almazor

Total hip and knee arthroplasties are effective surgical interventions for relieving pain and improving physical function caused by arthritis. Although the majority of patients substantially improve, not all report gains or are satisfied after receiving a total joint arthroplasty. This article reviews the literature on patient outcomes after total hip and knee arthroplasties for osteoarthritis and the evidence pertaining to factors that affect these patient-centered outcomes. Mounting evidence suggests that no one patient-related or peri-operative factor clearly predicts the amount of pain relief or functional improvement that will occur following total hip or knee arthroplasty.

Rheumatic Diseases in the Elderly: Dealing with Rheumatic Pain in Extended Care Facilities

Bill H. McCarberg

Rheumatic diseases representing over 100 conditions are common in elderly people, are increasing in frequency, and are undertreated. Extended care facilities have special needs and restrictions, making pain management more complicated. Understanding how to assess pain in a population at risk for poor pain control is vital. Treatment individualized to the patient's special circumstances where optimal care rarely means cure or complete relief of symptoms leads to improved function and quality of life.

FORTHCOMING ISSUES

PREVIOUS ISSUES

ELSEVIER
SAUNDERS

Clin Geriatr Med 21 (2005) xi–xiii

CLINICS IN
GERIATRIC
MEDICINE

Preface

Rheumatic Diseases in the Elderly: A "Perfect Storm"

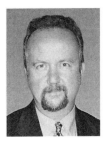

Arthur Kavanaugh, MD
Guest Editor

Rheumatic diseases have always been of great relevance to health care providers and patients. Representing more than a hundred distinct diseases and syndromes, these conditions account for about one in six of all visits to primary care providers, and affect a substantial proportion of the population. A recent estimate is that 27% of the United States population has physician-diagnosed arthritis [1]. This makes arthritis the leading cause of physical disability, and explains its tremendous economic toll, estimated at more than $85 billion annually.

It has long been recognized that arthritis and musculoskeltal conditions are of particular concern among older persons. Thus, a number of important rheumatic conditions (eg, osteoarthritis, osteoporosis, polymylagia rheumatica, and so on) typically arise among older persons. Also, for other diseases for which there is no cure (eg, rheumatoid arthritis, ankylosing spondylitis, gout, and so on), patients diagnosed at earlier ages carry the burden of disease into their later years. Other diseases (eg, gout, pseudogout, malignancy associated rheumatic conditions, and so on) are associated with both comorbid conditions whose prevalence increases with advancing age or with the use of various medications more commonly used by older persons. With the anticipated increase in longevity in the general population, both the prevalence, and hence the impact, of rheumatic conditions are predicted to increase dramatically in years to come. These considerations, along with the unique challenges associated with optimal diagnosis and therapy of such conditions among older persons suggest that we can expect to create a "perfect storm" of rheumatic diseases in the elderly. The challenge will fall to virtually all clinicians to be well versed in this important area.

In this volume, authors with a variety of backgrounds take on some of the important aspects of caring for older persons with rheumatic diseases. Some of the more common conditions are discussed in greater detail. Interestingly, for many of these conditions, there are difficult issues regarding accurate diagnosis in the elderly. For example, the prevalence of many autoantibodies, including rheumatoid factor and antinuclear antibodies increases among healthy older persons [2], reflecting alterations in B cell homeostasis and regulation associated with age [3]. Similarly, laboratory tests used to follow the acute phase response, such as the erythrocyte sedimentation rate, have a higher range of "normal" values among older persons, thus affecting their utility in identifying systemic inflammation often associated with various rheumatic diseases. Although there are well established classification criteria for several rheumatic diseases, these were established in most cases predominantly among younger persons. Therefore, such criteria may be inaccurate in the elderly, for whom the differential diagnosis may be broader, and diagnoses may be more difficult to establish [4]. Accurate diagnosis is of course critically important, as it is the cornerstone of effective therapy.

Therapeutic considerations for many disease states can be challenging among older persons, and this is certainly the case for rheumatic diseases. This important facet of caring for older persons with rheumatic diseases is covered in many articles in this volume. Issues such as polypharmacy, comorbid conditions that affect the pharmacokinetics or pharmacodynamics of medications, and even normal alterations in physiology must all be accounted for when choosing the optimal therapeutic approach to rheuamtic diseases in the elderly. These same factors also affect the impact of toxicity of medications. A common example is nonsteroidal anti-inflammatory medications (NSAIDs). NSAIDs are among the most widely used of all medications, and the elderly are very frequent consumers of these drugs for sundry forms of arthritis. Unfortunately, the elderly are at higher risk for several important untoward effects of these agents, including gastorintestinal bleeding and renal insufficiency. Illustrating the complexity of this problem is the current situation with cyclooxygenase-2 specific agents (COX-2 inhibitors) [5]. These agents, whose introduction to the clinic was widely anticipated based upon their more favorable gastrointestinal safety profile, are now under closer scrutiny concerning their potential association with cardiovascular complications. The population at greatest risk of such complications included persons with established cardiovascular disease or risk factors for such disease; this, of course, is relevant to the elderly! Confounding the discussions of optimal therapy of rheumatic diseases in older persons is that clinical trials of new arthritis treatments have largely excluded persons with substantial comorbidities and have had underrepresentation among older people.

A key undercurrent throughout the discussion of diagnosing and treating rheumatic diseases in the elderly is the impact of these conditions on the affected patient and their families. Although it is widely recognized that rheumatic diseases often have a significant deleterious affect upon functional status and are a major contributor to disability, this is particulary crucial among older persons. Comorbid illnesses and even normal physiologic changes associated with aging affect the ability of the patient to withstand the ravages of unchecked disease. Addressing functional status and alleviating pain are central to the care of persons with rheumatic diseases. In many cases, a multidisciplinary approach is beneficial. These important areas are reviewed in several articles in this volume.

There is hope for the future in the care of elderly patients with rheumatic diseases. Recognition of this "perfect storm" will facilitate research into the area. Already, there has been increasing interest delineating immunologic, physiologic, and psychosocial alterations that occur with normal aging. Greater understanding should allow the translation into better management for patients.

Arthur Kavanaugh, MD
Center for Innovative Therapy
Division of Rheumatology, Allergy and Immunology
University of California–San Diego
9500 Gilman Drive, La Jolla, CA 92093-0943, USA
E-mail address: akavanaugh@ucsd.edu

References

[1] MMWR 2004;53(18):383–6.

[2] Kavanaugh AF. Rheumatoid arthritis in the elderly: Is it a different disease? Am J Med 1997; 103(6A):40S–8S.

[3] Linton PJ, Dorshkind K. Age-related changes in lymphocyte development and function. Nat Immunol 2004;5:133–9.

[4] Rasch EK, Hirsch R, Paulose-Ram R, et al. Prevalence of rheumatoid arthritis in persons 60 years of age and older in the United States. Effect of different methods of case classification. Arthritis Rheum 2003;48:917–26.

[5] Bombardier C, Laine L, Reicin A, et al. Comparison of upper gastrointestinal toxicity of rofecoxib and naproxen in patients with rheumatoid arthritis. N Engl J Med 2000;343:1520–8:959–63.

ELSEVIER
SAUNDERS

CLINICS IN
GERIATRIC
MEDICINE

Clin Geriatr Med 21 (2005) 465–490

Perception, Assessment, Treatment, and Management of Pain in the Elderly

Robert L. Barkin, PharmD, MBA, DAPM, FCP, NHA[a,b,*],
Stacy J. Barkin, MA, MED, PsyD Candidate[c],
Diana S. Barkin, AB[d]

[a]Department of Anesthesiology, Family Medicine, Pharmacology, and Psychiatry,
Rush Medical College, Rush University Medical Center, 1653 West Congress Parkway,
Chicago, IL 60612, USA
[b]Rush Pain Center, North Shore Pain Center, Rush North Shore Medical Center,
9600 Gross Point Road, Skokie, IL 60076, USA
[c]St. Luke's Hospital, Scottsdale, AZ, USA
[d]American Journal of Therapeutics, 11-21 North Skokie Valley Highway, Suite 21-G3,
Lake Bluff, IL 60044, USA

Twenty to 50% of community elderly suffer from pain. Up to 80% of the institutionalized elderly report at least one pain problem (Appendix Box 1). Multiple pain etiologies that occur in elderly patients may be the occurrence of multiple chronic diseases: osteoarthritis, rheumatoid arthritis, cancer, degenerative joint disease, bone/joint disorders, osteoporosis, surgical pain, trauma, neuropathic pain, and nociceptive pain (Appendix Box 2). The incidence of unrelieved pain inhibits respiration, decreases mobility, and decreases their functional status, which may lead to iatrogenic events, which include pneumonia, constipation, and deep vein thrombosis. Prolonged inpatient stays and extended care facilities (ECF) or nursing homes may decrease the elderly patient's quality of life and initiate social isolation. There exists some roadblocks or barriers to the detection of pain in the elderly client. These include social, emotional, cognitive, and subjective issues with the patient. Pain is that which the patient states. Consider the experiential component of pain that includes physiologic and psychosocial issues, the history of the pain complaints and their presentation and past treatments. First consider their ability for coping mechanisms, their

* Corresponding author. 1211 Blackthorne Lane, Deerfield, IL 60015.
   E-mail address: rbarkin@rush.edu (R.L. Barkin).

expectations of treatment and management outcomes, and respective provisions, their educational level, socioeconomics, cultural, and personality of the patient. Consider also the signs and symptoms that are observed—the subjective manifestations of pain coupled with the objective sympathetic and autonomic indices of pain. Examine the grimacing, the moaning, changes in mental status, changes in appetite, agitation, rigidity, disorders of initiating and maintaining sleep. Patients demonstrate withdrawn affects, paucity of conversation, depression, allodynia, lack of adaption skills, and some without physiologic or behavioral signs (Appendix Box 3). A nonreport of pain does not mean there is no painful experience. This relates to the elderly in that the pain becomes undetected or misunderstood. The elderly patient must have the opportunity to achieve the goal that pain is not inevitable, concurrent with chronic illness, or the result of the aging process (Appendix Box 4). We must overcome the patient barriers of the fear of reporting pain. The elderly often accompany the fear of illness progression, which may bring them closer to a terminal event, and there may be no cure or no treatment (Appendix Box 5). Reporting pain by an elderly patient is not a sign of weakness. We encourage our elderly patients to discuss these issues with their health care providers. Some patients may also have fear of treatment costs due to fixed income or a lack of financial reserve or resources (Appendix Box 6). Barriers to a recognition of persistent pain in the elderly reflecting both health care professionals and the health care system are found in Appendix Boxes 6–8. Treatment goals should include enhanced functional status and augmented activities of daily living (ADLS).

Concurrent with initiating a treatment plan with the elderly patient, we consider multimodal or multiple pharmacotherapies accounting for age-related pharmacokinetic changes, age-related pharmacodynamic changes, and including the specific risks of each drug in each drug class and drug–drug, drug–disease, and drug–laboratory interactions. This patient-specific treatment plan begins with creating a comprehensive pain history including the location, distribution, time sequences in associative activities, and the quality of the pain, severity of pain, and the aggravating factors. Examine a complete medication history including the motor sensory, autonomic, and comorbidity evaluation (sleep, mood, functional status, complete metabolic profile) medications used over the past few months, prescription, over-the-counter drugs, phytopharmaceuticals, home remedies, the use quantitied/quantified alcoholic beverages and social recreational drugs, inquiring into which drugs have helped, which drugs have not helped, and initiating the behavioral assessments, concerns about the causes and beliefs of pain, family and other social relationships, and cultural background (see Appendix Boxes 6 and 7).

Factors that will affect drug dosing in the elderly include but are not limited to diminished renal function (creatinine clearance [Clcr] ≤ 30), which will create diminished renal excretion and higher serum levels, decrease in hepatic function, which will decrease in the already diminished microsomal oxidation (hepatic cytochrome P450) causing increase in serum level coupled with the age-related decreases in renal function. Additionally, there is a decrease in serum protein, especially albumin, for acidic drug binding, which will affect the serum binding and increase serum levels. Consider the alpha$_1$ acid glycoprotein (α_1 AGP) for binding of basic drugs, which will affect the serum binding and increased levels; compliance variations, which will alter serum levels, the changes in target organ sensitivity, the cytochrome P450; and interaction of multiple medications, which will diminish or increase renal excretion or hepatic metabolism including the active metabolites; and last, consider also genetic polymorphism (usually occurring a CYP450, 2C, 2D6), whether the patient may be classified as slow or poor metabolizer (see Appendix Box 8).

In selecting a pharmacotherapeutic agent or agents we have to review the etiology of the pain, such as nociceptive pain, neuropathic pain, visceral, ischemic, or combinations, multiple etiologies of pain that the patient presents with, and ultimately, an ongoing structured clinical evaluation of the treatment successes or failures, the need for augmentation, or for decremental and incremental changes. This intervention program leads to a dynamic process for evaluating elderly patients who present with painful episodes. Discussion of eudynia (symptom based acute pain) and malydynia (chronic pain syndrome based) is included.

Pain is among the most common reasons elderly patients present for medical care. Acute and chronic pain is debilitating, and diminishes functional status. Recovery is slow, interference with daily activities and personal care occurs, and manifests as a decremental change in the patient's quality of live, compounded by societal costs [1–11].

Acute pain (symptom-based eudynia, category I pain) is often associated with an identifiable injury or trauma, as a known antecedent, response to therapeutic options, and resolves in less than 1 to 3 months (Table 1). Acute pain/eudynia has known tissue damage etiology, serves biologic usefulness, is localized and transient, and displays a direct linear trauma injury or stimulus–response relationship. However, acute pain may be independent, concurrent with other multiple chronic pain etiologies, or be a flare of a chronic pain disease. Chronic pain of the elderly presents a treatment challenge because the multiple pathogenesis may be unclear (disorder syndrome-based maldynia category II pain) with less opportunity to predict the course of recovery. For patients experiencing psychosocial and financial stress, such nonspecific ambiguous prognosis is devastating (see Table 1).

Table 1
Factors that affect drug dosage in the elderly

Cause	Effect
↓ Renal function	↓ renal excretion parent compound and metabolites and ↑ serum levels of parent and metabolites
↓ Hepatic function	↓ metabolism; accumulation
↓ Serum protein (especially albumin)	Higher blood levels of unbound active drug
↓ Compliance	Therapeutic end points not achieved
↑ or ↓ target organ sensitivity	Iatrogenic effects
Interactions of multiple drugs (CYP 450)	↑ or ↓ in serum levels, AUC, CL, T1/2β

Table 2
Eudynia acute pain versus maldynia chronic pain

Eudynia acute pain category I symptom based	Maldynia chronic pain category II disorder syndrome based
A protective biologically useful unpleasant sensory and emotional experience associated with a known etiology or tissue damage, localized, transient, temporary, displays a direct linear stimulus/trauma response relationship.	A long-term pathologic experience that outlasts protective biologic utility invades and pervades the patient's life, affecting their behavior, vocation, avocation, daily tasks, function capacity, emotional state, social and family interactions.

Among the goals of the clinician is providing an opportunity for patients to regain some dominion control over their lives by providing the most effective and efficient pain treatment regimen possible [1–5,10,11]. There are multiple dimensions to pain that include depression, anxiety, anger, and frustration as emotional aspects and the somatic sources eliciting the sensory aspects (Tables 2,3).

Pain usually defined as chronic lasts longer than 1 to 3 months or exceeds the typical recovery time of an initial injury. Chronic pain may be continuous or episodic or a combination of both qualities or an acute flare of chronic pain, and involves central sensitization and neuroplasticity on a microlevel. Chronic pain is commonly accompanied by emotional stress, frustration, increased irritability, anger, anxiety, agitation, depression, social withdrawal, financial distress, loss of libido, disturbed sleep patterns, and diminished appetite or weight loss (see Table 2). Chronic pain can have a wide-ranging impact; its management must therefore focus on multiple aspects of the elderly patient's life and those close to them. Often the inappropriately treated acute pain for over a month may ultimately manifest as chronic pain. A multidisciplinary, comprehensive treatment plan is optimal, including (1) individual psychosocial counseling in conjunction with patient/family education; (2) noninvasive or minimally invasive procedures like massage therapy, physical therapy, transdermal or transcutaneous electrical nerve stimulation, or acupuncture; (3) up-to-date polymodal/polypharmacothera-

Table 3
Psychosocial and somatic aspects of pain which may surface in the elderly

Depression	Anger	Somatic source	Anxiety
Loss of social position	Bureaucratic	Symptoms of debility	Fear of hospitalization
Loss of job vocation	roadblocks,	Therapy adverse	or nursing home
Loss of role in family	Loneliness, aloneness,	reactions and side	Anticipatory fear
Chronic fatigue and	boredom	effects	of pain
insomnia	Delay in diagnosis	Noncancer pathology	Family and finance
Sense of helplessness,	Unavailable clinicians	Cancer	stressors Fear of death,
hopelessness,	Irritability	Neuropathic,	disfigurement
worthlessness,	Therapeutic failure	nociceptive, visceral,	Uncertainty about
disfigurement	Unavailable	ischemic, somatic	future
	pharmacotherapy		Unrealistic expectations
	Insurance limitation		

Box 1. Persistent pain in the elderly: consequences

Depression
Anxiety and agitation
Decreased socialization
Loss of appetite, weight loss, poor nutrition
Sleep disturbances (initiating, maintaining)
Decreased ambulation
Increased health care use
Increased health care cost
Deconditioning
Pathophysiology (deep vein thrombosis, pulmonary embolism,
    decubitus, infection, and so on)

---

peutic or anesthetic therapies, implant devices, or stimulators; and (4) if necessary, surgical intervention and physical medicine with rehabilitation focused to enhance the patient's functional status. Health care practitioners must consider uniting these various options in tailoring a patient-specific treatment plan, addressing both physiologic and psychologic symptoms [1,2,10–16]. Traditionally, the focus upon pain treatment was palliative. Today, the focus is directed at prevention of pain based upon pain etiologies in a patient-specific manner (Box 1).

An initial approach to persistent pain management in the elderly patient begins with acceptance of pain complaints as genuine, addressing both physiologic and psychosocial components. We attempt to focus upon the underlying multiple etiologies with patient specificity of analgesic and adjuvant therapeutic needs of invasive and noninvasive treatments. The goal is pain relief (analgesia), not complete pain ablation (anesthesia). The treatment plan is individually designed based upon blood chemistry profiles (including renal, liver, metabolic, hemologic electrolytes, and so on) pharmacokinetics, pharmacodynamics, pharmacologic, and drug interaction potentials (Table 4).

Table 4
Traditional versus modern treatment of acute pain

Traditional	Modern
Palliate pain	Prevent pain based upon etiology of pain(s)
Stay with a few "standard" analgesics	Try new drugs, combination drugs, use drugs concomitantly when appropriate (polymodal polypharmacy).
Stay with low dosages	Meet individual's physiologic (sensory) and psychologic (emotional) analgesic needs
Use prn dosing	Use time specific dosing: prevent drug-seeking behavior
	Use pharmacokinetics & pharmacodynamic design of treatment plan

A pharmacotherapeutic plan begins with a thorough pain medication history to identify the nature and characteristics of the patient's pain (acute-eudynia, chronic-maldynia, nociceptive, neuropathic, ischemic, and visceral). The patient and family interview should focus on patient-reported pain descriptors (example: exacerbation/modulation of pain; pain quality and intensity; pain sites as local, disseminated, or regional; characteristics and temporal relationship of pain) current pharmacotherapies (prescription, over-the-counter, phytopharmaceutical, or social/recreational agents, a quantified/qualified alcohol use pattern), and past treatments (including successes/failures, adverse effects, and true allergic reactions). A history should be developed of quantified ethanol use, tobacco use, caffeine use, and social recreational drugs (prescribed or illicit). A complete blood chemistry profile should be considered to determine if dosage changes are warranted based upon serum protein and renal/hepatic function. Health care practitioners should familiarize themselves with the pharmacodynamics, pharmacokinetics, potential drug–drug, drug–laboratory, drug–disease, or drug–food interactions and contraindications of any pharmacotherapy used by the patient [1,2,12,14] (see Appendix Boxes 6 and 7). Pharmacokinetics of the elderly affect pharmacologic activity including adipose tissues and body compartments (Fig. 1), serum albumin, α_1 AGP (increased during stress) renal/hepatic dysfunction, gender differences, and gender polymorphism (Box 2) [1,2,7,9,17–22].

A polypharmaceutical or other complex regimen may be jointly decided upon. Depending upon the nature of the specific pain complaint/etiology in a given patient, the combination of an opioid, nonsteroidal anti-inflammtory drugs (NSAIDs), antidepressants, anxiolytics, anticonvulsants (AEDs), centrally acting agents, peripheral analgesic anesthetic, muscle relaxants, or other analgesics may be considered. Health care practitioners should also take into consideration any

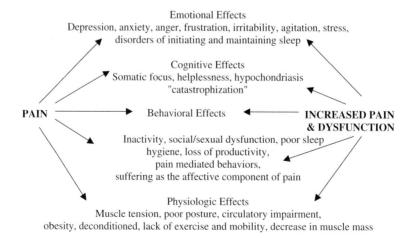

Fig. 1. Emotional, cognitive, behavior, and psyiologic effects manifested concurrently with increased pain and dysfunction.

Box 2. How pharmacokinetics affects pharmacologic activity

Pharmacokinetics in the Elderly Patient

Higher fat to lean body mass content, less skeletal muscle mass
Reduced serum albumin (for acidic drugs), total protein; α_1, acid glycoprotein (for basic drugs) (α_1 AGP)
Reduced renal glomerular filtration rate and tubular reabsorption, reduced creatine clearance
Reduced hepatic function, mixed function oxidases (CYP450)
Reduced first-pass gut metabolism (CYP450)
Genetic polymorphism
Gender differences

---

factors that affect the likelihood of compliance (age of patient, frequency/complexity of regimen, route of administration, tolerance of regimen, and so on) [1,2,9,15–22]. Elderly patient dose titrations may benefit from using an approximate estimated Clcr calculation that reflects the glomerular filtration rate (GRF). Does adjustments based upon this Clcr are indicated with many medications [22]. This calculation is found in Box 3.

The presence of adult chronic pain in the general population is estimated to occur in up to 40%, up to 80% in residents of ECF, and up to 75% in those patients with advanced terminal disease. The underreporting of pain by the elderly is multifactual, which includes addiction fears, side effects, adverse reaction, pharmacodynamic intolerance, perceived inevitable pain existence, fears of intrusiveness to others, inability to communicate painful events, and lack of family caregivers with involvement in pain management. Pain may be pathophysiology, may be nociceptive, neuropathic, visceral, or ischemic in combination with association of anxiety or depression. The goals of pain management should focus on enhanced functionality and performance of ADLS to improve the quality of life. Among extended care facility/nursing home patients, multi-

---

Box 3. Cockroft-Gault Formula

Clcr = (140 − patients age) × (ideal or lean body weight in kg)
× .85 if female ÷ 72 × stable serum creatinine(mg/dl)

Clcr (ml/min) − Renal Function
70 to 150 normal
30 to 70 mild impairment
10 to 30 advanced impairment
0 to 10 end stage renal impairment

---

pain states include lumbar sacral pain, arthritis, fracture, neuropathic, FMS CRPS types I and II, malignancy, cephalgia, and other chronic pain syndromes that gives rise to functional disability.

Chronic pain is a prominent health problem and among the common causes of long-term disability. Chronic pain presents as nociceptive insult to somatic and visceral tissues, and a neuropathic insult culmination in neurologic dysfunction due to neurologic lesion.

Common descriptors of musculoskeletal pain include pain upon motion, stiffness, somnolence, tender joints, and limited range of motion. Neuropathic descriptors include allodynia, hyperalgesia, hyperpathia, and pain paroxysm.

Neuropathic pain mechanism include peripheral mechanisms (membrane hyperexcitability, ectopic discharge, and peripheral sensitization from cell wall trauma) and central mechanisms (wind-up phenomenon, central sensitization, Aβ fiber reorganization, decremental loss of inhibition control mechanisms). Neuropathic pain symptoms including dysesthesia, paresthesia, continuous pain often "burning," intermittent shooting electric shock, lightening bolt, and lancinating. Autonomic system evaluation of neuropathic pain includes changes in temperature and color of skin, vasomotor, pseudomotor, pilomotor, tropic changes, hair, skin, and nails; postural hypotension is often present.

Pharmacologic agents

Nonopioid analgesics: aspirin, nonsteroidal anti-inflammtory drugs, acetaminophen

An extensive review of these agents has been published elsewhere [2]. Aspirin (ASA) is used to reduce inflammation, pain, and fever. It inhibits prostaglandin synthesis and acts on the hypothalamus to reduce fever, prevent the formation of platelet aggregation substance thromboxane, and inhibits vitamin K-dependent and independent clotting factors. Renal elimination of ASA is primarily as fee salicylic acids and conjugated metabolites. Use should be avoided in end-stage renal disease. The dose should be modified when aspirin is used for long-term therapy in the presence of hepatic compromise. Side effects of ASA include gastrointestinal (GI) irritation, nausea, vomiting, tinnitus, metabolic acidosis, acute respiratory distress syndrome, and occult GI blood loss. Both aspirin and salicylic acid enter the central nervous system (CNS), and effects such as dizziness, vertigo, fatigue, insomnia, lethargy, confusion, depression, and headache may occur [1,2,15,22–24].

Caution should also be taken in treating patients with platelet or bleeding disorders or renal dysfunction. All patients receiving ASA (81 to 325 mg) for TIAs stroke (due to fibrin platelet emboli) or MI who subsequently are prescribed a cyclooxygenase (COX) II agent must remain on the ASA (81 mg to 325 mg) for the ASA COX I effects. Patients with a history of nasal polyps, asthma, or rhinitis may exhibit aspirin intolerance, leading to severe exacerbation of allergic symptoms including potentially fatal bronchospasms. Elderly patients may exhibit dermatologic, GI, and hematologic effects even from low-dose ASA [22].

Acetaminophen (APAP) is an analgesic and antipyretic agent that lacks anti-inflammatory properties. APAP postulates of a central mechanism may be mediated through nitric oxide modulation by glutamate or substance P, central COX II mechanisms, serotonin, or other mechanisms yet to be identified. Metabolism occurs in the liver, primarily by cytochrome P-450 1A2, 3A5, and 2E1. A slight increase in the dosing interval may be needed when renal dysfunction is present. Prolonged use of APAP in patients with severe liver disease is not recommended. Hepatotoxicity may occur with daily chronic doses of more than 3000 mg to 4000 mg/d or an acute dose of 7 to 8 g or more, and is exacerbated in patients with a history of alcohol abuse or malnutrition (glutathione stores depletion). No more that 3 to 4 g of APAP daily is acutely recommended [1,2,22,25–29].

NSAIDs are antipyretic, anti-inflammatory, and analgesic agents that decrease prostaglandin production through their variable inhibition of COX I and II or NSAIDs carry the risk of severe GI, hepatic, hematologic, cardiovascular and renal adverse effects, which should be considered when contemplating their use long-term for pain. All NSAIDs have a dose ceiling effect. Drug monitoring should include, evaluation of cardiovascular risk factors of MI or stroke, complete blood count, Clcr calculation, urinalysis, potassium level, liver function tests, occult fecal, blood and urine testing for hematuria and proteinuria; GI ulceration, bleeding, and perforation occur, often without warning symptoms [1,2,24,30].

Other adverse effects associated with NSAID use include reduced renal blood flow and glomerular filtration, interstitial nephritis, acute tubular necrosis, papillary necrosis, nephrotic syndrome, sodium and water retention (edema), acute renal failure, hyperkalemia, and hypertension; NSAIDs also decrease the efficacy of diuretics, β-blockers, and angiotensin converting enzyme (ACE) inhibitors. Elderly patients, patients with diabetes mellitus, or those with mild to moderate renal insufficiency may be predisposed to hyperkalemia, as may patients receiving concomitant therapy with other hyperkalemia-induction (ACE inhibitors, potassium-sparing diuretics, salt substitutes) agents. Local as well as systemic injury is caused by prostaglandin synthesis inhibition of gastric mucosa defense and platelet function, respectively. Inhibition of platelet aggregation can lead to enhanced bleeding, a nonexistent feature of Coxibs (ie, Rofecoxib) [1,2,24,30].

The isoenzymes of oral COX have been identified: COX-I and COX-II. COX-3 maybe central, and identified possibly with the mechanism of action (MOA) of APAP. Only three COX II-specific agents (coxibs) are currently available in the United States, (eg, celecoxib, rofecoxib, valdecoxib) although others may be available shortly (eg, etoricoxib, lumaricoxib). A comparison of these three agents is seen in Table 1. Distribution, regulation, function of COX, along with a complete review of COX I/COX II agents, has been fully described elsewhere [2,13,14,25,26,31].

Acute sodium retention is Cox II inhibition mediated and clinically resolves with continuation of therapy. GFR is influenced due to inhibition of COX I.

COX II-specific agents spare the GFR that decrementally deteriorates in the elderly. Cardiovascular effects, edema, hypertension, hepatic effects, and hyperkalemia are of clinical significance in the elderly. As with all NSAIDs, the COX II agents should be used with caution in patients with preexisting fluid retention, hypertension, cardiovascular MI, stroke risk factors or heart failure. The COX I/II sites in the kidney include the macula densa, podocytes, thick ascending limb, efferent/afferent arterioles, and the glomerulus. Rofecoxib has been additionally studied to be opioid sparing in the postoperative treatment of pain. Rofecoxib has prominent pharmacologic, pharmacokinetic, pharmacodynamic, and pharmacotherapeutic advantage over the currently available COX II-specific agents [2,24,30]. Etoricoxib is a "third-generation" oral Coxib with 100% bioavailability to be released. Paracoxib is merely a parenteral prodrug for Valdecoxib.

Centrally acting agents

Tramadol

Tramadol is an atypical analgesic with a binary MOA. The MOA of this chiral compound combines centrally acting opioid (μ_1) activity with a secondary spinal mechanism of monoamine reuptake (serotonin [5-HT] and norepinephrine [NE]) inhibition. With its weak affinity for μ-opioid receptors (M1 metabolite binds more to the μ opiate receptor than parent tramadol), in conjunction with 5-HT and NE reuptake blockade (more affinity of parent tramadol than M1 metabolite), tramadol modulates multiple pathways that mediate pain. Tramadol is a racemate, and each enantiomer has differing pharmacology. Spinally and supraspinally, tramadol is associated with a lower degree of respiratory depression than opioids. It exhibits a low potential for tachyphylaxis and abuse, and is used for the chronic management of moderate to moderately severe pain acute pain [32]. The concomitant use of tramadol and NSAIDs (ie, rofecoxib) may offer the therapeutic benefits of both central and peripheral analgesia, although the requisite studies have not yet been concluded. Tramadol represents an option for patients who are at risk for the side effects of NSAIDs but are reluctant to take opioid analgesics. Only 20% of tramadol is bound to plasma proteins. The active metabolite M1 and the parent exhibits linear pharmacokinetics, and uses the CYP 450 2D6 and 3A4 hepatic enzyme substrate. Dialysis removes less than 7% of a given dose. For patients over the age of 75 years the dose is less than 300 mg/d, for a Clcr $\leq$30 mL/min the dose is 200 mg/d in equally divided doses, and for cirrhosis, the dosage is reduced to 100 mg/d in equally divided doses due to increased plasma concentrates and prolonged $t_{0.5\beta}$.

Tramadol has been additionally well studied in elderly populations and for a variety of conditions. It has been very acceptable, well tolerated overall, and has proven to be effective in musculoskeletal pain, fibromyalgia, acute pain/chronic pain, osteoarthritis, chronic low back pain, and neuropathic pain. Tramadol is available as 37.5 mg in combination with APAP (325 mg), and is becoming the preferred dosage form for the elderly for pain (acute, chronic flares) moderate to moderately severe intensity [1,2,13,33–46]. Tramadol 37.5 mg/APAP 325 mg combination has been shown to produce analgesic equal to or greater than meperidine, hydrocodone, and codeine [44–46].

Opiates and opioids

The most notable class of medications used to treat pain are the opiates and opioids. When opiates are used for management for chronic pain, both chemical and psychologic dependence may ensue. Both practitioners and patients can exhibit "opiophobia" (the patient fear of opiate use, the clinician's concern of "opiate addiction," and the pharmacist cautions about dispensing the prescription), which may lead to unnecessary under use of opiates in pain management. The analgesic effects appear to be a function of several factors, including affinity for specific receptor binding sites ($\mu_{1, 2}$, δ, κ), intrinsic activity at respective receptors, presence or absence of active metabolites, and the pharmacokinetics and pharmacodynamics of the specific agents genetic polymorphism: population variations of opioid receptors and gender differences. Opioids hyperpolarize the neuron due to enhancement of potassium influx and inhibit neurotransmitter release by calcium influx inhibition. A dose reduction is initially used in the elderly followed by retitration. The binding of μ receptors (m_2) produces euphoria, and μ_1 is associated with morphine-like analgesia; μ_2 is associated with respiratory depression, miosis, and inhibited GI motility. The μ_2 receptor has been associated with effects on GI motility, euphoria, respiratory depression, bradycardia, and psychologic aspects of chemical dependence. A brief comment upon each frequently prescribed opiate/opioid will follow. Codeine, a weak analgesic, is metabolized to morphine, while hydrocodone is metabolized to hydromorphone. This hepatic metabolism occurs through the CYP 450 2D6 pathway. For a Clcr of 10 to 50 mL/min administer $\leq$75% of the codeine dose and $\leq$50% of the dose when Clcr is 10 mL/min or less. Codeine may cause the release of antidiuretic hormone. This pathway may have decremental changes in the elderly, and is subject to genetic polymorphism, which may produce less than adequate analgesia. DNA-sequence variation (polymorphism) in CYP2D6 prevents O-demethylation of codeine to morphine with consequent decremental analgesia. Hydrocodone, a phenanthrene derivative, is a dehydrogenated ketone codeine derivative. Fixed hydrocodone analgesic combinations include APAP and ibuprofen. Hydrocodone has been associated with abuse, possibly due to μ_2-mediated euphoria and the active hydromorphone metabolite. The duration of action is 4 to 6 hours, with a $t_{0.5\beta}$ of 3.3 to 4.5 hours; withdrawal peaks 48 to 72 hours after last dose. Most opioids have side effects including sedation, nausea, vomiting, pruritus, and urinary retention. Constipation is an adverse effect to which tolerance does not develop, so a laxative or stool softener may be added to opiate/opioid therapy. Morphine as an opiate standard of comparison has the dosage administered according to pharmacodynamic effects and the patient's pharmacokinetic characteristics. Elderly patients are more sensitive to morphine and its two glucuronide metabolites (M-3-G, M-6-G). Dose adjustments are not necessary in mild hepatic disease, but excessive sedation occurs in cirrhotic patients. This is a function of the accumulation of the active analgesic metabolite, morphine-6 glucuronide (M-6-G), which is renally eliminated. Oxycodone is an analgesic metabolized by the CYP-450 2D6 isoenzyme and is excreted renally. Oxymorphone is a minor active metabolite of oxycodone created through hepatic CYP 450 metabolism, and ultimately, is itself metabolized by CYP450 3A4. Euphoria is noted with oxycodone, which may be a μ_2 event coupled with lipophilicity and the bolus dose release is about 38% in less than 2 hours postingestion in the extended release dosage forms; κ agonist activity is noted with oxycodone. The $t_{0.5}$ is 3.5 to 4 hours (single dose immediate release). Events noted in the elderly have been euphoria, diaphoresis, confusion, and memory deficits. The agent has been prominently associated with abuse and misuse. Oxycodone is contraindicated with hypercarbia and paralytic ileus. Oxymorphone is to be available in an oral sustained release and oral immediate release dosage form that complements the injectable and rectal dosage form. There is limited to no CYP450 events, and the agent is primarily μ_1 with limited or no euphorigenic effects demonstrated to date. This provides an excellent opportunity in well-selected elderly patients.

Opiates/opioids each uniquely produce a wide spectrum of pharmacologic effects including analgesia, dysphoria, euphoria, somnolence, respiratory depression, diminished GI motility, altered circulatory dynamics, histamine release, and physical dependence [1,2,10–12,14,37,47–51].

Morphine acts as a pure agonist, binding with and activating opioid receptors at sites in the periaqueductal and periventricular gray matter, the ventromudulla and the spinal cord to produce analgesia. The principal therapeutic actions of morphine on the CNS are analgesia, sedation, and alterations of mood. The pharmacologic activity is primarily due to the parent compound morphine. One metabolite, morphine-6-glucornide (M-6-G), has been shown to have analgesic activity, but poorly crosses the blood–brain barrier and may accumulate during renal dysfunction or excessive administration. Elimination of morphine is primarily via hepatic metabolism by phase II process to glucuronide metabolites (55–56%), which are then renally excreted. The terminal half-life of morphine is 2 to 4 hours, up to 15 hours, with linear pharmacokinetics over the dosage range of 30 to 100 mg. Following the administration of oral morphine, approximately 50% of the morphine, because of presystemic (CYP-450 metabolism first pass) elimination, only about 20% to 40% of the administered dose reaches the systemic circulation. Genetic polymorphism of MDR1 gene (pharmacogenomics) may predetermine morphine toxic administration events.

Morphine is 30% to 35% reversibly bound to plasma proteins. The major pathway of the detoxification of morphine is conjugation. Virtually all morphine is converted to glucuronide metabolites including morphine-3-glucuronide, M-3-G (about 50%), and morphine-6-glucuronide, M-6-G (about 5–15%). M-3-G has no significant analgesic activity but have some algesic properties. M-6-G has been shown to have opioid agonist and analgesic activity in humans.

Meperidine, a synthetic opioid produces normeperidine by CYP450 2D6 as an active nonopioid toxic metabolite, which is clinically important as it is not naloxone-reversible. The half-life ($t_{0.5\beta}$) of normeperidine is 15 to 30 hours, depending on the patient's renal function and the $t_{0.5}$ of meperidine is 3 to 4 hours. After repeated dosing, normeperidine accumulates, and the concentration may exceed that of meperidine in the plasma. Resultant effects of normeperidine include respiratory arrest and excitatory neurotoxicity (hyperreflexia, myoclonus, grand mal seizures, and agitation). These effects have been reported after less that 24 hours of dosing in patients at all ages and with in those exhibiting normal renal function, as well as in those with impaired renal function. Anticholinergic effects of meperidine are serious enough that the patient may have urinary retention and need catheterization; cardiac effects include a range of ventricular response to atrial flutter and superventricular tachycardia.

Meperidine also blocks the neuronal reuptake of norepinephrine and serotonin with a serotonin syndrome produced by monoamine oxidase inhibitor (MAOI) drug interactions. Deaths related to meperidine–MAOI interactions have been reported. Serotonin syndrome has also been reported with concomitant use of meperidine and fluoxetine. Meperidine use may aggravate preexisting seizure disorders. Meperidine withdrawal often lasts 4 to 5 days. Use of meperidine in chronic pain and acute pain is falling into disuse [1,2,11,23,24,47–50,52].

Methadone is a racemic mixture, a diphenylheptane μ_1 agonist, N-methyl-D-aspartate (NMDA) receptor antagonist (d-isomer), blocks specific calcium channels and lesser κ agonist with possible delta receptor activity. The d-isomer potentiates the L-isomer antinociceptive effects and decreases tolerance by NMDA antagonism. Following chronic exposure desensitization of μ and delta receptors may occur. Reuptake blockade of 5-HT and NE are also mechanisms of action. It has an analgesic duration of 4 to 6 hours and up to 8 hours with chronic dosing. The CYP450 2D6 and 3A4 are the substrates for methadone metabolism. The $t_{0.5\beta}$ is 15 to 25 hours with single dosing. If the Clcr is low, use 50% to 75% or less of the dose. Side effects include miosis, lower extremity edema, hypotension, dose-related bradycardia, histamine release, peripheral vasodilation, and choreic movements (clonazepam responseive). Methadone withdrawal may have a 6- to 7-week recovery.

Propoxyphene is a synthetic opiate analgesic having a $t_{0.5\beta}$ of 6 to 12 hours with chemical similarity to methadone. It is metabolized in the liver to norpropoxphyene, a toxic metabolite that is eliminated in urine. Norpropoxyphene is not an opioid but has local anesthetic proarrhythmic lidocaine-like effects and cardiac anesthetic effects similar to those of amitriptyline or quinidine. Because of its long half-life (30–36hours), norpropoxyphene accumulates if the parent drug is given repeatedly. Propoxyphene is associated with abnormal liver function tests. Norpropoxyphene accumulation is associated with seizures, arrhythmias, pulmonary edema, and it is poorly dialyzed. There have also been reports of apnea, cardiac arrests, and death. Naloxone does not reverse the effects of norproxyphene. Propoxyphene is not to be used in suicidal/addiction prone patients. Chronic use of this agent is highly discouraged, and use in elderly patients in not recommended. Propoxyphene is associated with jaundice and cholestatic jaundice. Caution is warned when prescribing this agent for patients using tranquilizers, antidepressants, or alcohol in excess. The United States General Accounting Office has listed propoxyphene among drugs "inappropriate for the elderly," and has emphasized, as has this author, that alternative analgesics are both more effective and safer; consequently, propoxyphene use in the elderly is discouraged [1,2,10–12,23,47,53,54].

Hydromorphone is a phenanthrene μ_1, μ_2, and lesser κ agonist using CYP450 2D6 to change the lipophilic parent compound to a glucuronide. Side effects include myoclonus (clonazepam responsive). The $t_{0.5\beta}$ is 2 to 3 hours; some dosage forms contain tartrazine, and caution is required in patients with renal or hepatic dysfunction. Duration of action is generally 4 to 5 hours or longer. Hydromorphone may also increase cerebral spinal fluid pressure and cause transient hyperglycemia. Sustained action dosage forms are to be available.

Fentanyl is a highly lipophilic opioid analgesic with agonist activity at the μ opioid receptors and less κ agonist activity in the brain, spinal cord, and smooth muscle. The $t_{0.5\beta}$ is averaged 2 to 4 hours and uses CYP 3A4 for metabolism. The transdermal semipermiable membrane patch is applied to the skin and is replaced every 3 days. Transdermal onset of analgesia is 8 to 24 hours, and absorption is a function of intracutaneous blood flow. One week should be allowed before altering the dose; equilibration is not reached until 6 days after a dosage change. The transdermal delivery system offers continuous transdermal fentanyl administration. Avoid transdermal system exposure to any external heat source, as an elevated skin temperature and augmented perfusion increases drug absorption. An increase in core temperature to $40°C$ ($104°F$) may increase serum fentanyl concentration by up to 33%. Decreased fat stores, elderly, muscle wasting, cachectic, debilitated, or altered clearance, should create a prescribing caution. Initiate to a dosage not greater than 12.0 to 25 µg/h, unless they are receiving greater than 135 mg/d of oral morphine or oral equivalent. If Clcr is 10 to 50, use 75% of the normal dose. Redistribution occurs from the CNS to muscle and fat. Adverse effects include hypotension, bradycardia, seizures, and rigidity of thoracic and skeletal muscles. Titration with tramadol 37.5 mg/APAP 37.5 mg tablets during achievement of fentanyl transdermal system steady state for as-needed dosing has been successful in practice without subjecting the patient to an increase in nontherapeutic opioid effects. A transmucosal (oral cavity) dosage form of fentanyl is also available. A generic substitute is highly discouraged in the transdermal dosage form.

Mixed agonist-antagonist

Pentazocine, nalbuphine, and butorphanol are the mixed opioid agonist-antagonist. Nalbuphine and pentazocine must be used with caution in patients receiving opioids, to avoid precipitating withdrawal, and consequently, increasing pain. Pentazocine is an agonist at both κ and σ receptor sites. Dysphoria, nightmares, confusion, depersonalization, seizures, visual hallucinations, and disorientation are other adverse effects caused by pentazocine if Clcr is 10 to

50 mL/min use less than 75% of the dose. Pentazocine use is discouraged, especially in the elderly patient [1,2,54].

Butorphanol is an antagonist-agonist at the μ receptor. Therapeutic effects also may occur via agonist effects on the κ receptor. Abstinence may occur with coadministration of propoxyphene and methadone. Negative side effects can be minimized with administration in small doses; a nasal delivery form is available. Nalbuphine has both κ and σ agonist and μ antagonist activity properties. The analgesic duration is 3 to 6 hours, and following n-dealkylation it is excreted renally and via bile as a glucuronide. The most common adverse reaction is sedation with a ceiling effect of analgesia.

Buprenorphine is a partial agonist at the μ receptors and an antagonist at the κ receptors. It may also have some antagonist activity at the σ receptor, but lacks dysphoric effects. Buprenorphine is available in combination for oral administration indicated for opioid dependence. Duration of action is 6 to 8 hours, $T_{0.5\beta}$ is 2 to 3.5 hours. Elimination is 70% in feces and 20% unchanged in the urine. Metabolism is by n-dealkylation. Slow dissociation from μ_1 receptor is noted. Buprenorphine has been used for analgesia without producing hemodynamic instability in the management of pain resulting from a myocardial infarction. It has lower incidence of nausea and vomiting than other opioids. Abstinence has not been a clinical event with any coadministered opiates in our clinical practice [1,2,10–12,23,47,48,50,53–56]. Use with cautions includes: the elderly or debilitated, severe hepatic, renal or pulmonary function; prostatic hypertrophy, urethral structure, acute alcoholism, delirium tremens, and/or kyphoscoliosis.

Antidepressants

5-HT (serotonin) selective reuptake inhibitors (SSRIs) have a limited receptor-specific pharmacokinetic and pharmacodynamic serotonergic side effect profile. Adverse effects most commonly reported include headache, insomnia, anxiety, dizziness, tremors, drowsiness, nausea, vomiting, diarrhea, dyspepsia, xerostomia, sexual dysfunction, anorexia, and diaphoresis. Serotonin syndrome can occur when using SSRIs in combination with other medications, that is, MAOIs, dihydroergotamine, tryptophan, dextromethorphan, lithium, or nefazodone or "tryptans" that block the reuptake of 5-HT. SSRIs inhibit the CYP-450 enzyme system and cause delayed clearance of certain medications. Use of CYP-450 1A2, 2D6, and 3A4 enzymes provide a substrate for their metabolism. All SSRIs can increase serum levels and decrease clearance of other substrate agents inhibiting these CYP450 (1A2, 2D6, 2C5, 34) hepatic enzyme systems. SSRIs exhibit a nonnegligible absolute risk of upper GI bleeding, and this causal relationship was confined to periods of SSRI use as opposed to periods of nonuse. Platelet 5-HT release plays on role in hemostasis. 5-HT is taken up from the blood circulation by 5-HT transporters similar to brain 5-HT transporters. Platelets are incapable of synthesizing 5-HT; therefore, 5-HT store depletion could induce hemorrhagic complications. The 5-HT role in hemostasis occurs by enhancement of effects upon adenosine diphosphate and thrombin. SSRIs in therapeutic doses consistently deplete 5-HT following several weeks of treatment [57]. The SSRIs are less effective than other antidepressants for the management of pain. Serotonin augments the rostral ventromedial medulla, and norepinephrine modulates the peripheral afferent fibers. A complete list of drug interactions involving the CYP 450 system and substrate drugs that may be used in the management of pain are provided elsewhere [1,2,11,12,14,15,22, 23,53,58–60].

Tricyclic antidepressants

Amitriptyline is hepatically converted to active metabolite, nortriptyline. Imipramine is transformed by the liver to desipramine. Trazodone (not a tricyclic antidepressant [TCA]) hepatically converted to *meta*-chlorophenyl piperazine (mCPP), a serotonin agonist, and is generally given at be bedtime because of its sedative properties. Trazodone is associated with orthostatic hypotension and use is discouraged in the elderly.

In general, the adverse effects of TCAs result mostly from cholinergic/muscarinic receptor blockade, α_2-adrenergic blockade, histaminergic (H_1 H_2) blockade, and dopaminergic blockade. Receptor blockade of cholinergic/muscarinic receptors can produce blurry vision, xerostomia, sinus tachycardia, constipation, urinary retention, and a memory dysfunction. Blockage of H_1 and H_2 receptors produces sedation, dizziness, weight gain, hypotension, and potentiation of CNS depressant agents. α_1 adrenergic blockade is often associated with postural hypotension and dizziness. Dopamine-receptor blockade has been associated with extra-pyramidal syndrome, dystonia, akathisia, rigidity, tremor, akinesia, neuroleptic malignant syndrome, tardive dyskinesia, and endocrine changes. Tachycardia and prolong the PR and QRS intervals with membrane stabilization occur. Orthostatic hypotension and, in patients who have impaired left ventricular function, congestive heart failure may occur. Bupropion blocks reuptake of both norepinephrine and dopamine, and also has relatively few cardiac side effects, minimal, if any, effects on cardiac conduction, and no production of orthostatic hypotension [1,2,10,12,14,58,59,61]. Metabolism of bupropion is by CYP450 2B6 and has produced CYP450 2D6 inhibition.

There are other receptor-specific antidepressants such as venlafaxine, nefazodone, and mirtazapine that do not currently fit into any broad antidepressant classification. Venlafaxine, an serotonin norepinephrine reuptake inhibitor (SNRI), has a complex MOA. It blocks the reuptake of serotonin at low doses, blocks the reuptake of norepinephrine at medium doses, and blocks the reuptake of dopamine at higher doses. Venlafaxine is, therefore, in effect three drugs in one due to such dose-related receptor-mediated events. Venlafaxine provided the therapeutic benefits of tertiary and secondary amine antidepressants without the TCA side-effect profile. Venlafaxine also is beneficial in chronic pain, as it lacks clinically relevant CYP 450 interactions, is easily titratable in an elderly patient, use is encouraged with the extended release dosage form, and is available in both immediate and action dosage form and has a curvalinear dose response curve, low plasma protein bindery, and without hepatic insults as is seen with duloxetine [1,2,61,62].

For patients receiving hemodialysis the venlafaxine dose should follow 4 hours after dialysis has been completed. Another SNRI duloxetine is to be released; this agent is a CYP450 2D6 inhibitor in which each of two active metabolites are CYP450 inducers. This agent has an indication that includes depression and diabetic peripheral neuropathic pain (about 25% better than a placebo).

Nefazodone, is another antidepressant that acts dually on 5-HT. Reuptake inhibition for 5-HT and NE occurs, coupled with 5-HT_2 receptor blockade. There is some α_1-adrenergic inhibition that produced orthostatic hypotension. This agent produces two active metabolites: the OH-nefazodone metabolite, which has activity similar to that of nefazodone, and the mCPP metabolite, which is the same metabolite found with trazodone. The MOA of mCPP is that of a 5-HT agonist coupled with mild 5-HT_2 and 5-HT_3 antagonism. This agent exhibits zero-order kinetics. There is also relevant CYP 450 3A4 inhibition [1,2,14]. A black box warning of potential hepatotoxicity accompanies this product.

Mirtazapine is an atypical antidepressant described as a noradrenergic 5-HT-specific antagonist. This agent produces therapeutic antagonism at α_2 auto- and hetero-receptors, thus facilitating enhanced noradrenergic and 5-HT, respectively. Mirtazepine's therapeutic benefits include negligible sexual dysfunction, a decrease in migraine headache, and a decrease in anxiety, agitation, depression, and insomnia are associated with 5-HT_2–5-HT_3–H_1–α_2-hetero, and α_2-autoreceptor blockade. Further antagonism occurs at 5-HT_2 receptors (decreasing anxiety and agitation) and at 5-HT_3 receptors (decreasing nausea and GI distress). H_1-receptor antagonism at low doses (≤ 30 mg) produces drowsiness, facilitating sleep and improving appetite. No clinically significant interactions are revealed on the CYP 450 system. Mirtazapine is a useful adjuvant agent in the management of chronic pain [23,61–66].

Anxiolytic agents

The principal modulatory site of the GABA receptor complex is found on its α subunit and is referred to as the benzodiazepine or ω receptor. Three subtype ω receptors have been identified, and it is thought that the ω_1 receptor is associated with sedation and the ω_2 is associated with AED, anxiolytic, and myorelaxant effects. The clinical effects of the ω_3 receptor have not been thoroughly investigated yet. The ω_2 receptors are associated with memory dysfunction such as forgetfulness or amnesia because of their anterograde amnesic effects, especially in some elderly patients.

Clonazepam offers a therapeutic option among other benzodiazepines. Lorazepam, temazepam, and oxazepam may be especially useful to patients with liver impairment, because these drugs do not have any active metabolites and are metabolized by phase II processes of glucuronidation [1,2,47,49,60,62,

67–69]. As with all benzodiazepines, falls and gait disturbances may occur in the elderly; an agent such as venlafaxine may be more beneficial for anxiety disorders comorbidity with pain or exclusive of pain.

Anticonvulsants

AEDs have produced therapeutic benefits in a variety of neuropathic painful syndromes. Such agents include carbamazepine, phenytoin, valproic acid, tiagabine, gabapentin, oxcarbazepine, vigabatrin, zonisamide, lamotrigine, and topiramate; these agents have been described elsewhere in the literature [1,2].

Topiramate has several mechanisms of action, all of which are not found with another single agent to date. Diminishing action potential by sodium channel blockade; increasing GABA frequency activation at GABA receptors, selectively antagonizing kainate activation at kainate/AMPA receptor sites, and providing glutamate antagonism (the only AED where glutamate antagonism is a prominent AED activity); additionally, some carbonic anhydrase inhibition occurs. Absorption is rapid with the bioavailability (f) about 80%. AMPA and kainate receptors have a role in mediating neuropathic pain. Pharmacokinetics linear steady state (Css) is achieved in about 4 days. Plasma protein binding is only 13% to 17%. Metabolism is minimal as a 70% of a dose is recovered unchanged in the urine; elimination half-life ($t_{0.5\beta}$) is 18 to 23 hours. The drug is cleared by hemodialysis. Clearance diminished in those patients exhibiting moderate renal impairment or hepatic impairment. Side effects seen in some patients include paresthesia or anorexia, to name a few. A $\leq 1\%$ incidence of renal calculi requires adequate hydration. CNS-related side effects are dose related, and are generally not observed at doses less than 200 mg/d. Cognitive motor slowing and speech or work finding difficulty are only seen in very minimal percent of patients when high doses are initiated, rapid incremental dose changes or with coprescribing with other AEDs. In our clinical practice with a large number of patents this CNS event occurrence was not a clinically relevant finding in the elderly patient. Clinical applications may be available for bipolar disorder, obesity treatment, bulimia, ethanol abuse, neuropathic pain syndromes, and migraine headache prophylaxis.

Skeletal muscle relaxants

Baclofen acts as a GABA$_B$ agonist and hyperpolarized membranes. Carisprodol is metabolized in the liver by CYP-450 2C19 to an active metabolite, meprobamate. It should be avoided in patients with renal or hepatic disease. With prolong use this drug is associated with dependence. Use of carisprodol is discouraged in the elderly.

Cyclobenzaprine, a frequently used muscle relaxant, is structurally similar to the tricyclic antidepressants. Side effects include drowsiness, dizziness, confusion, ataxia, xerostomia, and anticholinergic effects. Contraindications are similar to those of tricyclic antidepressants. Cyclobenzaprine should be avoided long term, and the manufacturer recommends that administration not exceed a 3-week period [1,2]. Use in the elderly patient is discouraged. Tizanidine, an α_2 adrenergic agent, may be titrated with very low doses. Side effects include xerostomia, drowsiness, dizziness, hypotension, and urinary frequency. Cautious use is suggested in elderly or those with impaired renal function. Tizanidine is hepatically metabolized and excreted in feces and urine. Metaxalone, a non-proprandol centrally acting muscle relaxant, may be administered on an empty stomach. Use caution in hepatic or renal dysfunction. Hemolytic anemia, leukopenia, and hepatotoxicity have been reported. Side effects include dizziness, drowsiness, paradoxical stimulation, nausea, and abdominal discomfort [1,2,22].

Topical analgesics

Capsaicin is a topical analgesic that may inhibit the synthesis, transport, and release of substance P, a peripheral neurotransmitter of pain. Capsaicin is used to treat pain associated with neuralgia, neuropathic pain, and arthritis.

Lidocaine topical patches (5%) are available for the relief of allodynia (painful hypersensitivity), chronic painful postherpetic neuralgia (PHN), and a variety of neuropathic pain conditions and nociceptive pain conditions; they are to be applied to intact skin cover in the painful area for 24 hours daily and 12 hours for PHN. The patch is placed over the intact skin painful areas (back, neck, joints, extremities) and left on for 24 hours daily. Lidocaine, aside from Na channel blockade, may affect A delta C-fiber on the dorsal horn of the spinal cord. Negligible systemic effects are seen in the elderly patients.

Sleep-promoting agents

Treating disorders of initiating and maintaining sleep secondary to pain requires pharmacologic intervention when sleep hygiene methods have proved less that satisfactory. Selection of a pharmacologic agent necessitates pharmacodynamic and pharmacokinetic decisions that address patient's specific needs. Zaleplon, a nonbenzodiazepine hypnotic, effects the $\omega 1$ receptor. Absorption is rapid, bioavailability is about 30%, and metabolism is primarily by aldehyde oxidase and by minor CYP 3A4 substrates forming inactive metabolites. The mean $t_{0.5}$ is about 1 hour. Therefore, the rapid onset, no active metabolites, no CYP 450 drug interactions of clinical consequence, rapid clearance from the body, and no major memory impairments make this agent highly suitable for use for patients with insomnia secondary to pain [1,2,70].

Miscellaneous agents

There are several other medications that can be used to relieved pain. Clonidine and tizanidine are both α agonists, and are believed to inhibit pain transmission by modulating NE and 5-HT release in the dorsal horn on the lamina of the spinal cord. Potentiation of μ-opioid receptors and a decrease in the wide

---

Box 4. Approach to persistent pain management

Respect and accept the complaint of pain as genuine
Address psychosocial components
Treat underlying disorder(s)
Address patient specific analgesics/adjuvant therapy needs
Relieve pain (not ablate pain)
Analgesics
Invasive interventions
Adjuvant agents
Nonpharmacologic methods
Customize treatment to patient-specific individual patient
    needs (pharmacokinetic pharmacodynamic, pharmacologic,
    drug interactions)

---

range of neuron excitability are additional mechanisms of the α_2 agonist; also, modulating specific calcium channels. Botulinum toxin type A has been used as an investigation ally for some painful syndromes [22,71,72].

Evaluation and reevaluations of the elderly patient by the health care provider promotes their decision to address emotional, cognitive, behavioral effects, and physiologic alterations that precipitate increased pain and dysfunction in the elderly (Box 4).

In conclusion, following this pharmacologic review the clinician is able to evaluate the pharmacotherapies for a specific patient's needs, basing the selection process upon personal clinical experiences, patient-specific concerns, side effects, adverse effects, drug interaction, pharmacodynamics, pharmacokinetics, and pharmacotherapeutics.

Appendix Box 1. Epidemiology of pain in the United States

- Over 20% of Americans >60 years of age have persistent pain related to arthritis, joint pain, or back pain
- Over 50 million Americans suffer from persistent pain
- Approximately 25 million Americans experience acute pain related to injuries or surgery

Appendix Box 2. Development of persistent pain in the elderly

Degenerative disease
Rheumatoid arthritis or osteoarthritis

Low back disorders
Arthropathies
Osteoporosis
Neuropathic pain (diabetic neuropathy, postherpetic neuralgia, trigeminal or
    occipital neuralgia)
Headaches
Oral pathology
Chronic leg cramps
Peripheral vascular disease
Poststroke syndromes
Improper positioning, use of restraints
Immobility, contractures
Pressure ulcers
Amputations
Chronic regional pain syndrome (I&II)

Appendix Box 3. Presence of pain in the elderly: nonspecific signs and symptoms

Frowning, moaning, grimacing, fearful facial expressions, grinding of teeth
    (bruxism)
Sighing, groaning, fearfulness, breathing heavily, withdrawn
Bracing, guarding, rubbing
Fidgeting, increasing or recurring restlessness
Striking out, increasing or recurring agitation
Eating or sleeping poorly
Mental status change
Decreasing activity levels
Depressed affect sudden onset
Resistant certain movements during care, rigidity
Change in gait or behavior
Paucity of interaction, speech
Loss of function—lack of adaptation skills

Appendix Box 4. Recognition of persistent pain in the elderly setting: patient-related behaviors

Cognitive and sensory impairment
Fear of addiction
Depression/anxiety
Lack of education regarding available treatment options
Underused pharmacotherapy

Pain is not inevitable with aging or chronic illness
Nonreport of pain does not equal no painful experience

Appendix Box 5. Recognition of persistent pain in the elderly setting: patient-related behaviors

Reluctance to report pain or take pain medications
Pain—undetected, misunderstood
Coexisting medical conditions
Coping expectations, experience
Multiple medications
Multiple pain etiologies
Sensory, emotional, cognitive impairments
Fear of reporting pain as a sign of weakness, fear of illness progression, no "cure," no treatments, close to terminal event

Appendix Box 6. Persistent pain in the elderly: common misconceptions

Is a sign of personal weakness to acknowledge
Is a punishment for past actions
A terminal event is impending
It always indicates the presence of a serious disease
Acknowledgment will lead to loss of independence and dependency upon others
They have a higher tolerance for pain (especially cognitive impaired)
They cannot accurately self-report pain (especially cognitive impaired)
Pain as an attention getting device
They are more likely to become "addicted" to pain medications

Appendix Box 7. Recognition of persistent pain in the elderly: setting health care professional barriers

Inadequate knowledge of pain treatment management
Lack of documented baseline and ongoing assessments
Lack of a standardized pain assessment tool(s) patient specific
Reliance solely upon pain scales (subjective)
Fear of resident or patient "addiction"
Temporal limitations
Concern about side effects of analgesic(s)
Insufficient retitration

Renal and hepatic dysfunction dose alterations
Concern about residents becoming intolerant to analgesics
Discriminating subjective and objective pain indices
Fear of regulatory scrutiny/sanctions
Pharmacotherapy knowledge deficits (pharmacokinetics, pharmacodynamics, pharmacotherapeutics, knowledge deficits of neuropathic and nociceptive pain interventions)
Priority given to pain management by facility (nursing home, hospital, and so on)
Inadequate reimbursements
Limited onsite pharmacy services
Staff education and evaluation progress (ineffective, nonexistent)
Pharmacotherapy options availability

Appendix Box 8. Elements of a pain history

Specific location of pain(s)
Distribution of pain (Dermatome)
Time sequences of pain
Associated events or activities that precipitate pain
Describe quality of pain
Burning, stabbing, spasms, dull, aching, throbbing
Laboratory data
Complete medication history
All medications over the past 6 months prescribed
Prescription and OTC drugs
Phytopharmaceuticals and home remedies
Alcohol and social drug use/abuse (prescribed/illicit) quantified/qualified
Drugs that have provided relief
Drugs that have not provided relief
Family and other interested third parties
Type of pain
    Nociceptive
    Neuroceptive
Severity of pain (objective, subjective)
Aggravating factors identified
Collateral pain mediated events
Insomnia, anxiety, depression, agitation, frustration, anger
Diagnostic tests performed
Behavioral assessment
All health care providers
Beliefs about pain relationships cause, meaning
Religious beliefs
Cultural background

References

[1] Barkin RL, Lubenow TR, Bruehl S, et al. Management of chronic pain, Part I and Part II. Disease-a-month, Vol. 42. St. Louis (MO): Mosby; 1996. p. 385–456.

[2] Barkin RL, Barkin D. Pharmacologic management of acute and chronic pain: a focus on drug interactions and patient specific pharmacotherapeutic selection. South Med J 2001;94:756–70.

[3] Merksey H, Bogduk N. Classification of chronic pain. 2nd ed. IASP Task Force on taxonomy. Seattle (WA): IASP Press; 1994.

[4] Decker MW, Meyer M. Therapeutic potential of neuronal nicotinic acetylcholine receptor agonists as novel analygesics. Biochem Pharmacol 1999;58:917–23.

[5] Katz B, Helme RD. Pain problems in old age. In: Tallis RC, Fillit HM, Brocklehurst JC, editors. Brocklehurst's textbook of geriatric medicine and gerontology. London: Harcourt Brace; 1998. p. 1423–30.

[6] Gloth III MF, editor. Hand book of pain relief in older adults: an evidence based approach. Totowa, NJ: Humanna Press; 2004.

[7] Loeser JD, Butler SH, Chapman CR, et al, editors. Bonica's management of pain. Phildelphia (PA): Lippincott Williams & Wilkins; 2001.

[8] Vrinten DH, Warfield CA, Bajwa ZH, et al. Principles and practice of pain medicine. Eur J Pharmacol 2001;429:61–9.

[9] Barkin RL, Oetgen J, Barkin SJ. Pharmacotherapeutic management opportunities utilized in chronic nonmalignant pain, supplement to drug topics. Montvale (NJ): Medical Economics Publishers; 1999.

[10] Schwer WA, Barkin RL, Katz WA, et al. The management of chronic pain in the elderly. Langhorn (PA): Education Medical Communications; 2000.

[11] McCarberg B, Barkin R. Long acting opioids for chronic pain: pharmacotherapeutic opportunities to enhance compliance, quality of life, and analgesia. Am J Ther 2001;8:181–6.

[12] Barkin RL, Barkin DS. Pharmacotherapeutic challenges in the elderly: polypharmacy, drug interactions, compliance and side-effects/adverse effects predictions. Anesthesia Today 1998;9:12–9.

[13] Barkin RL. Pharmacotherapy for nonmalignant pain. Am Fam Phys 2001;63:848.

[14] Barkin RL, Schwer WA, Barkin SJ. Recognition and management of depression in primary care: a focus on the elderly. A pharmacotherapeutic overview of the selection process among the traditional and new antidepressants. Am J Ther 2000;7:205–26.

[15] Barkin RL, Fawcett J. The management challenges of chronic pain: the role of antidepressants. Am J Ther 2000;7:31–47.

[16] Gibson SJ, Katz B, Corran TM, et al. Pain in older persons. Disabil Rehab 1994;16:127–39.

[17] Masoro EJ. Physiology of aging. In: Brocklehurst's textbook of geriatric medicine and gerontology. London: Harcourt Brace; 1998;6:85–96.

[18] Woodhouse K. The pharmacology of aging. In: Brocklehurst's textbook of geriatric medicine and gerontology. London: Harcourt Brace; 1998;11:169–78.

[19] Sarkozi L. Biochemical tests. In: Brocklehurst's textbook of geriatric medicine and gerontology. London: Harcourt Brace; 1998;16:217–26.

[20] Mann DMA. Neurobiology of aging. In: Brocklehurst's textbook of geriatric medicine and gerontology. London: Harcourt Brace; 1998;29:385–422.

[21] Harkins SW, Price DD. Assessment of pain in the elderly. In: Turk DC, Melzack R, editors. Handbook of pain assessment. New York: The Guilford Press; 1992.

[22] Beebe F, Barkin RL, Barkin SJ. Clinical and pharmacologic review of skeletal muscle relaxants for muscalosketal conditions. Amer J Therap 2005;12(2):151–71.

[23] Barkin RL, Chor PN, Braun BG, et al. A trilogy case review highlighting the clinical and pharmacologic applications of mirtazapine in reducing polypharmacy for anxiety, agitation, insomnia, depression, and sexual dysfunction. Primary care companion. J Clin Psychiatry 1999; 1:142–5.

[24] Barkin RL, Barkin DS, Barkin SJ, et al. Opiate, opioids, and centrally acting analgesics and

drug interactions: the emerging role of the psychiatrist. Medical Update for Psychiatrists 1998; 3:172–6.

[25] Barkin RL. Applying principles of science to the selection of COX-2 nonsteroidal anti-inflammatory drug. Pain Clin 2002;14:41–7.

[26] Barkin RL. Events associated with nonsteroidal anti-inflammatory, COX-1 and COX-2 drug use in patients with renal and hepatic insufficiency. Pain Clin 2002;14:24–7.

[27] Barkin RL, Sable KS. Caution recommended for prescribing and administering COX-1, COX-2 and COX-2 specific NSAIDs. Pharmacy and Therapeutics 2000;25:196–202.

[28] Barkin RL. Acetaminophen, aspirin or ibuprofen in combination analgesic products. Am J Ther 2001;8:433–42.

[29] Latta KS, Ginsberg B, Barkin RL. Meperidine: a critical review. Am J Ther 2002;9:53–68.

[30] Barkin R, Buvanendran A. Utilization of the COX-2 inhibitors (COXIBS) in the management of acute, postoperative pain and an overview of COX-1 NSAID agents. In: Eisenkraft JB, editor. Danne Miller Memorial Education Foundation. Progress in Anesthesiology. 2004.

[31] Agrawal NGB, Porras AG, Matthews CZ, et al. Single and multiple dose pharmacokinetics of etoricoxib, a selective inhibitor of cyclooxygenase-22, in man. J Clin Pharmacol 2003;43: 268–76.

[32] Cicero TJ, Adams EH, Geller A, et al. Assessment of tramadol abuse from April 5 1995 until March 31, 2000; progress report of the Independent Steering Committee, USA. ISC; 2000.

[33] Gaynes BL, Barkin RL. Analgesics in ophthalmic practice: a review of the oral non-narcotic agent tramadol. Optom Vis Sci 1999;76.

[34] Barkin RL. Three challenging, diverse pain patients' requirements for patient-specific treatment, economic and therapeutic implications of analgesia in hospital pharmacy. A poster Symposium at the 32 Annual ASHP Mid-year Clinical Meeting, Atlanta, GA, December 1997.

[35] Barkin RL. Focus on tramadol: a centrally acting analgesic for moderate to moderately severe pain. Analgesic Digest 1996;1:11–2.

[36] Barkin RL. Cancer pain treatment insights. Pharmacotherapy 1997;17:397–8.

[37] Barkin RL. Focus on tramadol: a centrally acting analgesic for moderate to moderately severe pain. Formulary 1995;30:321–5.

[38] Barkin RL. Alternative dosing for tramadol aids effectiveness. Formulary 1995;30:542–3.

[39] Katz WA. Pharmacology and clinical experience with tramadol in osteoarthritis. Drugs 1996; 52:39–47.

[40] Roth SH. Efficacy and safety of tramadol HCl in breakthrough musculoskeletal pain attributed to osteoarthritis. J Rheumatol 1998;25:1358–63.

[41] Schnitzer TJ, Gray WL, Paster RZ, et al. Efficacy of tramadol in treatment of chronic low back pain. J Rheumatol 2000;27:772–8.

[42] Moulin D, Harati Y. Tramadol for the treatment of the pain of diabetic neuropathy. Neurology 1999;52:1301.

[43] Russell IJ, Kamin M, Bennett RM, et al. Efficacy of tramadol in treatment of pain in fibromyalgia. J Clin Rheum 2000;6:250–7.

[44] Moore PA, Crout RJ, Jackson DL, et al. Tramadol hydrochloride: analgesic efficacy compared with codeine, aspirin with codeine, and placebo after dental extraction. J Clin Pharmacol 1998;38:554–60.

[45] Tarradell R, Pol O, Farre M, et al. Respiratory and analgesic effects of meperidine and tramadol in patients undergoing orthopedic surgery. Methods Find Exp Clin Pharmcol 1996; 18:211–8.

[46] Fricke Jr JR, Karim R, Jordan D, et al. A double-blind, single-dose comparison of the analgesic efficacy of tramadol/acetaminophen combination tablets, hydrocodone/acetaminophen combination tablets, and placebo after oral surgery. Clin Ther 2002;24:953–68.

[47] Huff J, Barkin RL, Lagatuta F. A primary care clinician's and consultants guide to medicating for pain and anxiety. Associated with outpatient procedures. Am J Ther 1994;1:186–90.

[48] Loh VT, Barkin RL. Appropriate use of opiates/opioids in migraine headache pain management. Continuing pharmacy education. Princeton (NJ): Bristol-Myers Squibb Company; 1998.

[49] Barkin RL, Richtsmeier AY. Alternative agents in pharmacologic management of sickle cell pain crisis complicated by acute pancreatitis. Am J Ther 1995;2:819–23.

[50] Leiken J, Barkin RL. Nalbuphine vs. meperidine in sickle cell anemia DICP. Ann Pharmacother 1990;24:781–2.

[51] Barkin RL. Pain management update: IV. Morphine infusions in children. Resident Staff Physician 1988;34:11–3.

[52] Richtsmeier A, Barnes SD, Barkin RL. Ventilatory arrest with morphine patient-controlled analgesia in a child with renal failure. Am J Ther 1997;4:255–7.

[53] Barkin RL, Iusco AM, Barkin SJ. Opoids used in primary care for the management of pain; A pharmacologic, pharmacotherapeutic, pharmacodynamic overview. Weiners pain management: A practical guide for clinicians. 7th edition. 2005;54:779–94.

[54] Barkin RL, Schwer WA, Barkin SJ. Recognition and management of depression in primary care: a focus on the elderly. A pharmacotherapeutic overview of the selection process among the traditional and new antidepressants. Am J Ther 2000;7:205–26.

[55] Barkin RL. Alternative dosing for tramadol aids effectiveness. Formulary 1995;30:542–3.

[56] Barkin RL. Withdrawal syndrome is not precipitated when butorphanol is added to opiate or opioid therapy: a comment on intranasal butorphanol-induced apraxia reversed by naloxone. Pharmacotherapy 1996;16(5):969.

[57] Dalton SO, Johansen C, Mellemkjaer L, et al. Use of selective serotonin reuptake inhibitors and risk of upper gastrointestinal tract bleeding. Arch Intern Med 2003;163:59–64.

[58] Barkin RL, Braun BG, Kluft RP. The dilemma of drug therapy for multiple personality disorder patients. In: Braun BG, editor. Treatment of multiple personality disorders. Washington (DC): American Psychiatric Press; 1986. p. 107–32.

[59] Braverman B, O'Connor C, Barkin RL. Pharmacology, physiology and anesthetic management of antidepressants in updated in pharmacology and physiology in anesthesia. Philadelphia: Lippincott Health Care.

[60] Bone RC, Levine RL, Barkin RL, et al. Recognition assessment, and treatment of anxiety in the critical care patient. Disease-a-month, vol. XL1. St. Louis (MO): Mosby; 1995. p. 5–95.

[61] Fawcett J, Barkin RL. Efficacy issues with antidepressants. J Clin Psychiatry 1997;58:32–9.

[62] Bhatia S, Bhatia S, Barkin R. Letters to the editor mirtazapine revisited. Am Fam Phys 1997; 56:2190–2.

[63] Fawcett J, Barkin RL. A meta-analysis of eight randomized, double-blind, controlled clinical trials of mirtazapine for the treatment of patients with major depressions and symptoms of anxiety. J Clin Psychol 1998;59:123–7.

[64] Davis J, Barkin RL. Clinical pharmacology of mirtazapine revisited. Am Fam Phys 1999; 60:1101.

[65] Fawcett J, Barkin RL. Review of the results from clinical studies on the efficacy, safety and tolerability of mirtazapine for the treatment of patients with major depression. J Affect Disord 1998;51:267–85.

[66] Barkin R. Mirtazapine: a multireceptor pharmacologic agent addressing multiple needs in the cancer patient. J Terminal Oncol 2003;2:39–41.

[67] Bone R, Levine R, Barkin RL. Recognition, assessment and treatment of anxiety in the critical care patient. Dis Mon 1995;41(5):293–360.

[68] Barkin RL, Leikin JB, Barkin SJ. Noncardiac chest pain: A focus upon psychogenic causes. Am J Ther 1994;1:321–6.

[69] Richtsmeier HA, Barkin RL, Alexander M. Benzodiazepines for acute pain in children. J Pain Symptom Manage 1992;7:492–5.

[70] Barkin RL. Pain management and the effects of pain on sleep. In: Golbin AZ, Kravitz HM, Keith LG, editors. Sleep Psychiatry. London: Taylor & Francis; 2005.

[71] Devers A, Galer BS. Topical lidocaine patch relieves a variety of neuropathic pain conditions: an open-label study. Clin J Pain 2000;16:287–94.

[72] Power I, Barratt S. Analgesic agents for the postoperative period. Nonopioids. Surg Clin North Am 1999;79:275–95.

ELSEVIER
SAUNDERS

Clin Geriatr Med 21 (2005) 491–511

CLINICS IN
GERIATRIC
MEDICINE

Crystal-Associated Arthritis in the Elderly

Christopher M. Wise, MD

Internal Medicine Division of Rheumatology, Allergy, and Immunology, Medical College of Virginia,
Virginia Commonwealth University Health System, 417 North 11th Street, Box 980647,
Richmond, VA 23298, USA

The two best-recognized forms of crystal-induced joint disease are caused by the deposition of monosodium urate (MSU) and calcium pyrophosphate dihydrate (CPPD). Although initially described by Sir Alfred Garrod in the eighteenth century, the first modern association of articular crystal deposition with arthritis was established in 1961 with the identification of MSU crystals in the synovial fluid of patients with acute gout [1]. This was followed shortly by the recognition of "pseudogout" associated with CPPD crystals [2]. Since then, a great deal has been learned about these two common types of arthritis, both of which are seen frequently in elderly patients. In addition, the role of other crystals, particularly basic calcium phosphate crystals, in the pathogenesis of osteoarthritis has been further explored.

Gout and pseudogout usually present as acute, self-limited episodes of mono-arthritis but may be associated with polyarticular attacks, chronic arthritis, and destructive changes in cartilage and bone. MSU and CPPD crystals can be found in synovial tissue and fluid from asymptomatic patients or during acute attacks of arthritis associated with a marked inflammatory response. The factors responsible for the inflammatory response to crystals are not completely understood [3]. The phlogistic properties of crystals seem to be linked to their ability to bind immunoglobulins and other proteins. These complexes bind to surface receptors on macrophages and mast cells, leading to activation and release of proinflammatory cytokines, chemotactic factors, and other mediators. An influx of phagocytic cells—particularly neutrophils—follows. Crystals are engulfed, and subsequent disruption of lysosomes releases arachidonate metabolites, collagenases, and oxygen radicals. Factors that contribute to the self-termination of attacks include digestion of crystals by myeloperoxidase; increased heat and

---

E-mail address: cmwise@hsc.vcu.edu

blood flow leading to dissolution and removal of crystals from the joint; alteration of the crystal properties by the inflammatory process itself; and downregulation that occurs with crystal phagocytosis by more mature macrophages later in the attack [4,5].

Gout typically has an onset in middle-aged adults, but has an increasing prevalence in older age groups, often with unique and atypical features. Pseudogout, on the other hand, is more often associated with onset in elderly patients and has more predictable features in this population. The recognition of crystal-induced arthritis in elderly patients should lead to the avoidance of unnecessary diagnostic tests and therapies in many patients with acute and chronic arthritis and allow more optimal management of two conditions that usually have a favorable outcome.

Gout

Epidemiology and pathogenesis of gout and hyperuricemia

Gout has been classically recognized as a disease affecting middle-aged men, but in fact has an increasing frequency in men and women in older age groups. The annual incidence of gout in men in most studies is in the range of 1 to 3 per 1000, but is much lower in women [6]. In the Framingham Study, for example, the 2-year incidence of gout was 3.2 per 1000 for men compared with 0.5 per 1000 for women [7]. The epidemiology of gout may have changed in various population groups over the past 10 to 20 years. For example, recent studies of gout in the United States over the past 2 decades has suggested that the incidence of gout may be increasing, with most of this increase coming in men and women over the age of 65 [8,9]. On the other hand, the average age of onset of gout appears to have decreased in a recent study of patients in Taiwan [10].

The overall prevalence of self-reported gout in the general population is 0.7% to 1.4% in men and 0.5% to 0.6% in women. In people over 65, this prevalence increases to 4.4% to 5.2% in men and 1.8% to 2.0% in women [6,11–13]. In male populations in particular, gout reaches a high prevalence by the fifth decade. For example, the prevalence of gout in a study of United States physicians was 5.8% among Caucasians and 10.9% among in African Americans who had been surveyed for a mean of 28 years after graduation from medical school [14]. Thus, most patients with gout are men, even in older age groups. However, among patients with the onset of gout after the age of 60, the distribution between men and women is almost equal, and in those with onset after 80, women seem to predominate [15,16].

The incidence and prevalence of gout is parallel to that of hyperuricemia in the general population. Serum urate levels increase by 1 to 2 mg/dL in men at the time of puberty, but women exhibit little change in urate levels until after menopause, when concentrations approach those seen in men [17]. Hyperuricemia is clearly associated with an increased risk of developing gout, although most patients with elevated serum uric acid levels do not have gout [18]. Persons with serum urate levels greater than 10 mg/dL have an annual incidence of gout of 70 per 1000 and a 5-year prevalence of 30%, whereas those with levels less than 7 mg/dL have an annual incidence of only 0.9 per 1000 and prevalence of 0.6%. Additional factors that correlate strongly with serum urate levels and the prevalence of gout in the general population include serum creatinine levels, body weight, height, and blood pressure. Most of the renal disease in patients with gout is believed to be the result of nephrosclerosis related to hypertension. However, a direct pathogenetic role for uric acid in the development of renal disease and hypertension is still possible [19,20]. Recent studies have also demonstrated that the development of gout is associated with higher levels of alcohol, meat, and seafood consumption but not with higher levels of vegetable purine intake, and the risk of gout is decreased in those with higher levels of dairy product consumption [21,22].

Hyperuricemia can result from decreased renal excretion or increased production of uric acid. In 80% to 90% of patients with primary gout, hyperuricemia is caused by renal underexcretion of uric acid, even though renal function is otherwise normal. The defect in renal excretion of uric acid in patients with primary gout may be attributed to reduced filtration, enhanced reabsorption, or decreased secretion, but it is unclear which of these mechanisms is most important. Patients with secondary gout related to renal disease are hyperuricemic because of a decreased filtered load and decreased tubular secretion of uric acid. Patients with lead nephropathy seem to be particularly prone to the development of gout, and recent studies have suggested that subclinical exposure to environmental lead may contribute to some of the hyperuricemia and gout seen in the general population [23,24]. The hyperuricemia associated with diuretic therapy, seen frequently in older populations, results from volume depletion, which leads to a decreased filtered load as well as enhanced tubular reabsorption [25]. A renal mechanism is also the cause of hyperuricemia associated with most other drugs, including low-dose aspirin and cyclosporine. About 40% of patients report a family history of gout in most series, and the hereditary component for serum uric acid levels in the general population has been estimated to be approximately 40% [17,26]. Most available data suggests that the genetic component of hyperuricemia and gout is related to multiple genes involving production and excretion of uric acid.

Typical clinical features

In typical gout, occurring most often in middle-aged men, the usual initial attack of gout occurs after years of sustained hyperuricemia and deposition of monosodium urate in the synovial tissue (Table 1). The initial attack of gout is monoarticular in 85% to 90% of patients [17]. Lower-extremity joints are usually affected, with approximately 60% of first attacks involving the first metatarsophalangeal (MTP) joints. Attacks may last from a few days to 2 to 3 weeks, with a gradual resolution of all inflammatory signs and a return to apparent normalcy.

Table 1
Clinical features of gout: typical versus elderly onset gout

Feature	Typical gout	Elderly onset gout
Age of onset	Peak in mid-40s	Over 65
Sex distribution	Men >> women	Men = women
Presentation	Acute monoarthritis	Polyarticular onset more often
	Lower extremity	Upper extremity more often
	(Podagra 60%)	Finger involvement more often
Tophi	After years of attacks	May occur early or without history
	Elbows > fingers	of prior attacks
		Possibly more often over fingers
Associated features	Obesity	Renal insufficiency
	Hyperlipidemia	Diuretic use, especially in women
	Hypertension	Alcohol use less common
	Alcohol use, heavy	

An "intercritical" period lasting weeks to months may elapse before a new attack occurs in the same or another joint. Without specific therapy, a second attack will occur in 78% of patients within 2 years, and in 93% within 10 years. Over subsequent years, attacks occur more frequently and may be polyarticular and associated with fever and constitutional symptoms [27–29]. Tophaceous deposits become apparent over the elbows, fingers, or other areas over the years, and chronic polyarticular arthritis may develop, sometimes resembling rheumatoid arthritis or degenerative joint disease.

Clinical features of gout in the elderly

The recognition of gout in elderly patients may be complicated by a tendency for patients in this age group to present differently than younger patients (see Table 1). Clinical observations have suggested several areas where gout in elderly patients differs from gout in younger age groups, as follows:

1. Polyarticular gout is more common in older patients and appears earlier in disease.
2. Women make up a larger proportion of older patients with gout.
3. Gout involves the small joints of the fingers in older patients more frequently.
4. Tophi occur earlier in the course of gout in older patients, often in atypical locations.
5. Diuretic use and renal disease are more frequent in older populations with gout.

Polyarticular gout

Patients with polyarticular gout tend to be older than those with monoarticular attacks, with a mean age of 60 to 64 years reported in previous series [27–29]. About 10% to 39% of these patients give a history of a polyarticular onset of their disease. One series of 36 patients with the onset of gout after the age of 60 noted a polyarticular onset in 18 (50%), a much higher incidence than that seen in typical middle-aged patients with gout [16]. The higher frequency of polyarticular involvement in older patients is likely to result from multiple factors. Elements that likely contribute to this phenomenon include more patients with chronic concomitant cardiac and renal disease, and medications such as low-dose aspirin and diuretics that contribute to the development of chronic hyperuricemia. A delay in diagnosis and treatment of gout in younger age groups may result in more older patients with a more indolent inflammatory component that may be difficult to distinguish from rheumatoid arthritis [16,30,31]. In such patients, the history of illness at onset is often difficult to obtain, and a prior history of acute intermittent arthritis or podagra may not be recalled.

Increased female frequency

An increased frequency of female patients is noted among older patients with gout, particularly in those with elderly onset gout. Most women, possibly up to 85%, have the onset of disease after menopause [32]. In a recent series of Korean women with gout, 75% developed the first symptomatic episode of gout after the onset of the menopause, and most of those with gout before menopause had renal disease or were taking cyclosporine for renal transplantation [33]. The mean age of women with gout in most series tends to be about 10 years older than in men, with a shorter duration of disease at the time of study [32]. Women constitute about 50% to 60% of patients with the onset of gout over the age of 60 [15,34,35], and almost all of the patients with the onset of disease over the age of 80 [15,36].

Small-joint finger involvement

Gouty inflammation of the small joints of the fingers in elderly patients has been noted more frequently in recent years (Fig. 1). Osteoarthritis of the distal and proximal interphalangeal (IP) joints is common in elderly patients, particularly women, and the typical inflammatory exacerbations seen in this condition are attributed to basic calcium phosphate crystals or other factors. The first convincing series of patients experiencing acute gout in previously osteoarthritic distal IP joints was reported by Simkin et al in 1983 [37]. In this series of five patients (four women and one man, ages 67 to 77), attacks of acute inflammation occurred in previously osteoarthritic joints, with urate crystals demonstrated in four of the involved joints. Most of these patients had a history of previous attacks of gout and obvious tophaceous deposits in the involved joints or elsewhere. Subsequent series have described a predilection for involvement of the small joints of the hands in elderly patients with gout, particularly women (see references [15,16,32,34,35]). In one of the larger series of patients with elderly onset gout, initial symptoms beginning in the fingers was noted in 25% of women, but none of the men [16]. Another series of women with gout noted

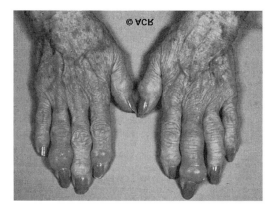

Fig. 1. Acute gout in the distal interphalangeal joints, mimicking a flare of osteoarthritis. (Courtesy of the Clinical Slide Collection on the Rheumatic Diseases, American College of Rheumatology, 1996.)

upper extremity involvement, usually in the finger joints, in about 30% [32]. Two larger series of patients with gouty involvement of the proximal and distal IP joints have been published [34,35]. In both studies, most patients were women with a mean age in the 70s. Distal IP joint involvement was a little more common than proximal IP involvement. Roentgenographic differentiation from the typical changes of erosive osteoarthritis was sometimes difficult, but the presence of soft tissue densities, large intraarticular and nonmarginal erosions, and osteolysis were more characteristic of gouty involvement. In addition, both series noted a high frequency of diuretic use in patients with IP joint involvement with gout.

Early atypical tophaceous gout

The early development of tophi, often in atypical locations, has been described frequently in elderly patients with gout, again particularly in women (Fig. 2). One early series reported that 44% of elderly women with gout had tophi compared with 8% of men, even though the women had a shorter duration of illness and

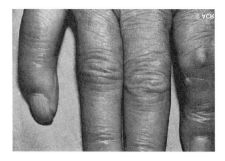

Fig. 2. A tophaceous gouty deposit over the index finger, with early ulceration. (Courtesy of the Clinical Slide Collection on the Rheumatic Diseases, American College of Rheumatology, 1996.)

fewer previous attacks [15]. In addition, at least three patients in this series had developed tophi on the fingers without any history of previous gouty attacks. The potential for the development of tophi without a prior history of gout was reported in another series of four elderly women with finger pad tophi seen over a 1-year period of time [36], and in a subsequent series of larger numbers of patients [38]. Another series of mostly postmenopausal women noted the presence of tophi in 27%, with localization to the fingers in 90% and no tophi noted on the elbows [32]. However, a more recent series of 22 women and 18 men with elderly onset gout did not demonstrate a tendency for an atypical distribution of tophi [16], and another series did not find any difference in age or sex between patients with finger pad tophi compared with those without [39]. Thus, observations of frequent atypical tophi in older patients may be the result of some element of observer bias.

Increased association with diuretic use

A high association with diuretic use and renal insufficiency has been noted in most elderly populations with gout [25]. Diuretic use has been reported in over 75% of patients with elderly onset gout, with a frequency of 95% to 100% in women [15,16,32]. In addition, most small series of elderly patients with atypical finger joint disease or tophaceous deposits report a consistent majority of patients taking diuretics [34–37]. A recent retrospective cohort study documented an almost twofold increase in the risk for initiating antigout therapy in patients within 2 years of starting thiazide diuretics for hypertension compared with nonthiazide therapy [40]. However, the recent increasing prevalence of gout in older populations in one recent study did not find that this increase was associated with diuretic use [8]. The association of gout and alcohol use appears to be less in elderly patients, particularly among women. Finally, some degree of renal insufficiency appears to be a regular phenomenon in most series of elderly patients with gout. Due to a lack of direct comparison to other elderly patients, it is unclear whether this decrease in renal function is peculiar to patients with gout, or merely reflects the trend seen in elderly populations in general.

Diagnosis and differential diagnosis

In younger patients, gout is often suspected on the basis of a typical attack of podagra in a male, or the development of tophi after many years of recurring attacks. In elderly patients, many of the presenting elements often relied on as surrogates for diagnosis are not present, and identification of crystals in synovial fluid or tissue becomes even more important in confirming a diagnosis.

In elderly patients, gout should be considered when attacks of acute pain and swelling are seen in osteoarthritic IP joints of the fingers, especially in patients with renal disease or on chronic diuretic therapy. Gout should be suspected when enlargement of these joints seems out of proportion to that seen with typical Heberden's or Bouchard's nodes. In patients with long-standing symptoms or in

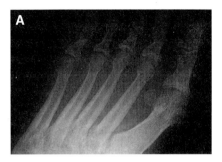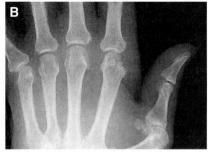

Fig. 3. Radiographic features of gout, showing characteristic well-defined lytic and erosive lesions of the metatarsal-phalangeal joints of the foot (*A*) and metacarpal-phalangeal joints of the hand (*B*).

elderly patients where tophaceous disease may appear early in the illness, radiographs may reveal well-defined gouty erosions in or around joints, particularly in the hands and feet, with characteristic overhanging edges (Fig. 3A and B) [41]. Most patients with gout have chronically elevated uric acid levels. However, serum uric acid levels may be normal at the time of an attack in up to half of patients, probably as an indirect result of the inflammatory process itself.

The detection of needle-shaped, negatively birefringent urate crystals under polarized light microscopy is the definitive diagnostic test for gout. Although this is best done by arthrocentesis in the setting of an acute attack, aspiration of synovial fluid from previously affected joints or aspiration of a subcutaneous nodule suspected of being a tophus is often helpful [42,43]. An examiner experienced in crystal identification should examine the synovial fluid, since inexperienced observers may miss their presence.

Alternative diagnoses should be considered in all patients suspected of gout. Acute arthritis can be caused by infection, other crystal induced arthropathies, particularly pseudogout (CPPD deposition disease). Because of a tendency for polyarticular attacks, sometimes associated with fever, gout should be considered in patients with suspected acute bacterial arthritis with negative cultures [27–29]. In addition, gout and infection can coexist in the same joints, making therapeutic decisions difficult in individual cases [44]. Synovial fluid cultures are essential in any patient with suspected gout having fever, comorbid conditions, or purulent-appearing synovial fluid.

Management

The goals of therapy in gout include termination of the acute attack, prevention of further attacks in the subsequent several weeks, assessment for associated and contributing factors, and consideration of long-term hypouricemic therapy (Table 2) [45–47]. The therapy of gout in older patients is often influenced by the presence of comorbid conditions, which dictate different approaches to the acute and chronic therapy [48].

Table 2
Management of gout: therapeutic options in elderly patients

Treatment options	Treatment notes
Acute attack:	
Nonsteroidal antiinflammatory drugs (NSAIDs) (Indomethacin and others)	With caution, low doses, limited periods, normal renal function, avoid Indomethacin in elderly; use selective COX-2 inhibitor
Corticosteroids (intraarticular, oral, parenteral)	Preferable in patients with comorbid conditions, with caution in diabetes
Corticotropin (ACTH) (parenteral)	Similar to corticosteroids, availability limited in some
Colchicine (oral)	With extreme caution, low doses, healthy patients only, consider avoidance of IV preparation
Short-term prophylaxis:	
Colchicine-low dose	With caution, low dose or avoid with renal insufficiency
NSAIDs-low dose	With caution, low dose, or avoid with renal or peptic ulcer disease; use selective COX-2 inhibitor
Long-term hypouricemic therapy:	
Uricosuric agents (Probenecid and others)	Seldom effective in elderly patients due to renal dysfunction
Allopurinol	Reduce dosage based on creatinine clearance

Management of acute gout

Treatment of acute gout should be initiated as early into the attack as possible to achieve optimal results. Agents available for terminating acute gout include colchicine, nonsteroidal antiinflammatory drugs (NSAIDs), corticotropin (ACTH), and corticosteroids. Because of the variable toxicities of these therapies, the choice among agents should be based on the patient's age and overall health, with underlying renal and gastrointestinal disease often limiting factors for NSAID and colchicine use. In recent years, corticosteroids have been used more often in older patients with multiple comorbid conditions because of their low toxicity profile.

Colchicine has been used for centuries to treat acute attacks of gout. Unfortunately, most patients experience nausea, vomiting, and abdominal cramps, and diarrhea when given doses needed to control severe attacks. Colchicine should be given more cautiously in elderly patients (at the minimal dose required to control the acute attack) and avoided in those with renal or hepatic insufficiency or in patients already on chronic maintenance colchicine [49]. Intravenous colchicine was used more in the past for acute gout, but increasing recognition of the potential for bone marrow suppression and other systemic toxicities has resulted in guidelines for restricting dosage or availability, and this form of colchicine should not be used in elderly patients or should be used with extreme caution [50,51]. Because of these multiple limitations, colchicine has a limited role in the therapy of acute crystal induced arthritis in elderly patients.

NSAIDs remain the agents of choice for acute gout in young, healthy patients without comorbid diseases. The use of all NSAIDs is limited by the risks of

NSAID gastropathy (eg, gastric ulceration and gastritis), other GI bleeding, acute renal failure, fluid retention, interference with antihypertensive therapy, and, in older patients, problems with mentation. The risks of toxicity of all types are increased in elderly patients, particularly those with renal dysfunction [45,52,53]. Indomethacin, in particular, though notorious for its efficacy, is also notorious for its poor tolerability in elderly patients. Thus, in most elderly patients with acute gout, indomethacin should be avoided and other NSAIDs should be used only in low doses for short periods of time. Careful monitoring of renal function is particularly important in patients with decreased renal function or edematous states before starting therapy. The newly available selective cyclo-oxygenase-2 (COX-2) inhibitory NSAIDs (celecoxib, valdecoxib) have potential as safer therapy for acute gout, as these agents have a decreased risk of serious gastro-intestinal toxicity and do not inhibit platelet function [54]. However, selective COX-2 inhibitors still have potential to interfere with renal function and cause edema, and should be used with caution in patients with renal insufficiency, hypertension, and edema.

Corticosteroids have become increasingly popular in acute gout in recent years in elderly patients [55–61]. Intraarticular steroids after arthrocentesis are extremely useful in providing relief, particularly in large effusions where the aspiration of as much fluid as possible will result in rapid improvement in pain and tightness of the affected joint. The dosage of steroid varies depending on the size of the joint, ranging from 5 to 10 mg of triamcinolone for small joints of the hands or feet to 40 to 60 mg for larger joints such as the knee [62]. Systemic corticosteroids may also be useful in patients where colchicine or NSAIDs are inadvisable, or in patients with polyarticular attacks. Tapered doses of oral prednisone, starting at 40 to 60 mg daily, and single intramuscular injections of ACTH (40 units) or triamcinolone (40 to 60 mg) have all been shown to be as effective as NSAIDs in acute gout. In most studies of systemic steroids for acute gout, only a small proportion of patients have required repeat therapy or experienced "rebound" attacks in the first several days after therapy.

Intercritical gout

Patients remain at increased risk for another attack for several weeks after resolution of an acute attack of gout. For this reason, prophylaxis with small doses of colchicine or NSAIDs may be considered to prevent further attacks in selected patients. Colchicine in a dose of 0.6 mg twice daily will prevent attacks in over 80% of patients. Prophylaxis should be continued for 1 to 2 months after an acute attack or for several months in patients with a history of frequent attacks, as well as when urate lowering drugs are initiated. The dose of colchicine should be reduced to 0.6 mg every day to every other day, or duration limited in patients with reduced renal function, because bone marrow suppression and myoneuropathy have been reported in patients on chronic low-dose colchicine with a creatinine clearance of less than 50 mL per minute [63,64].

A 24-hour urine collection or spot urinary urate/creatinine determination to determine whether a patient is an "overproducer" or "underexcretor" of uric acid is seldom useful in elderly patients [65,66]. Because most elderly patients with gout have decreased renal function and many have tophaceous disease, uricosuric drugs would not be indicated in management, and information obtained from this determination is usually of no help in making decisions regarding long-term hypouricemic therapy. Dietary factors are not likely to have a major impact on elderly patients with gout, and even a strict purine-free diet has only a small effect on serum urate levels. However, some patients may have a mild reduction in serum urate levels with dietary restrictions designed to improve lipid profiles [67,68]. Heavy alcohol use appears to be less common in elderly women, but may be a correctable factor in older men. A history of homemade whiskey (moonshine) ingestion and possible chronic lead intoxication should be considered in male gout patients with renal insufficiency [69]. A review of concomitant medications, with special attention to diuretic use, is essential in all elderly patients with gout. In patients with tophaceous disease or recurrent attacks, the need for diuretics should be assessed, and discontinuation considered in those patients where alternatives are available for managing comorbid hypertension and cardiac disease. In addition, the effect of low-dose aspirin on urate excretion in this population should be considered when treatment is initiated in elderly patients with gout [70].

Chronic hypouricemic therapy

Therapy with drugs to lower urate levels should be considered in patients who have had crystal proven gout with recurrent attacks and in those with tophaceous gout. In addition, patients with a history of gout and renal insufficiency may have improvement in renal function with hypouricemic therapy, possibly due to reduction in renal urate deposition or reduced use of NSAIDs [71]. Because of the high frequency of comorbid conditions and decreased life expectancy in elderly patients, it may be less important to institute urate-lowering therapy than in younger patients with many years of cumulative attacks and joint damage in their future [72].

Most patients who have had more than two to three attacks, those with coexistent renal disease, or those with tophi and evidence of radiographic joint damage should be treated with hypouricemic therapy. Reduction of serum urate levels well into the normal range (ie, below 6.0 mg/dL) will eventually lead to prevention of further attacks and resorption of tophi [73]. As noted previously, low-dose colchicine or NSAIDs may be used to prevent attacks that can occur for several months after beginning therapy, but still should be used with caution in older patients with reduced renal function [74].

Uricosuric drugs are seldom used in elderly patients due to the high frequency of renal insufficiency in this population, but may be considered in patients with a creatinine clearance greater than 50 mL per minute, no history of nephrolithiasis, and a 24-hour excretion of urate less than 700 mg daily. Probenecid in doses of

1 to 2 g daily is the most commonly used agent in this class, but carries a risk of precipitating renal stones, which may be reduced by high urine volume and alkalinization with bicarbonate intake. Overall, up to 25% of patients are not well controlled on currently available uricosuric drug therapy. Benzbromarone, a uricosuric agent currently available in Europe, has been shown to be comparable to allopurinol in lowering urate levels in patients with moderate renal insufficiency, but has also been associated with severe hepatoxicity in some patients [13,75]. In addition, recent studies demonstrating a uricosuric effect with the lipid-lowering agent, fenofibrate, and the angiotensin receptor blocker, losartan, suggests that these agents could be used in selected patients to lower serum urate levels [76,77].

Allopurinol, the only currently available inhibitor of xanthine oxidase, will reduce serum urate levels in almost all compliant patients [46,78]. In practice, the dosage of allopurinol prescribed is often inappropriately high or low in elderly patients, but compliance among elderly patients tends to be better than in younger patients [79,80]. A dose of 300 mg daily is standard in younger patients with normal renal function, but this should be reduced to 200 mg in patients with glomerular filtration rates (GFR) below 60 mL per minute, and to 100 mg in those with a GFR below 30 mL per minute. Patients with a GFR less than 10 mL per minute can be treated with 100 mg every 2 to 3 days. The dose of some other drugs, particularly azathioprine, needs to be reduced in patients on allopurinol because of common pathways of metabolism. Approximately 2% of patients taking allopurinol develop a hypersensitivity rash that can progress to a severe exfoliative dermatitis in a small number of patients [78]. This is more likely to occur in patients taking ampicillin or in those with renal insufficiency. Severe rashes may be accompanied by a syndrome of vasculitis, hepatitis, and interstitial renal disease, with a risk of mortality of 20% in some series. Because of this, allopurinol should be discontinued in any patient developing a rash, and re-institution considered only in patients with mild rashes and a clear-cut need for allopurinol therapy. In addition, a regimen of slow oral desensitization, starting with doses of 50 mcg daily and increasing to 100 mg daily over a 4-week period has been shown to be safe and successful in allowing most patients with prior hypersensitivity reactions to restart allopurinol therapy [81]. Other nonpurine agents capable of inhibiting xanthine oxidase and thereby lowering uric acid are in development (eg, febuxostat).

Calcium pyrophosphate dihydrate deposition disease (pseudogout)

The term "pseudogout" was first used to describe patients with goutlike attacks of arthritis, CPPD crystals found in synovial fluids, and radiographic intra-articular cartilage calcification (chondrocalcinosis) [2]. Since that time, other clinical presentations and patterns of joint disease have been associated with CPPD crystals, and the term "CPPD deposition disease" has been used.

CPPD deposition disease is generally a disease of the elderly with an average age of patients in most series of around 70 years. The metabolic basis for CPPD formation and deposition is less well understood than that for urate crystals. CPPD crystal formation occurs almost exclusively in the articular and peri-articular tissue, usually near the surface of chondrocytes [82]. Crystal formation is enhanced by locally elevated levels of either calcium or pyrophosphate (PP_i) or factors in the cartilage matrix that promote crystal formation. An abnormal substrate of matrix collagen and proteoglycan, as well as variations in mineral content, may promote crystal deposition. Local elevations of PP_i levels appear to be related to overactivity of a cell surface enzyme (ectoenzyme) known as nucleoside triphosphate pyrophosphohydrolase (NTPPH), which catalyzes the extracellular hydrolysis of ATP, and the extracellular transport of PP_i by a trans-membrane protein (ANK) [83]. In addition, some of the excess PP_i production may take place intracellularly through NTPPH or as a by-product of cellular proteoglycan and protein synthesis. Other factors that may contribute to excess PP_i and crystal formation include decreased activity of pyrophosphatase, degenerating cellular debris, abnormal matrix collagen, and even the local influence of growth factors (transforming growth factor and insulin-like growth factor). The mechanisms by which CPPD crystals induce inflammation are believed to be similar to those observed in gout.

The role of calcium containing crystals (both CPPD and basic calcium phosphate) in the development of osteoarthritis has been supported by clinical observations and by experimental evidence of the effects of these crystals on cartilage in vitro [84–86]. Both crystals have been associated with exaggerated forms of osteoarthritis, and are more commonly seen in osteoarthritic joints than in normal joints or those affected by inflammatory forms of arthritis. In addition, calcium-containing crystals have been shown to promote synovial hyperplasia, induce collagenase and metalloproteases, and lead to the generation of pro-inflammatory prostaglandins and cytokines [87].

The radiographic correlate of CPPD deposition disease (chondrocalcinosis) is a common finding in older individuals; it may be an incidental finding or associated with arthritis. The prevalence of chondrocalcinosis in the general population is as high as 10% to 15% in those age 65 to 75, and increases to over 40% in patients over 80 years of age [30,88,89]. In most of these older individuals, concomitant osteoarthritis is present. Because osteoarthritis is common in the elderly, the role each process plays in the pathogenesis of the other is not completely understood. Most cases of CPPD are idiopathic. However, familial occurrence has been reported. Most of the familial forms have shown an autosomal-dominant transmission but have displayed various clinical presentations, and most appear to involve single gene mutations [90]. An association with various endocrine and metabolic conditions is well accepted (Box 1). These include hyperparathyroidism in up to 5% of cases, hypophosphatasia, hypo-magnesiemia, and hemochromatosis. Schumacher first described a distinct form of arthritis in association with hemochromatosis in 1964 [91]. This arthropathy has some similarities to osteoarthritis and rheumatoid arthritis and may be the

---

Box 1. Clinical associations with CPPD deposition disease

Aging

- Asymptomatic chondrocalcinosis or associated
  with osteoarthritis

Idiopathic
Familial
Endocrine and metabolic diseases

- Hyperparathyroidism
- Hemochromatosis
- Hypophosphatasia
- Hypomagnesemia

---

initial presenting feature in some patients [92]. Arthritis is a common clinical feature at the time of diagnosis of hemochromatosis, and patients with arthropathy tend to be older [93].

Clinical features

CPPD deposition disease may have many clinical presentations mimicking gout, rheumatoid arthritis, osteoarthritis, or neuropathic joint disease [94]. In addition, CPPD may coexist in symptomatic or asymptomatic form with any of these conditions. The three most common clinical forms of the disease present as acute attacks of mono or polyarthritis (pseudogout), as a chronic arthropathy associated with osteoarthritis or as an incidental asymptomatic process. The joints most frequently involved in pseudogout are the knee, wrist, shoulder, and hip. In fact, knee involvement is so characteristic of CPPD deposition that it is often said that the knee joint is to pseudogout what the MTP joint is to gout.

Acute pseudogout is similar to acute gout, with acute monoarticular swelling, particularly prominent in the knee, wrist, or over the dorsum of the hand and wrist. Attacks may be precipitated by trauma and have been noted to occur after acute medical illness or after surgery, [95]. Polyarticular attacks have been reported, but are not as well described, and probably not as common as in gout. Other systemic features, such as fever, confusion, disorientation, nuchal rigidity, and leucocytosis have been reported in individual cases [96].

Diagnosis and differential diagnosis

The main differential diagnosis is with other crystal-induced processes, primarily gout, and with infection, which should always be included in the dif-

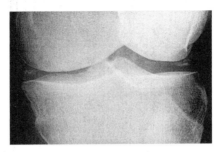

Fig. 4. Radiograph of a knee, showing typical articular chondrocalcinosis in the areas of the medial and lateral meniscus. (*From* Rheumatic Disease Clinics of North America 2000;26(3):527–46.)

ferential diagnosis. Thus, synovial fluid aspiration and examination for crystals is essential to the diagnosis. The synovial fluid in pseudogout is usually inflammatory and may occasionally be hemorrhagic. A leucocyte count of 10,000 to 20,000/mm^3 cells is the rule, but in the small joints, as in the wrist, high counts may be seen. CPPD crystals are pleomorphic, and may be intracelluar or extracellular. These crystals can be visualized under regular microscopy as square or rectangular intracellular inclusions, and give a weakly positive birefringence under polarized microscopy. Because of this weak birefringence, many laboratories may miss CPPD crystals, emphasizing the importance for an observer experienced in crystal identification to examine the fluid.

Occasionally, infection or other crystals, such as MSU or BCP, may coexist with CPPD. Radiographic studies of affected joints often reveal chondrocalcinosis of the articular cartilage (Figs. 4 and 5). Bilateral calcifications of the menisci in the knees or of the triangular ligament at the radioulnar joint at the wrist are characteristic. Other features include narrowing and sclerosis of the radiocarpal and patellofemoral joints. Rarely, extra-articular calcifications involving tendons or "tophaceous" deposits occur. Other clinical presentations include a "pseudorheumatoid" type with polyarticular joint swelling, morning

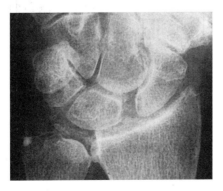

Fig. 5 Radiograph of a wrist, showing typical articular chondrocalcinosis in the triangular cartilage distal to the ulna, and in the radiocarpal and intercarpal joints. (*From* Rheumatic Disease Clinics of North America 2000;26(3):527–46.)

stiffness, pain, and high sedimentation rate. Because of the high prevalence of wrist involvement in CPPD and the increased prevalence of positive rheumatoid factor tests in older populations, it may be difficult to distinguish a patient with CPPD arthropathy from a patient with early rheumatoid arthritis. The radiologic findings of chondrocalcinosis, the absence of erosive disease, and the synovial fluid findings of CPPD crystals help differentiate CPPD deposition from true rheumatoid arthritis. Because CPPD deposition disease and osteoarthritis are both common in elderly patients, it is not surprising that they often coexist in the same patient.

In individual patients with pseudogout, studies to evaluate for underlying associated metabolic conditions may include calcium, phosphorous, alkaline phosphatase, and iron studies, in addition to radiographic studies of affected joints. However, these studies are less likely to reveal an associated condition in older populations, where idiopathic CPPD deposition is extremely common.

Management

With the exception of therapeutic strategies aimed specifically at uric acid metabolism, the management of the patient with pseudogout is similar to the management of the patient with acute gout (see discussion under gout), with the main goal of therapy being control of the acute inflammatory reaction [46]. Rest of the inflamed joint(s), NSAIDs, or intraarticular corticosteroid preparations are the mainstay of therapy. Because many attacks are of short duration, complete aspiration of the joint may be sufficient to significantly relieve pain and discomfort in some patients. Colchicine is effective in acute pseudogout but should be used with caution because of the risk of toxicity in elderly patient at the doses required to control the acute attack (see discussion under gout). At lower doses of 0.6 mg once or twice daily, colchicine can be helpful in preventing further attacks [97]. In some patients, intramuscular or subcutaneous ACTH (40 units) or intramuscular triamcinolone (60 mg) can control the acute inflammatory reaction [60]. For those with chronic pain and inflammation, physiotherapy, analagesics, colchicine, and NSAIDs are alternatives for management. For patients with chronic pseudorheumatoid CPPD deposition disease, hydroxychloroquine in doses of 200 to 400 mg per day has been shown to be superior to placebo in one small controlled study [98].

Basic calcium phosphate (bcp)-hydroxyapatite deposition disease

A group of apatite-like (basic calcium phosphate or BCP) crystals has been identified in pathologic synovial fluids and articular and periarticular tissues in various musculoskeletal disorders [99]. Because of their smaller size and lack of easily available detection methods, the identification of these crystals is much more difficult than for CPPD crystals. For these reasons, most of the information on the role of BCP crystals in arthritis is based on the use of x-ray diffraction or infrared spectroscopy. BCP crystals may be found in 30% to 60% of synovial fluids from patients with osteoarthritis and may contribute to the low-grade inflammatory process and cartilage destruction seen in typical osteoarthritis and seem to be associated with more severe osteoarthritis [85,87]. In other patients, periarticular soft tissue calcifications may be associated with an acute inflammatory reaction, clinically recognized as acute calcific periarthritis-tendinitis-bursitis. Shoulder involvement is common, and involvement of the first metatarsophalangeal joint ("pseudopodagra"), primarily affecting young women, has been described. Subcutaneous or periarticular calcifications have been found as well in patients with chronic renal failure and secondary to connective tissue disorders, such as in patients with inflammatory myopathies.

A severe destructive arthropathy of the shoulder and of the knee associated with BCP crystals has been described primarily in older women [100–103]. This entity, the "Milwaukee shoulder-knee syndrome," is often bilateral and in most patients leads to significant functional impairment and pain. It is associated with rotator cuff degeneration and glenohumeral joint instability. Radiologic changes include glenohumeral degeneration, periarticular calcification, rotator cuff degeneration and rupture, and superior displacement of the humeral head.

The synovial fluid may be serosanguineous and contains few cells. Under regular light microscopy, hydroxyapatite crystals may appear as clumps or as intracellular "shiny coins" and are not birefringent under polarized microscopy. Radiograph diffraction and biochemical analysis may be needed for definitive identification of these crystals. The treatment of these patients is frequently unsatisfactory. Joint aspirations and intra-articular corticosteroid injections have been helpful in some. For those patients with acute periarthritis, analgesics, NSAIDs, corticosteroid injections, and physiotherapy are the choices in therapy.

References

[1] McCarty DJ, Hollander JL. Identification of urate crystals in gouty synovial fluids. Ann Intern Med 1961;54:452–60.

[2] McCarty DJ, Kohn NN, Faires JS. The significance of calcium phosphate crystals in the synovial fluid of arthritis patients: the "pseudogout syndrome." I. Clinical aspects. Ann Intern Med 1962;56:711–37.

[3] Schiltz C, Liote F, Prudhommeaux F, et al. Monosodium urate monohydrate crystal-induced inflammation in vivo: quantitative histomorphometric analysis of cellular events. Arthritis Rheum 2002;46(6):1643–50.

[4] Landis RC, Yagnik DR, Florey O, et al. Safe disposal of inflammatory monosodium urate monohydrate crystals by differentiated macrophages. Arthritis Rheum 2002;46(11):3026–33.

[5] Yagnik DR, Hillyer P, Marshall D, et al. Noninflammatory phagocytosis of monosodium urate monohydrate crystals by mouse macrophages. Implications for the control of joint inflammation in gout. Arthritis Rheum 2000;43:1779–89.

[6] Roubenoff R. Gout and hyperuricemia. Rheum Dis Clin North Am 1990;16:539–50.

[7] Abbott RD, Brand FN, Kannel WB, et al. Gout and coronary artery disease. The Framingham study. J Clin Epidemiol 1988;41:237–42.

[8] Arromdee E, Michet CJ, Crowson CS, et al. Epidemiology of gout: Is the incidence rising? J Rheumatol 2002;29(11):2403–6.

[9] Wallace KL, Riedel AA, Joseph-Ridge N, Wortmann R. Increasing prevalence of gout and hyperuricemia over 10 years among older adults in a managed care population. J Rheumatol 2004;31(8):1582–7.

[10] Yu KH, Luo SF. Younger age of onset of gout in Taiwan. Rheumatology (Oxford) 2003;42(1). 166–70.

[11] Lawrence RC, Hochberg MC, Kelsey JL, et al. Estimates of the prevalence of selected arthritic and musculoskeletal diseases in the United States. J Rheumatol 1989;16:427–41.

[12] Lawrence RC, Helmick CG, Arnett FC, et al. Estimates of the prevalence of arthritis and selected musculoskeletal disorders in the United States. Arthritis Rheum 1998;41(5): 778–99.

[13] Bieber JD, Terkeltaub RA. Gout: on the brink of novel therapeutic options for an ancient disease. Arthritis Rheum 2004;50(8):2400–14.

[14] Hochberg MC, Thomas J, Thomas DJ, et al. Racial differences in the incidence of gout. Arthritis Rheum 1995;38:628–32.

[15] MacFarlane DG, Dieppe PA. Diuretic-induced gout in elderly women. Br J Rheumatol 1985; 24:155–7.

[16] Ter Borg E, Rasker J. Gout in the elderly, a separate entity? Ann Rheum Dis 1987;46:72–6.

[17] Wortmann RL, Kelley WN. Gout and hyperuricemia. In: Ruddy S, Harris ED, Sledge CB, editors. Textbook of rheumatology. Philadelphia: Saunders; 2001. p. 1339–76.

[18] Campion ES, Glynn RJ, DeLabry LO. Asymptomatic hyperuricemia: risks and consequences in the Normative Aging Study. Am J Med 1987;82:421–6.

[19] Lin KC, Tsao HM, Chen CH, Chou P. Hypertension was the major risk factor leading to development of cardiovascular diseases among men with hyperuricemia. J Rheumatol 2004; 31(6):1152–8.

[20] Johnson RJ, Kang DH, Feig D, et al. Is there a pathogenetic role for uric acid in hypertension and cardiovascular and renal disease? Hypertension 2003;41(6):1183–90.

[21] Choi HK, Atkinson K, Karlson EW, et al. Purine-rich foods, dairy and protein intake, and the risk of gout in men. N Engl J Med 2004;350(11):1093–103.

[22] Choi HK, Atkinson K, Karlson EW, et al. Alcohol intake and risk of incident gout in men: a prospective study. Lancet 2004;363(9417):1277–81.

[23] Shadick NA, Kim R, Weiss S, et al. Effect of low level lead exposure on hyperuricemia and gout among middle aged and elderly men: the normative aging study. J Rheumatol 2000;27: 1708–12.

[24] Lin JL, Tan DT, Ho HH, Yu CC. Environmental lead exposure and urate excretion in the general population. Am J Med 2002;113(7):563–8.

[25] Scott JT, Higgins CS. Diuretic induced gout: a multifactorial condition. Ann Rheum Dis 1992;51:259–61.

[26] Wilk JB, Djousse L, Borecki I, et al. Segregation analysis of serum uric acid in the NHLBI Family Heart Study. Hum Genet 2000;106(3):355–9.

[27] Hadler NM, Franck WA, Bress NM, Robinson DR. Acute polyarticular gout. Am J Med 1974; 56:715–9.

[28] Lawry GV, Fan PG, Bluestone R. Polyarticular versus monoarticular gout: a prospective comparative analysis of clinical features. Medicine 1988;67:335–43.

[29] Raddatz DA, Mahowald ML, Bilka PJ. Acute polyarticular gout. Ann Rheum Dis 1983;42: 117–20.

[30] Doherty M, Dieppe P. Crystal deposition in the elderly. Clin Rheum Dis 1986;12:97–116.

[31] Sewell KL, Petrucci R, Keiser HD. Misdiagnosis of rheumatoid arthritis in an elderly woman with gout. J Am Geriatr Soc 1991;39:403–6.

[32] Puig JG, Michan AD, Jimenez ML, et al. Female gout: clinical spectrum and uric acid metabolism. Arch Intern Med 1991;151:726–32.

[33] Park YB, Park YS, Song J, et al. Clinical manifestations of Korean female gouty patients. Clin Rheumatol 2000;19(2):142–6.

[34] Fam AG, Stein J, Rubenstein J. Gouty arthritis in nodal osteoarthritis. J Rheumatol 1996;23: 684–9.

[35] Lally EV, Zimmermann B, Ho Jr G, Kaplan SR. Urate-mediated inflammation in nodal osteoarthritis: clinical and roentgenographic correlations. Arthritis Rheum 1989;32:86–90.

[36] Shmerling RH, Stern SH, Gravallese EM. Tophaceous deposition in the finger pads without gouty arthritis. Arch Intern Med 1988;148:1830–2.

[37] Simkin PA, Campbell PM, Larson EB. Gout in Heberden's nodes. Arthritis Rheum 1983; 26:94–7.

[38] Wernick R, Winkler C, Campbell S. Tophi as the initial manifestation of gout: report of six cases and review of the literature. Arch Intern Med 1992;152:873–6.

[39] Holland NW, Jost D, Beutler A, et al. Finger pad tophi in gout. J Rheumatol 1996;23(4):690–2.

[40] Gurwitz JH, Kalish SC, Bohn RL, et al. Thiazide diuretics and the initiation of anti-gout therapy. J Clin Epidemiol 1997;50(8):953–9.

[41] Nakayama DA, Barthelemy C, Carrera G, et al. Tophaceous gout: a clinical and radiographic assessment. Arthritis Rheum 1984;27:468–71.

[42] Agudelo CA, Weinberger A, Schumacher HR, et al. Definitive diagnosis of gout by identification of urate crystals in asymptomatic metatarsophalangeal joints. Arthritis Rheum 1979; 22:559–60.

[43] Pascual E, Batlle-Gualda E, Martinez A, et al. Synovial fluid analysis for diagnosis of intercritical gout. Ann Intern Med 1999;131(10):756–9.

[44] Yu KH, Luo SF, Liou LB, et al. Concomitant septic and gouty arthritis—an analysis of 30 cases. Rheumatology (Oxford) 2003;42(9):1062–6.

[45] Emmerson BT. The management of gout. N Engl J Med 1996;334:445–51.

[46] Agudelo CA, Wise CM. Crystal deposition diseases. In: Weisman MH, Weinblatt ME, Louie J, editors. Treatment of rheumatic disease. Philadelphia: Saunders; 2001. p. 447–60.

[47] Terkeltaub RA. Clinical practice. Gout. N Engl J Med 2003;349(17):1647–55.

[48] Fam AG. Gout in the elderly. Clinical presentation and treatment. Drugs Aging 1998;13(3): 229–43.

[49] Roberts WN, Liang MH, Stern SH. Colchicine in acute gout: reassessment of risks and benefits. JAMA 1987;257:1920–2.

[50] Wallace SL, Singer JZ. Systemic toxicity associated with the intravenous administration of colchicine—guidelines for use. J Rheumatol 1988;15:495–9.

[51] Bonnel RA, Villalba ML, Karwoski CB, Beitz J. Deaths associated with inappropriate intravenous colchicine administration. J Emerg Med 2002;22(4):385–7.

[52] Griffen MR, Piper JM, Daugherty JR, et al. Nonsteroidal anti-inflammatory drug use and increased risk for peptic ulcer disease in elderly persons. Ann Intern Med 1991;114:257–63.

[53] Gurwitz JH, Avorn J, Ross-Degnan D, et al. Nonsteroidal anti-inflammatory drug-associated azotemia in the very old. JAMA 1990;264:471–5.

[54] Fam AG. Treating acute gouty arthritis with selective COX 2 inhibitors. BMJ 2002;325(7371): 980–1.

[55] Alloway JA, Moriarty MJ, Hoogland YT, et al. Comparison of triamcinolone acetonide with indomethacin in the treatment of acute gouty arthritis. J Rheumatol 1993;20:111–3.

[56] Axelrod D, Preston S. Comparison of parenteral adrenocorticotropic hormone with oral indomethacin in the treatment of acute gout. Arthritis Rheum 1988;31:803–5.

[57] Fam AG. Current therapy of acute microcrystalline arthritis and the role of corticosteroids. J Clin Rheumatol 1997;3:35–40.

[58] Groff GD, Franck WA, Raddatz DA. Systemic steroid therapy for acute gout. Semin Arthritis Rheum 1990;19:329–36.

[59] Ritter J, Kerr JD, Valeriano-Marcet J, et al. ACTH revisited: effective treatment for acute crystal induced synovitis in patients with multiple medical problems. J Rheumatol 1994;21: 696–9.

[60] Roane DW, Harris MD, Carpenter MT, et al. Prospective use of intramuscular triamcinolone acetonide in pseudogout. J Rheumatol 1997;24:1168–70.

[61] Siegel LB, Alloway JA, Nashel DJ. Comparison of adrenocorticotropic hormone and triamcinolone acetonide in the treatment of acute gouty arthritis. J Rheumatol 1994;21: 1325–7.

[62] Fernandez C, Noguera A, Gonzalez JA, et al. Treatment of acute attacks of gout with a small dose of intraarticular triamcinolone acetonide. J Rheumatol 1999;26(10):2285–6.

[63] Kuncl RW, Duncan G, Watson D, et al. Colchicine myopathy and neuropathy. N Engl J Med 1987;316:1562–8.

[64] Wallace SL, Singer JZ, Duncan GL, et al. Renal function predicts colchicine toxicity; guidelines for the prophylactic use of colchicine in gout. J Rheumatol 1992;18:264–9.

[65] Gonzalez EB, Miller SB, Agudelo CA. Optimal management of gout in older persons. Drugs Aging 1994;4:128–34.

[66] Simkin PA. When, why, and how should we quantify the excretion rate of urinary uric acid? J Rheumatol 2001;28(6):1207–10.

[67] Fam AG. Gout, diet, and the insulin resistance syndrome. J Rheumatol 2002;29(7):1350–5.

[68] Snaith ML. Gout: diet and uric acid revisited. Lancet 2001;358(9281):525.

[69] Bautman V, Maesako JK, Haddad B, et al. The role of lead in gout nephropathy. N Engl J Med 1981;304:520–3.

[70] Caspi D, Lubart E, Graff E, et al. The effect of mini-dose aspirin on renal function and uric acid handling in elderly patients. Arthritis Rheum 2000;43:103–8.

[71] Perez-Ruiz F, Calabozo M, Herrero-Beites AM, et al. Improvement of renal function in patients with chronic gout after proper control of hyperuricemia and gouty bouts. Nephron 2000; 86(3):287–91.

[72] Michet CJ, Evans JM, Fleming KC, et al. Common rheumatologic diseases in the elderly. Mayo Clin Proc 1995;70:1205–14.

[73] Shoji A, Yamanaka H, Kamatani N. A retrospective study of the relationship between serum urate level and recurrent attacks of gouty arthritis: evidence for reduction of recurrent gouty arthritis with antihyperuricemic therapy. Arthritis Rheum 2004;51(3):321–5.

[74] Bull PW, Scott JT. Intermittent control of hyperuricemia in the treatment of gout. J Rheumatol 1989;16:1246–8.

[75] Perez-Ruiz F, Calabozo M, Fernandez-Lopez MJ, et al. Treatment of chronic gout in patients with renal function impairment: an open, randomized, actively controlled study. J Clin Rheumatol 1999;5:49–55.

[76] Feher MD, Hepburn AL, Hogarth MB, et al. Fenofibrate enhances urate reduction in men treated with allopurinol for hyperuricaemia and gout. Rheumatology (Oxford) 2003;42(2): 321–5.

[77] Takahashi S, Moriwaki Y, Tamamoto T, et al. Effects of combination treatment using antihyperuricaemic agents with fenofibrate and/or losartan on uric acid metabolism. Ann Rheum Dis 2003;62(6):572–5.

[78] Hande KR, Noone RM, Stone WJ. Severe allopurinol toxicity: description and guidelines for prevention in patients with renal insufficiency. Am J Med 1984;76:47–56.

[79] Smith P, Karlson N, Nair BR. Quality use of allopurinol in the elderly. J Qual Clin Pract 2000;20(1):42–3.

[80] Riedel AA, Nelson M, Joseph-Ridge N, et al. Compliance with allopurinol therapy among managed care enrollees with gout: a retrospective analysis of administrative claims. J Rheumatol 2004;31(8):1575–81.

[81] Fam AG, Dunne SM, Iazzetta J, et al. Efficacy and safety of desensitization to allopurinol following cutaneous reactions. Arthritis Rheum 2001;44:231–8.

[82] Reginato AJ, Reginato AM. Diseases associated with deposition of calcium pyrophosphate or hydroxyapatite. In: Ruddy S, Harris ED, Sledge CB, editors. Textbook of rheumatology. Philadelphia (PA): WB Saunders; 2001. p. 1377–90.

[83] Hirose J, Ryan LM, Masuda I. Up-regulated expression of cartilage intermediate-layer protein and ANK in articular hyaline cartilage from patients with calcium pyrophosphate dihydrate crystal deposition disease. Arthritis Rheum 2002;46(12):3218–29.

[84] Ryan LM, Cheung HS. The role of crystals in osteoarthritis. Rheum Dis Clin N Am 1999;25: 257–67.

[85] Jaovisidha K, Rosenthal AK. Calcium crystals in osteoarthritis. Curr Opin Rheumatol 2002; 14(3):298–302.

[86] Nalbant S, Martinez JA, Kitumnuaypong T, et al. Synovial fluid features and their relations to osteoarthritis severity: new findings from sequential studies. Osteoarthritis Cartilage 2003; 11(1):50–4.

[87] Morgan MP, McCarthy GM. Signaling mechanisms involved in crystal-induced tissue damage. Curr Opin Rheumatol 2002;14(3):292–7.

[88] Wilkins E, Dieppe P, Maddison P. Osteoarthritis and articular chondrocalcinosis in the elderly. Ann Rheum Dis 1983;42:280–4.

[89] Neame RL, Carr AJ, Muir K, et al. UK community prevalence of knee chondrocalcinosis: evidence that correlation with osteoarthritis is through a shared association with osteophyte. Ann Rheum Dis 2003;62(6):513–8.

[90] Timms AE, Zhang Y, Russell RG, et al. Genetic studies of disorders of calcium crystal deposition. Rheumatology (Oxford) 2002;41(7):725–9.

[91] Schumacher HRJ. Hemochromatosis and arthritis. Arthritis Rheum 1964;7:41–50.

[92] Tanglao EC, Stern MA, Agudelo CA. Arthropathy as the presenting symptom in hereditary hemochromatosis. Am J Med Sci 1996;312:306–9.

[93] Faraawi R, Harth M, Kertesz A, et al. Arthritis in hemochromatosis. J Rheumatol 1993;20: 448–52.

[94] McCarty DJ. Diagnostic mimicry in arthritis: patterns of joint involvement associated with calcium pyrophosphate dihydrate crystals. Bull Rheum Dis 1975;25:1438–40.

[95] Ho GJ, DeNuccio M. Gout and pseudogout in hospitalized patients. Arch Intern Med 1993; 153:2787–90.

[96] Bona D, Bennett R. Pseudogout mimicking systemic disease. JAMA 1981;246:1438–40.

[97] Alvarellos A, Spilberg I. Colchicine prophylaxis in pseudogout. J Rheumatol 1986;13:804–5.

[98] Rothschild B, Yakaobov LE. Prospective 6 month double blind trial of hydroxychloroquine treatment of CPPD. Compr Ther 1997;23:327–30.

[99] Molloy ES, McCarthy GM. Hydroxyapatite deposition disease of the joint. Curr Rheumatol Rep 2003;5(3):215–21.

[100] Halverson PB, Carrera GF, McCarty DJ. Milwaukee shoulder syndrome: fifteen additional cases and a description of contributing factors. Arch Intern Med 1990;150:677–82.

[101] McCarty DL, Halverson PB, Carrera CF, et al. "Milwaukee shoulder"—association of microspheroids containing hydroxyapatite crystals, active collagenase, and neutral protease with rotator cuff defects. I. Clinical aspects. Arthritis Rheum 1981;24:464–73.

[102] Halverson PB. Crystal deposition disease of the shoulder (including calcific tendonitis and milwaukee shoulder syndrome). Curr Rheumatol Rep 2003;5(3):244–7.

[103] Antoniou J, Tsai A, Baker D, et al. Milwaukee shoulder: correlating possible etiologic variables. Clin Orthop 2003;407:79–85.

ELSEVIER
SAUNDERS

Clin Geriatr Med 21 (2005) 513–525

CLINICS IN
GERIATRIC
MEDICINE

Rheumatic Disease in the Elderly: Rheumatoid Arthritis

Zuhre Tutuncu, MD[a],*, Arthur Kavanaugh, MD[b]

[a]Division of Rheumatology, Allergy and Immunology, University of California–San Diego,
9500 Gilman Drive, La Jolla, CA 92093-0943, USA
[b]Center for Innovative Therapy, Division of Rheumatology, Allergy and Immunology,
University of California, San Diego, 9500 Gilman Drive, La Jolla, CA 92093-0943, USA

Arthritic complaints in the elderly are most frequently associated with degenerative, noninflammatory arthritis. Not uncommonly, however, forms of inflammatory arthritis may be seen. A major concern is that arthritic disorders may diminish elderly patients' functional status, and therefore, their independence. Pain, stiffness, and constitutional symptoms can contribute to immobility, weakness, and increased falls, and in fact, decreased life span. As the population of people who are over the age of 60 years is growing, the prevalence of disability from arthritis is also increasing.

Rheumatoid arthritis

Rheumatoid arthritis (RA) is now known to increase in incidence and prevalence up to approximately age 85. The prevalence of RA in persons 60 years of age and older is reported to be around 2% [1]. The issue of whether RA arising in the elderly population is a distinct disease from younger onset RA (YORA) is not still settled. Differences in demographic and disease features such as sex, type of onset, involvement of large versus small joints, disease activity, and the rate of progression and functional decline have been described [2,3]. However, there are difficulties in definitely establishing the diagnosis of RA in this popu-

---

* Corresponding author.
E-mail address: ztutuncu@ucsd.edu (Z. Tutuncu).

0749-0690/05/$ – see front matter. Published by Elsevier Inc.
doi:10.1016/j.cger.2005.02.009

lation [4]. Therefore, some of the previously reported heterogeneity of RA in the elderly population may relate to diagnostic imprecision.

Current classification criteria, which rely on the presence of clinical signs and symptoms, laboratory, and radiographic findings, lack the ability to differentiate RA from similar rheumatic conditions, especially in elderly persons [5]. Other diseases with similar clinical features may be incorrectly classified when these criteria are applied [6–8]. Patients in the early stages of disease and those with mild RA may not be correctly identified using these criteria.

Etiology and pathogenesis

Despite extensive research, the cause of RA is unknown. It is believed that it is multifactorial, with genetic and environmental factors playing important roles. RA is strongly associated with major histocompatibility complex class II allele human leukocyte antigen (HLA)-DR4, and to a lesser extent to HLA-DR-1 and DR14.

Activated T cells, macrophages, and fibroblasts produce pro-inflammatory cytokines that play a key role in synovitis and tissue destruction in RA. Tumor necrosis alpha (TNF-α) and Interleukin 1 (IL-1) are two of the main cytokines that enhance synovial proliferation and stimulate secretion of matrix metalloproteinases, other inflammatory cytokines, and adhesion molecules [9].

Two clinical presentations of RA can be defined in the elderly population [2]. The first, referred to as elderly onset RA (EORA), is the de novo development of RA in persons older than age 60 to 65 years. Some studies suggest a dimunition of the female predominance in EORA [4]. Within the EORA population, acute onset of disease, and prominent elevations in the erythrocyte sedimentation rate (ESR) have been reported as being more common than for YORA [10,11]. Clinically, EORA is characterized by disabling morning stiffness and marked pain predominantly affecting the upper extremities. The physical examination is remarkable for pronounced synovitis of the shoulders and the wrists as well as the metacarpophalangial (MCP) joints and proximal interphalangial joints, with marked limitation of motion and severe soft tissue swelling. The reviews on this arthritis type have stressed that involvement of large joints, in particular shoulder joints, is a striking feature of arthritis in the elderly [12,13]. The second presentation of RA encountered in elderly patients is RA that developed before the age of 65 and persists. Most of these patients have had several decades of disease activity. As a result, they commonly have an advanced stage of the disease, and have often received therapy with multiple agents. Not uncommonly, they have undergone elective joint surgery. The physical examination of these patients usually reveals varying degrees of active polyarticular synovitis and deformities in both the upper and lower extremities. Ulnar deviation, elbow contractures, wrist subluxation, swan-neck, and Boutonniere deformities are common deformities that are encountered. Systemic manifestations such as rheumatoid lung, vasculitic ulcers, peripheral neuropathy, and secondary amyloid, all reflecting longstanding inflammatory disease may complicate the care of this population of RA patients.

Diagnosis

The accuracy of rheumatologic laboratory tests may also differ in older versus younger patients. Rheumatoid factor (RF) is an antibody that recognizes the Fc portion of the IgG molecule. Most of the RFs that are measured clinically are of the IgM isotype. The prevalence of both organ- and nonorgan-specific auto-antibodies, including RF, increases with advancing age. Therefore, the diagnostic value of this test has limitations especially among aged [2,4]. Anticyclic citrullinated antibody, which reacts with a common epitope identified by anti-fillagrin, antiperinuclear, and antikeratin antibodies, has been suggested to be more specific among the elderly [14].

Elevations in the ESR and C reactive protein levels provide a surrogate measure of active inflammation, and may be useful in establishing the activity of disease, estimating the prognosis, and gauging the response to therapy. Monitoring the ESR can sometimes be misleading in the elderly population where elevated ESR levels are not uncommonly related to other factors such as infection, congestive heart failure, hypercholesterolemia, or malignancy. Radiographic evaluation is seldom helpful as a diagnostic test in older patients with a recent onset of symptoms. In the early stages of the disease, soft tissue swelling and periarticular osteopenia are common. Uniform joint space loss, marginal erosions, and intraarticular deformities may be seen in advanced disease.

Prognosis

The outcome of EORA has been reported to be both better [12,14], and worse [13] than YORA. Prognostic factors have not been studied extensively in EORA. A frequent feature of EORA, acute onset, has been associated with a worse [15], equal [16], and a better [17] prognosis than EORA with a more insidious onset. In several reports, EORA patients who are seropositive for RF have been demonstrated to have either similar or worse prognosis when compared with younger seropositive RA patients [11,18]. However, longitudinal studies of RA patients not stratified for age have shown that high positive titers of RF, radiographic evidence of bony erosions, arthritis of more than 20 joints, rheumatoid nodules, HLA-DR4 allele, and elevated acute phase reactants are associated with more aggressive disease [19]. In interpreting results in the elderly it is necessary to consider that the prevalence of positive RF test results and the rate of ESR increase with age. Disease duration may contribute to a poor prognosis in the elderly by having a negative impact on the functional status of elderly patients. Comorbidity is another factor that contributes to the apparent worse prognosis among older patients. Intercurrent illnesses and therapies might cause patients to be less tolerant of the inflammation and other burdens caused by RA itself.

Differential diagnosis

The presence of clear-cut stigmata of one musculoskeletal disease does not necessarily mean that the symptoms are due to that disorder. As mentioned, the differential diagnosis of RA in the elderly may be complicated, as a variety of entities with similar signs and symptoms are prevalent in this population. Some of these conditions are polymyalgia rheumatica (PMR), calcium pyrophosphate deposition disease (CPPD), gouty arthritis, and osteoarthritis (OA). In addition, occult malignancy, thyroid disease, or other conditions can also manifest as an arthritis reminiscent of RA [20,21].

Therapy

It is important to realize that requirements change with aging, and symptomatology is often misleading; therefore, there must be flexibility regarding treatment of the aged. The management of rheumatologic disorders in elderly patients is complicated by diagnostic uncertainty, the presence of comorbid conditions, changes in pharmacokinetics and tissue responsiveness, and an increased frequency of adverse drug events [2,4]. The efficacy and toxicity of drugs commonly used in RA may differ among young and aged population. The primary objectives of therapy are to control pain, stop disease progression, and improve functional status.

New agents for the treatment of RA are being investigated in clinical trials. Although the prevalence of RA among the elderly is increasing, the elderly population is not well represented in the clinical trials. In general, treatment is becoming more aggressive for RA, and early intervention is becoming more common. Current strategies include early aggressive treatment with one or more disease-modifying antirheumatic drugs (DMARD), along with symptomatic therapy with nonsteroidal anti-inflammatory drugs (NSAIDs) and low-dose prednisone.

In elderly patients, a major consideration with the use of NSAIDs is the increased risk of toxicity. Risk factors for upper gastrointestinal bleeding in patients treated with NSAIDs include age over 65 years, a history of peptic ulcer disease or gastrointestinal bleeding, concomitant use of oral glucocorticoids or anticoagulants, and the presence of comorbid conditions. Risk factors for renal failure include age over 65 years, hypertension or congestive heart failure, and concomitant use of diuretics and angiotensin-converting enzyme inhibitors. Side effects including upper gastrointestinal toxicity, renal insufficiency, and central nervous system dysfunction are more serious in elderly than in younger patients [22]. Routine monitoring for toxicity from NSAIDs remains controversial, and the side effects can be unpredictable.

Over the last couple of years, cyclo-oxygenase-2 (COX-2) specific inhibitors (COXIBs) have been shown have comparable efficacy to traditional NSAIDs [22]. Although proven to be safer compared with nonselective NSAIDs from the gastrointestinal standpoint, the COXIBs' impact on renal function and blood pressure is comparable to nonselective NSAIDs, and careful monitoring of blood pressure is warranted after initiation after these agents [23,24]. COXIBs can be the preferred agents in situations where bleeding may be a concern, for example, on patients who are on anticoagulant therapy or during the perioperative period; as they do not interfere with platelet function. However, there is recent data that suggest COXIBs may increase the rate of thrombotic and cardiovascular events [25]. COXIB and NSAID usage is advised to be initiated with the lowest recommended dose, especially in low-weight subjects, because higher plasma may be detected in elderly patients [26].

Some patients may require low-dose oral steroids (often defined as ≤ 5 to 10 mg prednisone equivalent per day) when there is a period of flare of their RA or when initiating a new DMARD therapy. In fact, in the past, the use of low-dose prednisone was advocated as the second-line therapy in elderly patients with RA based on their rapid mode of action and elderly patients' predisposition to functionally deteriorate faster than younger population [27,28]. A moderate to excellent improvement with prednisone therapy was reported in 80 of 91 patients with EORA [28]. However, this therapy can be hazardous, especially in elderly patients, because it poses an increased risk for osteoporosis, infection, glucose intolerance, gastrointestinal erosive disease, and hypertension. There are data that suggest that with the long-term use of low-dose prednisone, the risk of osteoporosis may outweigh the clinical benefit [29]. Therefore, bone-protective agents and close monitoring of bone density are warranted with chronic usage of steroids.

DMARD therapy changes the course of RA, resulting in on sustained improvement in physical function, decreased inflammatory synovitis, and potentially slowing or prevention of structural joint damage. Most DMARDs take several months to achieve significant response. Methotrexate (MTX) has been the most effective antirheumatic therapy, but when used alone seldom leads to complete remission [30]. Hydroxychloroquine and sulfasalazine are generally preferred in slowly progressing disease. Because they carry a less toxic profile and need less frequent monitoring, they can be preferred agents in elderly patients with significant underlying medical problems. Leflunomide is a novel drug; its efficacy was found to be comparable to MTX. Leflunomide can be used in combination with MTX or in patients who cannot tolerate or have incomplete response to MTX [31]. Cyclosporin and Azathioprine are reserved for refractory patients who have failed other agents. Combination DMARD regimens, for example, MTX + hydroxychloroquine + sulfasalazine or MTX + Cyclosporin have shown significant clinical improvement when compared with single therapy or placebo [31,32]. Close follow-up and repeated evaluations are required for patients on DMARDs (Table 1). Some studies including patients older than 65 years of age have found no significant effect of age on termination of DMARD

Table 1
Disease-modifying antirheumatic drugs

	Side effects	Precautions and monitoring
Methotrexate	GI irritation	Addition of oral Folate supplement
	Oral ulcers	Monitor LFT, CBC, and diff and creatinine levels
	LFT elevation	Contraindicated in alcoholism, pregnancy
	BM suppression	Caution in impaired renal function
	Pneumonitis	Avoid using in Hepatitis B and C
	(uncommon)	Well-tolerated in elderly
	Nodulosis	
	(uncommon)	
Hydroxychloroquine	GI irritation	Retinal toxicity increases with > 70 years of age,
	Rash	800 mg of cumulative dose, > 6 mg of daily dose
	Headache	Ophthalmological test q 6–12 months
	Skin discoloration	Caution in hepatic disease, porphyria, psoriasis
	Retinal toxicity	
	(uncommon)	
Sulfasalazine	GI irritation	Caution in impaired renal function
	Rash	Monitor CBC and diff
	Itching	Monitor LFT q 3–6 months
	Dizziness	Enteric coated tablets can be better tolerated
	Headache	
	BM suppression	
Leflunomide	GI irritation	Monitor LFT, creatinine
	Rash	Avoid using in hepatic impairment
	BM suppression	Contraindicated in pregnancy
	LFT elevation	Cholestyramine is used to reduce plasma levels
Cylosporin	Hypertension	Contraindicated in renal failure
	Increased creatinine	Avoid in malignancy
	Hirsutism	Monitor BP and creatinine closely
	Nausea	Monitor K and uric acid, LFTs
	Tremor	
	Gingival hypertrophy	
Azathioprune	Fever, chills	Caution in hepatic and renal impairment
	GI intolerance	Monitor CBC and diff
	BM suppression	Check TMT enzyme deficiency before
	LFT elevation	initiating therapy

Abbreviations: BM, bone marrow; BP, blood pressure; CBC, complete blood count; GI, Gastrointestinal; LFT, liver function test; TMT, thiopurine methyltransferase.

treatment [33,34]. In addition, a tendency toward less efficacy and greater toxicity of DMARDs has been reported in older compared with younger patients [33,34]. However, in these studies prolonged disease duration might be the factor for early discontinuation of therapy rather than age, because it is well documented that patients fail to remain long term on any given DMARD. In some instances, pathophysiologic changes and comorbidity may make the use of particular agents problematic. For example, impaired baseline renal function makes it difficult to consider cyslosporine A as a therapeutic agent.

With better understanding of the pathogenesis of autoimmune diseases and advancing developments in biopharmaceutical technology, biologic therapeutic

Table 2
Comparison of biologic agents

	Etanercept	Infliximab	Adalimumab	Anakinra
Half-Life	3–4.8 days	8–9.5 days	10–13.6 days	4–6 hours
Binding target	TNF-α/LT-α	TNF-α	TNF-α	Type 1 IL-1r
Administration	Twice weekly, sc	Every 4–8 weeks, iv	Every other week, sc	Daily, sc
Side effects	Risk of increased infection, drug-induced SLE, autoantibody formation, demyelinating disease, injection side reaction, cytopenias, congestive heart failure			Injection site reaction, headache, neutropenia, risk of infection

Abbreviations: iv intravenous.; LT-α, lymphotoxin-alpha; sc, subcutaneous.

agents have been introduced (Table 2). These agents target specific components of the immune response considered central to the etiology of RA. Currently, there are three anti-TNF-α agents available for clinical use: infliximab, a chimeric anti-TNFα monoclonal antibody (mAb); etanercept, a soluble TNF-receptor construct; and adalimumab, a human anti-TNFα mAb. Different studies including patients with chronic refractory RA, patients with active disease, with or without concurrent MTX therapy, and patients with early RA showed rapid and sustained improvement with all three agents [35–37]. Joint damage as measured by X-ray progression, appeared to be slowed by these drugs [38–40].

Etanercept was found to be safe and effective in elderly patients with RA in a retrospective analysis of results from clinical trial. One hundred ninety-seven of 1128 patients enrolled in four double-blind, randomized and five open-label trials were 65 years of age and older. It was reported that 55% of patients showed improvement in American College of Rheumatology 20 criteria comparable to results in young patients. Treatment was generally well tolerated. This age group showed a lower rate of injection site reactions, headaches, and rash compared with younger patients. Death and cancer diagnosis in patients over 65 treated with Etanercept were similar to the estimated for this age group within the general population [41].

These agents represent a major advance in the treatment of severe inflammatory arthritis. However, the greater frequency of contraindications (eg, tuberculosis, malignancy, chronic infection) that are found in the older population may limit their usage [41].

Anakinra is an IL-1 receptor antagonist. It is commonly used in patients who are refractory to other treatments and are not good responders to TNF blockers. The overall magnitude of reductions in clinical symptoms and signs (20–30%) were relatively modest when compared with those reported in TNF-α blocking agents (60–70%) [35,36,42]. Anakinra is not recommended to be taken together with TNF blockers. Injection site reactions are the most frequently reported adverse event with anakinra [43].

In a study where EORA patients were matched with YORA patients based on their disease duration and compared to assess the types of treatment measures used in the two groups, it was shown that EORA patients received biologic therapy and combination DMARD therapy less frequently than YORA patients, despite identical disease duration and comparable disease severity and activity [44]. This suggests that there may be a need to use more aggressive therapeutic regimens in the geriatric population.

Differential diagnosis of RA in the elderly

Polymyalgia rheumatica

PMR may be an overlapping syndrome with seronegative EORA [3]. Although the diagnosis of PMR frequently is straightforward, it can be elusive. Elderly patients may have musculoskeletal complaints related to underlying degenerative disease or neurologic syndromes as other causes that can obscure the diagnostic picture. Patients with PMR are classically older than 50 years of age (90% are older than 60), and most are White [45]. It is a syndrome characterized by pain and morning stiffness in the neck, shoulder girdle, and pelvic girdle, with constitutional symptoms such as malaise and fatigue being common. Typically, the ESR is higher than 50 and frequently higher than 80. PMR can occur as a separate entity or in association with temporal arthritis. Patients with PMR dramatically improve with low doses of prednisone (10–15 mg/d). Once symptoms have resolved and the ESR has normalized, the dose of prednisone may be tapered slowly, while the patient is closely monitored for recurrence of symptoms or an elevation of ESR.

Calcium pyrophosphate deposition disease

CPPD includes arthritic syndromes associated with calcium pyrophosphate dihydrate crystal deposition in articular structures. The prevalence of CPPD increases with age; it may exceed 60% among persons over age 70 [46]. Chondrocalcinosis, the most common presentation of CPPD, is calcification of articular cartilage, generally an incidental finding in elderly patients. Acute pseudogout is caused by an inflammatory reaction by the shedding of crystals into synovial fluid, and often begins as self-limited acute arthritic attacks lasting from 1 day to 4 weeks; it may be as severe as, and resemble gout attacks. The most commonly affected joints are the knees, wrists, shoulders, ankles, and elbows. Patients tend to be symptom free between attacks. The diagnosis is suggested by the clinical presentation and confirmed by the presence of CPPD crystals in synovial fluid analysis. Chronic CPPD is often a symmetric arthritis affecting the knees, wrists, joints, hips, spine, shoulder, elbows, and ankles. Although the small joints of the hands and feet are generally spared, the second and third MCP joints can occasionally be involved. Symptoms are generally restricted to a few joints, and some patients have episodic pseudogout. A plain radiograph of an inflamed joint that shows chondrocalcinosis may be helpful in distinguishing CPPD from other inflammatory arthritis. Therapy includes NSAIDs, intra-articular steroid injections, oral colchicine, and systemic short-term steroids.

Gout

Gout is a disease caused by the deposition of monosodium urate crystals in the tissues and around joints. The prevalence increases substantially with age and increasing serum urate concentration. The incidence of clinical gout increases with time, especially after approximately 20 years of continued hyperuricemia [47]. In men, the first attacks generally occur between the fourth and sixth decades of life. In women, the age of onset is older and occurrence after menopause is almost invariably associated with diuretic usage. Because of increased longevity and frequent use of thiazide-diuretics, the prevalence of gout is increased in the elderly. The natural course of classic gout passes through distinct stages: asymptomatic hyperuricemia, acute intermittent gout, and chronic tophaceous gout. In a classic gouty attack, patients experience exquisite pain accompanied by warmth, swelling, and erythema around the affected joint. The initial attack is usually monoarticular and in one half of the patients involved the first metatarsophalangeal joint, which is referred as "podagra." In the elderly population, the joints previously damaged by OA or other conditions provide particularly favorable sites for subsequent involvement by gout. This includes involvement of interphalangeal joints. Over time, the attacks can become more frequent, longer in duration, and involve more joints. Eventually, the patient may enter a phase of chronic polyarticular gout with no pain-free intercritical periods. At this stage, inflammation of the involved joints is occasionally seen, and it may be easily confused with other types of inflammatory arthritis such as RA [48]. Tophaceous gout is the consequence of the chronic inability to eliminate urate as rapidly as it is produced. As the urate pool expands, deposits of urate crystals appear in cartilage, synovial membranes, tendons, soft tissues. The therapy of gout can be challenging in aged persons. Colchicine is an effective agent for the treatment of acute gout, but it carries the potential of causing diarrhea or other toxicities. Short-term NSAID usage is also effective in controlling the attack, but as discussed above, it needs to be used in caution in patients with peptic ulcer disease and in patients with renal insufficiency. Corticosteroids are usually reserved for patients in whom other treatments are contraindicated. Aspiration and intra-articular corticosteroid injection is a useful alternative in a patient with one or two involved joints. Uric acid-lowering agent therapy should be limited to patients with chronic tophaceous gout or severe and frequent attacks of acute gout. Allopurinol is the agent of choice for patients who have urate overproduction. Its dose needs to be adjusted when glomerular filtration is reduced.

Osteoarthritis

OA is the most common form of arthritis and accounts for more disability among the elderly than any other disease. Both the prevalence and severity parallel age in most individuals. Over one half of all people older than age 65 have radiographic changes of OA in the knees [49], and virtually everyone has such changes in at least one joint by age 75. In addition to age, obesity, repetitive trauma, race, and gender play roles in the prevalence and the severity of the disease. The pathogenesis and the determinants of OA progression are not fully understood. According to current views, OA is a slowly progressing inflammatory process, not a simple "wear and tear phenomenon." The main feature in the pathogenesis of OA is the cartilage breakdown due to slowly progressing inflammatory reaction. In this process, cytokines, such as IL-1 and TNF-α act as significant destructive mediators [50].

Most OA patients note the insidious onset of pain in affected joints. The pain is worsened by activity and improved at rest. Bony swelling/hypertrophy may develop and interfere with normal range of motion of the joints. Bony hypertrophy in distal interphalangeal (DIP) joints (Heberden's nodes), and proximal interphalangial joints (Bouchard's nodes) are found more commonly in women. In addition to the hands, the knees, hips, cervical, and lumbar spine are affected the most. Frequently, despite the distinctive pathogenesis and course of OA and RA, OA can be accompanied by inflammatory manifestations that make the two entities difficult to distinguish in the elderly. Generally, DIP and the first carpometocarpal joints are most commonly involved. However, unlike RA, this disease is not accompanied by systemic symptoms; and does not generally involve the MCPs, wrists. Laboratory tests and imaging may help in distinguishing from inflammatory arthritis. Typical X-ray findings of OA include loss of joint space, subchondral sclerosis, bony cysts, and reactive osteophyte.

No medication has been shown to stop or reverse the disease process underlying OA. Medications are therefore used to alleviate symptoms and increase function. Acetaminophen and NSAIDs are widely used. Weight loss, exercise for muscle strengthening, local corticosteroid injections, physical therapy, and hydrotherapy are other measures that can play a significant role in controlling pain and improving range of motion.

Glucosamine and chondroitin sulfate are classified as dietary supplements in the United States. A recent study suggests that glucosamine sulfate may slow cartilage space loss [51]. Viscosupplementation is a therapy for moderate OA for which standard management fails. The therapy consists of injecting hyaluronan into affected joints (currently approved only for knees). Hyaluronic acid forms the central axis of various proteoglycan aggregates necessary for functional integrity of cartilage and other extracellular matrices. There is evidence that repeated intra-articular injections of hyaluronan in OA of the knee might delay structural progression of disease [52]. For those with advanced disease, joint replacement surgery may dramatically improve the quality of life.

Summary

In old age, physiologic deterioration complicates the presentation of pathologic processes and handling of therapeutic substances. Despite developments in science and technology controversies in understanding and managing arthritis in the elderly still exist. The impact of musculoskeletal problems on the function and life style of elderly should stimulate the clinicians to focus on improving diagnostic and therapeutic interventions that will minimize the sequela of RA in the geriatric population. Greater involvement of elderly persons in clinical research and trials would provide helpful information, and should be promoted [53]. Advances in this area will have a great impact on reducing disability and improving quality of life among older patients.

References

[1] Rasch EK, Hirsch R, Paulose-Ram R, et al. Prevalence of rheumatoid arthritis in persons 60 years of age and older in the United States. Effect of different methods of case classification. Arthritis Rheum 2003;48:917–26.

[2] van Schaardenburg D, Breedweld FC. Elderly-onset rheumatoid arthritis. Semin Arthritis Rheum 1994;23(6):367–78.

[3] Nesher G, Moore TL. Rheumatoid arthritis in the aged. Incidence and optimal management. Drugs Ageing 1993;3:487–501.

[4] Kavanaugh AF. Rheumatoid arthritis in the elderly: Is it a different disease? Am J Med 1997; 103(6A):40S–8S.

[5] Sangha O. Epidemiology of rheumatic diseases. Rheumatology (Oxford) 2000;39(Suppl 2):3–12.

[6] Dugowson CE, Nelson JL, Koepsell TD. Evaluation of the 1987 revised criteria for rheumatoid arthritis in a cohort of newly diagnosed female patients. Arthritis Rheum 1990;33:1042–6.

[7] Pincus T, Callahan LF. How many types of patients meet classification criteria for rheumatoid arthritis? J Rheumatol 1994;21:1385–9.

[8] Arnett FC, Edworthy SM, Bloch DA, et al. The American Rheumatism Association 1987 revised criteria for the classification of rheumatoid arthritis. Arthritis Rheum 1988;31:315–24.

[9] Feldman M, Brennan FM, Maini RN. Role of cytokines in rheumatoid arthritis. Annu Rev Immunol 1996;43:28–38.

[10] Deal CL, Meenan RD, Goldenberg DL, et al. The clinical features of elderly-onset rheumatoid arthritis. Arthritis Rheum 1985;28:987–94.

[11] Ferraccioli GF, Cavelieri F, Mercadanti M, et al. Clinical features, scintiscan characteristics and X-ray progression of late onset rheumatoid arthritis. Clin Exp Rheumatol 1984;2: 157–61.

[12] Glennas A, Tore KK, Oddvar A, et al. Recent onset arthritis in the elderly: a five year longitudinal observational study. J Rheumatol 2000;27:101–8.

[13] van der Heijde DM, van Riel PL, van Leeuwen MA, et al. Older versus younger onset rheumatoid arthritis: results at onset and after 2 years of a prospective follow-up study of early rheumatoid arthritis. J Rheumatol 1991;18:1285–9.

[14] Palosuo T, Tilvis R, Strandberg T, et al. Filaggrin related antibodies among the aged. Ann Rheum Dis 2003;62:261–3.

[15] Oka M, Kytila J. Rheumatoid arthritis with the onset in old age. Acta Rheum Scand 1957; 6:280–3.

[16] Terkeltaub R, Esdaile J, Decary F, et al. A clinical study of older age rheumatoid arthritis with comparison to a younger onset group. J Rheumatol 1983;10:418–24.

[17] Corrigam AB, Robinson RG, Terenty TR, et al. Benign rheumatoid arthritis of the aged. BMJ 1974;1:444–6.

[18] van Schaardenburg D, Hazes JMW, de Boer A, et al. Outcome of rheumatoid arthritis in relation to age and rheumatoid factor at diagnosis. J Rheumatol 1993;20:45–52.

[19] Wagner U, Kaltenhauser S, Sauer S, et al. HLA markers and prediction of clinical course and outcome in rheumatoid arthritis. Arthritis Rheum 1997;40(2):341–51.

[20] Stummvoll GH, Aringer M, Machold KP, et al. Cancer polyarthrtis resembling rheumatoid arthritis as a first sign of hidden neoplasms. Report of two cases and review of the literature. Scand J Rheumatol 2001;30(1):40–4.

[21] Reilly PA. The differential diagnosis of generalized pain. Baillieres Best Pract Res Clin Rheumatol 1999;13(3):391–401.

[22] Bijlsma JWJ. Analgesia and the patient with osteoarthritis. Am J Ther 2002;9:189–97.

[23] Rahme E, Marantette MA, Kong SX, et al. Use of NSAIDs, COX-2 inhibitors, and acetaminophen and associated coprescriptions of gastroprotective agents in an elderly population. Arthritis Rheum 2002;47(6):595–602.

[24] Whelton A, White WB, Bello AE, et al. Effects of celecoxib and rofecoxib on blood pressure and edema in patients > or = 65 years of age with systemic hypertension and osteoarthritis. Am J Cardiol 2002;90(9):959–63.

[25] Bombardier C, Laine L, Reicin A, et al. Comparison of upper gastrointestinal toxicity of rofecoxib and naproxen in patients with rheumatoid arthritis. N Engl J Med 2000;343:1520–8.

[26] Alsalameh S, Burian M, Mahr G, et al. Review article: the pharmaceutical properties and clinical use of valdecoxib, a new cyclo-oxygenase-2-selective inhibitor. Aliment Phamacol Ther 2003; 17:489–501.

[27] Healey LA, Sheets PK. The relation of polymyalgia rheumatica to rheumatoid arthritis. J Rheumatol 1988;15:750–2.

[28] Lockie LM, Gomez E, Smith DM. Low dose adrenocorticosteroids in the management of elderly patients with rheumatoid arthrtitis. Semin Arthritis Rheum 1983;12:373–81.

[29] van Schaardenburg D, Valkeme R, Dijkmans BAC, et al. Prednisone for elderly-onset heumatoid arthritis: efficacy and bone mass at one year. Arthritis Rheum 1993;36:S269.

[30] Weinblatt ME, Weisman RF, Holdworth DE, et al. Long-term prospective study of methotrexate in the treatment of rheumatoid arthritis. Arthritis Rheum 1992;35:721–30.

[31] Kremer JM, Genovese MC, Cannon GW, et al. Concomitant leflunomide therapy in patients with active rheumatoid arthritis despite stable doses of methotrexate. Ann Intern Med 2002;137: 726–33.

[32] O'Dell JR, Haire CE, Erikson N. Treatment of rheumatoid arthritis with methotrexate sulfasalazine and hydroxychloroquine alone, or a combination of all three medications. N Engl J Med 1996;334:1287–91.

[33] Pincus T, Marcum SB, Callahan LF, et al. Long term drug therapy for rheumatoid arthritis in seven rheumatology private practices. Second line drugs and prednisone. J Rheumatol 1992;19:1885–94.

[34] Wolfe F, Hawley DJ, Cathey MA. Termination of slow acting anti-rheumatic therapy in rheumatoid arthritis: a 14 year prospective evaluation of 1017 consecutive starts. J Rheumatol 1990;17:994–1002.

[35] Maini R, St. Clair EW, Breedweld F, et al. Infliximab (chimeric anti-tumour necrosis factor α monoclonal antibody) versus placebo in rheumatoid arthritis patients receiving concomitant methotrexate: a randomized phase III trial. Lancet 1999;354:1932–9.

[36] Moreland LW, Baumgartner SW, Schiff MH, et al. Treatment of rheumatoid arthritis with a recombinant human tumour necrosis factor receptor (p75)-Fc fusion protein. N Engl J Med 1997;337:141–7.

[37] Weisman MH, Moreland LW, Furst DE, et al. Efficacy, pharmacokinetic, and safety assessment of adalimumab, a fully human anti-tumor necrosis factor-alpha monoclonal antibody, in adults with rheumatoid arthritis receiving concomitant methotrexate: a pilot study. Clin Ther 2003; 25(6):1700–21.

[38] Lipsky PE, Desiree MFM, van der Heijde DM, et al. Infliximab and methotrexate in the treatment of rheumatoid arthritis. N Engl J Med 2000;343:1594–602.

[39] Genovese MC, Bathon JM, Martin R, et al. Etanercept versus methotrexate in patients with early rheumatoid arthritis: two year radiographic and clinical outcomes. Arthritis Rheum 2002;46: 1443–50.

[40] Keystone E, Kavanaugh A, Sharp J, et al. Adalimumab (D2E7), a fully human anti-TNFα monoclonal antibody, inhibits the progression of structural damage in patients with active rheumatoid arthritis despite concomitant methotrexate therapy [abstract]. Arthritis Rheum 2002; 46(Suppl 9):S205.

[41] Fleischman RM, Baumgartner SW, Tindall EA, et al. Response to etanercept (enbrel) in elderly patients with rheumatoid arthritis: a retrospective analysis of clinical trials. J Rheumatol 2003; 30(4):691–6.

[42] Moreland LW, Baumgartner SW, Schiff MH, et al. Treatment of rheumatoid arthritis with a recombinant human tumour necrosis factor receptor (p75)-Fc fusion protein. N Engl J Med 1997;337:141–7.

[43] Bresnihan B, Alvaro-Garcia JM, Cobby M, et al. Treatment of rheumatoid arthritis with recombinant human interleukin-1 receptor antagonist. Arthritis Rheum 1998;41:2196–204.

[44] Tutuncu ZN, Kavanaugh A, Reed G, et al. Older onset rheumatoid arthritis patients receive biologic therapies less frequently than younger patients despite similar disease activity and severity: Analysis from the CORRONA Database [abstract]. Arthritis Rheum 2004;50:S402.

[45] Michet CJ, Evans JM, Fleming KC, et al. Common rheumatologic diseases in elderly patients. Mayo Clin Proc 1995;70:1205–14.

[46] Derfus BA, Kurian JB, Butler JJ, et al. The high prevalence of pathologic calcium crystals in pre-operative knees. J Rheumatol 2002;29(3):570–4.

[47] Lawrence RC, Hochberg MD, et al. Estimates of the prevalence of selected arthritic and musculoskeletal diseases in the United States. J Reumatol 1989;16:427–41.

[48] Cobb KL, Mendez EA, Espinoza LR. Gouty arthritis mimicking rheumatoid arthritis. J Clin Rheumatol 1998;4:225.

[49] Peyron JG. Epidemiologic and etiologic approach to osteoarthritis. Semin Arthritis Rheum 1979; 8:288–306.

[50] Goldring MB. The role of chondrocyte in osteoarthritis. Arthritis Rheum 2000;43:1916–26.

[51] Dodge GR, Jimenez SA. Glucosamine sulfate modulates the levels of aggrecan and matrix metalloproteinase-3 synthesized by cultured human osteoarthritis articular chondrocytes. Osteoarthritis Cartilage 2003;6:424–32.

[52] Listrat V, Ayral X, Francesca P, et al. Arthroscopic evaluation of potential structure modifying activity of hyaluronan (Hyalgan) in osteoarthritis of the knee. Osteoarthritis Cartilage 1997;5: 153–60.

[53] Studenski SA. Rheumatology, geriatrics, and a way forward. J Am Geriatr Soc 2002;50:1737–8.

CLINICS IN
GERIATRIC
MEDICINE

ELSEVIER
SAUNDERS

Clin Geriatr Med 21 (2005) 527–541

Total Joint Arthroplasties: Current Concepts of Patient Outcomes after Surgery

C. Allyson Jones, PhD[a,b,c,*], Lauren A. Beaupre, PhD[d],
D.W.C. Johnston, MD, FRCS(C)[d],
Maria E. Suarez-Almazor, MD, PhD[e]

[a]*Department of Physical Therapy, Faculty of Rehabilitation Medicine, University of Alberta,
2-50 Corbett Hall, Edmonton, Alberta T6G 2G4, Canada*
[b]*Department of Public Health Sciences, Faculty of Medicine and Dentistry, University of Alberta,
Edmonton, Alberta, Canada*
[c]*Institute of Health Economics, Edmonton, Alberta, Canada*
[d]*Division of Orthopaedics, Department of Surgery, Capital Health, Edmonton, Alberta, Canada*
[e]*Baylor College of Medicine, Houston, TX, USA*

Arthritis causes pain and dysfunction which then impacts health-related quality of life (HRQL), and is reflected in substantial health care resource use and costs. When conservative treatment fails to alleviate hip and knee joint pain and dysfunction caused by arthritis, total joint arthroplasty is an elective surgical option that can provide significant pain relief and improved function with proven cost-effectiveness [1–3].

Primary or secondary osteoarthritis accounts for the largest proportion of total joint arthroplasties performed. In excess of 168,000 total hip arthroplasties and 267,000 total knee arthroplasties are performed annually in the United States [4]. As surgery for total joint arthroplasties has evolved and the population aged, utilization rates for total joint arthroplasty have steadily increased [4–9].

Surgical rates are higher among older age groups (up to age 79 years) and women, reflecting the higher prevalence of osteoarthritis in these demographic groups. Despite substantial benefits after surgery, disparities in access are also widely reported, which cannot be attributed to clinical need. Racial, gender, and

* Corresponding author. Department of Physical Therapy, Faculty of Rehabilitation Medicine, University of Alberta, 2-50 Corbett Hall, Edmonton, Alberta T6G 2G4, Canada.
E-mail address: Allyson.Jones@ualberta.ca (C.A. Jones).

doi:10.1016/j.cger.2005.02.003

socioeconomic status disparities have been reported in the use of total joint arthroplasties [10–14].

Total joint arthroplasties are effective interventions, with low mortality rates and few severe adverse outcomes. In-hospital death rates are less than 1% for total joint arthroplasty [12,15–18]. Risk factors for mortality following total knee arthroplasty include older age, primary arthroplasty compared with revision, use of cement, preexisting cardiopulmonary disease, and simultaneous bilateral total knee arthroplasties [18]. Older age, men, patients with lower socioeconomic status, comorbid conditions, and patients with osteonecrosis are reported to have a greater risk of death following total hip arthroplasty [12].

Many different types of outcomes have been used to evaluate joint arthroplasties. For the most part, the assessment of effectiveness has focused on the surgical and technical aspects. Measurement of patient reported health outcomes has provided an alternate source of valuable information. Information gathered by patient health measures has been used to evaluate patient satisfaction, supplemental health care resources such as rehabilitation and allied health care services, and modification of surgical techniques. Because total joint arthroplasties are elective surgeries, knowledge about long-term patient-centered outcomes can also assist individuals in the decision-making process when considering future surgery.

A fundamental shift toward patient-centered outcomes has been advocated, and is reflected in much of the recent literature on joint arthroplasties. This article briefly reviews the literature on patient outcomes after total hip and knee arthroplasties for osteoarthritis and possible determinants of pain, function and HRQL.

Outcomes

Pain and function

Favorable gains reported for joint pain and functional status following total hip and knee arthroplasties are well established within the orthopedic literature. Treatment effectiveness entails within-patient change over time or longitudinal measurement. The recovery pattern is one of improvement occurring within the first few weeks after surgery, with the largest gains seen within the first 3 to 6 months [19–24]. Patients with total hip arthroplasties report significant pain relief within a week after surgery, while patients with total knee arthroplasties report less pain relief during this period [23]. Significant pain relief following surgery for total knee arthroplasty occurs much later, often not until 6 to 12 weeks postoperatively. Moreover, a significant proportion of patients still report marked pain at 3 months [25].

Functional gains are typically seen later than pain relief with larger gains reported for total hip arthroplasty than total knee arthroplasty [19,20,26,27]. Patients often report dysfunction during the initial recovery phase [28], with functional improvement seen over the subacute phase of recovery. This pattern of recovery has clinical relevance, given the discordance between limited function and the trend towards earlier discharges from the hospital. That is, patients are discharged home at an earlier phase of recovery when their immediate postoperative functional status is most likely lower than their preoperative status.

A key factor in postoperative recovery is the ability to rapidly regain an adequate level of functional independence in activities of daily living [29,30]. This is achieved by encouraging early and active physical therapy.

A primary treatment goal to attain functional independance includes joint range of motion. Limited range of joint motion after surgery is multifactorial. Improvement in hip flexion greater than 90° was seen within the first year after total hip arthroplasty, with gains reported up to the fifth year [31]. Because few studies statistically control for other factors such as comorbidities and contralateral joint involvement, the extent to which hip range of motion attained immediately postarthroplasty directly affects long-term functional outcomes remains ambiguous.

Knee range from 0° to 105° is optimal, given that 65° is required to ambulate and approximately 105° is needed to rise from sitting with ease. A distinct relationship between knee range of motion and self-reported functional status, however, has not been clearly defined. Miner and colleagues [32] reported a modest correlation between knee mobility and functional items of the Western Ontario and McMaster Universities (WOMAC) Arthritis Index, a disease-specific questionnaire for arthritis [33,34]. Knee mobility after total knee arthroplasty is not dependent upon gender, age, other joint involvement, preoperative deformity, or the use of a continuous passive motion machine (CPM) [30]. Postoperative range of motion is reported to be dependent on the preoperative range of motion, body mass index, prosthetic design, postoperative pain, and activity [30,35–37]. Evidence suggests that patients with the most restricted range preoperatively had the greatest relative improvements, typically occurring within 1 to 3 years after surgery [35,38,39].

The use of CPM machines for total knee arthroplasty has been shown to improve early knee range of motion. Most studies, however, reporting improved early range of motion were undertaken when hospital length of stay exceeded 1 week [40]. Studies that have used short-duration CPM with reduced hospital length of stay have not shown any advantages [41–44]. As hospital length of stay continues to decrease, the focus of rehabilitation is early mobilization, promoting independent patient transfers and ambulation, which precludes the use of passive treatment such as CPM as a therapy adjunct. The optimal management of stiff knees after surgery, however, remains unclear.

Health-related quality of life

Although condition-specific measures are usually more sensitive to change than generic measures, generic measures play an important and complementary role. Generic measures provide information on overall health status, and have the ability to capture side effects and the effects of comorbidities. Coexisting medical conditions that are typically seen in this elderly patient population, in turn, affect improvements reported in the hip and knee. Not only are improvements seen with joint pain and function, but marked short- and long-term gains are also reported in other dimensions of HRQL [11,19,45–49]. Positive benefits are seen after surgery in such HRQL dimensions as social function, mental health, and vitality [20,22,45,48–52].

Despite improvements in these dimensions, patients who have recovered from total joint arthroplasty may still fall short of population norms adjusted for age and sex. Our 6-month follow-up study of a community-based prospective cohort (276 patients who received knee arthroplasties and 228 who received hip arthroplasties) found the largest gains in bodily pain and physical function, with moderate improvement in social function, vitality, and mental health [45]. We used the SF-36, a generic health measure, which has established age–sex norms for the United States population [53–55]. The SF-36 physical function and pain scores achieved at 6 months were still lower than the age–sex-matched United States population norms. Similar findings were reported at 12 months following total joint arthroplasty by March and colleagues in a study of Australian patients [47]. Although documented improvement in health status is seen in total joint arthroplasties, total knee arthroplasties do not reach comparable levels as total hip arthroplasties. Both studies reported that patients who received total hip arthroplasties had SF-36 scores closer to the norm than those who underwent total knee arthroplasties. These findings suggest total knee arthroplasties provide pain relief and improve function, but not to a level comparable to the general population, nor to the degree reported with total hip arthroplasties [45].

Patient satisfaction

Although the measurement of pain and functional outcomes has been a primary focus of health outcomes research in total joint arthroplasty, preliminary work has also examined patient satisfaction of these outcomes. The measurement of satisfaction is a complex construct that is based on a number of commonly held assumptions [56]. One assumption is that patient satisfaction is influenced by health status. Within the joint arthroplasty literature, little evidence was found to delineate the relationship between patient satisfaction and health status. Moreover, patient expectations, demographic characteristics such as age and education, gender, and ethnicity, and psychosocial variables likely influence patient satisfaction. Further evaluation of the components affecting patient satisfaction may provide valuable insight into the relationship between patient satisfaction and the pain and functional gains reported in this patient population.

In light of limited evidence, it is most likely that many factors influence patient satisfaction. Moderate correlations between patient satisfaction and WOMAC scores have been reported with total knee arthroplasties, suggesting other factors such as patient expectations may influence satisfaction [57]. Documented predictors of overall satisfaction of total hip arthroplasty are older age, not living alone, worse preoperative hip scale score, and shorter length of stay [58].

Patient overall satisfaction with the outcome of total joint arthroplasties is generally considered good to excellent for the majority of patients [45,59–61]. The level of patient satisfaction, however, is influenced by whether the surgeon or patient reports the satisfaction. Surgeon satisfaction tends to be greater than patient satisfaction with greater discrepancies associated with higher levels of pain [57,62]. Disagreement between patient and surgeon is likely due to different perspectives. Orthopaedic surgeons primarily evaluate physical impairment, while patients consider the impact of total joint arthroplasty on their overall quality of life.

Determinants of pain function and HRQL outcomes

The clinical decision to undergo surgery for a total joint arthroplasty involves potential risks weighed against the benefits for each patient. Pain, function, prosthetic/technical issues, as well as medical and surgical factors need to be considered. Although revision and mortality rates are known for this patient population, there remains uncertainty regarding how a given health state affects the outcomes of this surgical procedure. Thus, the patient–physician decision-making process may not always be guided by the best evidence at patient level.

Despite the encouraging results, anywhere from 15% to 30% of patients receiving total joint arthroplasties report little or no improvement after surgery or are unsatisfied with the results after a few months [25,45,59,61,63]. Although surgeons and referring physicians agree that the primary indications for total joint arthroplasty are pain and dysfunction [64], the effects of secondary patient characteristics on pain and function are undetermined. Determinants of poor pain and functional outcomes have seldom been examined [20,25,46,63,65,66]. Because little is known about the determinants for total hip or knee arthroplasty, indications and contraindications for total joint arthroplasties are poorly defined.

Investigations of possible determinants have been primarily directed toward perioperative surgical complications, prosthetic-related factors, and nonsurgical medical factors. More recently, investigators have focused on psychologic factors as possible predictors of pain and functional outcomes. Mounting evidence suggests that no one patient-related or perioperative factor currently available to the orthopaedic surgeons or clinicians can clearly predict the amount of pain relief or functional improvement.

Perioperative surgical complications

Surgical or medical complications within the first few days after surgery can hinder recovery and joint mobility. Fortunately, severe complications are uncommon, and their relative contribution to the overall outcome of patients undergoing total joint arthroplasties is minimal.

The incidence of major complications following total joint arthroplasties is low [67–70]. Technical complications (eg, bleeding, fracture or nerve injury) during surgery or within the immediate postoperative period can have an impact on the outcome of the joint arthroplasty. Other medical complications include deep vein thrombosis, superficial infections, peripheral nerve damage, pulmonary embolism, and deep infections [60,71]. Dislocation of the prosthesis is an additional concern in total hip arthroplasty, with incidence rates varying by age, gender, surgical approach, and prosthesis orientation [69,72,73].

The role of surgical complications in the overall outcome of patients undergoing total joint arthroplasties is probably very small because the incidence is low. Furthermore, current guidelines and standards of practice in relation to anticoagulant and antibiotic therapy during the perioperative period have further reduced the occurrence of medical complications [74–76].

Prosthesis-related factors

The revision rate for total hip and knee arthroplasties is low, and ranges between 2% and 8% over 10 years [60,77–82].

A number of complications related to the prosthesis may result in prosthetic failure. Primary indications for revision of total hip arthroplasty include aseptic loosening (55%), osteolysis (33%), poly wear (30%), and instability (17%) [9]. Aseptic loosening (39%), poly wear (36%), instability (26%), and osteolysis (20%) are the common reasons for revision of total knee arthroplasty [9]. The literature is replete with investigations examining implant fixation, prosthesis design, and bearing surfaces. Although these factors appear to have little impact on short-term outcomes, they may have a greater effect on the longevity of the implant itself. Currently, there is little consensus in the literature on optimal prosthesis design [83,84], implant fixation [85–87], or bearing surfaces [83, 88–90].

Activity level, which is indirectly related to age, may also impact long-term survival of the prosthesis [91]. Total hip and knee arthroplasties can be safely done with acceptable outcomes in healthy older patients [92,93]. There is, however, a growing trend for joint arthroplasties to be performed in persons less than 60 years of age to improve quality of life during the most productive years of life. This may affect the longevity of the implant, as younger individuals will place higher and more frequent loads on the implant [91]. Further, a greater number of revisions will be expected in younger patients, as current implants may not survive the patient's lifespan.

Measuring the success of specific prostheses is a challenge, as manufacturers frequently modify prostheses designs before long-term outcomes are known from current models. This "planned obsolescence" will continue to provide many challenges to orthopedic surgeons and health care providers in ensuing decades. Joint registries are one approach to provide ongoing monitoring of implants so that widespread adoption of poor-quality implants may be avoided [94–98].

Nonsurgical medical factors

Evidence concerning potential risk factors is lacking, and subsequently, few explicit prognostic factors of total joint arthroplasties have been identified in the literature. The identification of determinants is a challenge because of the multidimensional construct of health status. Nonsurgical medical factors appear to have a small impact on the short-term outcomes of total joint arthroplasty.

Preoperative pain and function

Persuasive evidence suggests that preoperative pain and functional status predict pain and functional ability after surgery for both total knee and hip arthroplasties, but not to a large extent [20,46,99,100]. Although patients with greater preoperative pain and dysfunction report comparable improvements as patients with less preoperative pain and dysfunction, they do not reach similar postoperative levels. These differences are significant, and may have clinical relevance with respect to prolonged waiting times or preoperative interventions that may improve pain and function before surgery.

A small number of studies have evaluated the effectiveness and efficacy of preoperative exercise programs for patients waiting to receive either hip or knee arthroplasties. Preliminary evidence reported limited positive gains with pre-operative exercise programs [101,102]; however, others [103–105] have reported that exercise programs can produce pain relief in patients with knee osteoarthritis. Studies that assessed preoperative exercise in total joint arthroplasties have reported results from small cohorts of patients, and have also often failed to stratify on preoperative pain and functional scores. None of these studies specifically focused on patients who reported the lowest preoperative function, who may be expected to benefit most from a preoperative intervention.

Comorbid conditions

A greater number of comorbid conditions have been associated with worse short-term pain and functional outcomes in patients undergoing total knee or hip arthroplasties [20,46,93]. This is not a surprising observation because comorbid conditions are also predictive of postoperative complications [106] and longer hospital stays [107]. Quantitative evidence suggests that comorbid conditions exert a certain degree of influence on pain and functional outcomes. Given the magnitude of the observed effects, the overall impact appears to be small.

A number of studies have also shown that increasing age per se does not appear to have an independent effect on pain or functional outcomes [92,93,108]. Older age, however, is associated with more comorbid conditions, which may result in poorer outcomes. Investigators have reported that visual problems and musculoskeletal conditions such as chronic low back pain and contralateral joint involvement were influential comorbid conditions associated with postoperative dysfunction in total hip arthroplasty [20,63].

The small magnitude of effect may be due to methodologic difficulties in measuring comorbidities. No gold standard exists regarding the measurement of comorbid conditions. A frequently used measure of comorbid conditions is the identification of conditions from a predefined list. The coexisting conditions are then summed to generate a single summative score. This method likely does not represent the true effect of comorbidities on recovery after total joint arthroplasties because it summarizes a complex construct in a simple manner. A simple summative score may dilute important effects of certain conditions, masking the true effect of certain conditions on functional recovery. For instance, hypertension is a medical condition that may affect mortality; however, it most likely will not affect the functional recovery. Furthermore, summing a long list of comorbid conditions, some of which may not be relevant to the outcome, may generate a spurious estimate of comorbidity [109]. Single summative scores, however, are of interest when analyzing large administrative databases and for exploratory purposes because the identification of individual medical conditions has clinical value.

The type of data source is another methodologic issue that affects the measurement of comorbid conditions. Traditionally, comorbidities have been extracted from the medical chart, retrieved from an administrative database, or based on patient self-report. Findings from our earlier work indicate that comorbidities extracted from the medical chart perform better in predicting variables of health service use, whereas self-reported comorbid conditions perform better with the use of HRQL outcomes [110]. In general, there is a consensus among investigators of clinical health outcomes that better methods are needed to assess the impact of comorbid conditions.

Obesity

Clinical disagreement exists on the effect of obesity in these patients [111]. The effect of body weight in patients with total joint arthroplasties remains unresolved in the literature [112–115]. Concern about obesity is expressed in the literature regarding the high mechanical failure of the prosthesis over the long-term [113] and potential increased postoperative complications [115,116]. Investigators have postulated that obesity is related to lower activity levels that may reduce the rate of loosening in this patient subgroup. Although a higher body mass index was reported to be associated with greater postoperative pain and dysfunction in a retrospective cohort of patients with total hip arthroplasties [65], others have discounted obesity as an adverse factor [50,113,117,118]. Although obesity is of clinical concern, obesity alone does not appear to be a factor that affects HRQL outcomes after total joint arthroplasty.

Psychologic factors

Causal models that attempt to define relationships between clinical variables and HRQL outcomes after total joint arthroplasties have not defined any strong relationships. Evidence from our earlier work and others corroborate that demographic variables, comorbidities, preoperative health status, type of prosthesis, and surgical complications do not contribute largely to the explanation of pain and functional outcomes [20,46,99]. The aforementioned suggests that medical and surgical factors do not largely contribute to the longer term functional outcomes of total joint arthroplasty. The relationships may be influenced by both internal and external sources such as psychosocial attributes.

In a double-blind, placebo-controlled trial 180 veterans with knee osteoarthritis were randomly assigned to arthroscopic debridement, arthroscopic lavage alone, or placebo arthroscopy. Psychologic variables, including expectation for improvement, depression, optimism, anxiety, stress, satisfaction with general health, social functioning, vitality, and somatization together accounted for 7% to 21% of the variance in the change scores for all of the pain and function outcomes [119]. Although sparse research has examined psychologic determinants in total joint arthroplasties, early work suggests that psychologic determinants contribute more than medical and baseline variables in predicting pain and functional outcomes after total knee arthroplasties [25,66]. These psychologic determinants, which include both affective and cognitive factors, influence total joint arthroplasty outcomes through patients' expectancies about surgical outcomes as well as through expectations regarding their own sense of self-efficacy.

Summary

Focus of outcome research for total joint arthroplasties has been directed toward understanding the surgical and technical aspects. More recent evaluations of total joint arthroplasties have used patient-centered outcomes. The lack of success reported by some patients can be attributed to surgical-related factors or complications, but in others, no specific reason can be identified. Little is known about the causal inferences of clinical variables on these outcomes; however, several patient characteristics may, indeed, affect the pain and functional outcomes after total joint arthroplasties.

The role that comorbid conditions exert on pain and functional outcomes is not clearly defined. The effect of comorbid conditions as they relate to pain and functional outcomes requires further examination. Standardized measures of comorbid conditions are typically weighted with respect to mortality, an infrequent endpoint in total joint arthroplasty surgery. If specific comorbidities and patient-related factors that affect pain and functional recovery can be readily identified, orthopaedic surgeons and clinicians would then be able to present evidence-based risks to patients during preoperative planning stages. Because little is known about the type of comorbid conditions and other patient-related factors that affect outcomes after total joint arthroplasty, indications and contraindications are poorly defined and utilization rates vary among geographic regions.

The relationship between psychosocial variables and pain and functional outcomes is one of particular interest because so little investigation has explored this plausible model. It is known that patients with high levels of anxiety or depression tend to have a worse outcome; however, the extent to which it affects their understanding and expectations about the surgery and behaviors in relation to recovery, rehabilitation, and return to their usual daily activities has yet to be ascertained.

With an aging population that is expected to live a longer and more active life, coupled with increasing technical and surgical advancements the demand for total joint arthroplasties will increase. Inasmuch as these procedures have a positive outcome on most patients' function and HQRL, younger patients with arthritis are receiving total joint arthroplasties. This demographic subgroup will likely continue to increase. To date, we have relatively little information regarding long-term patient outcome and prosthesis survivorship in these more active patients. Further work is required to determine implant longevity and subsequent outcomes following revision surgery in young patients.

Improvement seen with pain and function after total joint arthroplasties, for the most part, remains unexplained by clinical factors. No one patient-related or perioperative factor that is available to the orthopaedic surgeon or clinician can clearly predict the amount of pain relief or functional improvement. A myriad of factors most likely affect the outcomes of pain and function. Most arthroplasties are appropriately performed because the majority of patients improve, but health status data available to surgeons and clinicians are not helpful in identifying those patients who will not improve. For more explicit answers to emerge, alternative factors such as psychosocial factors and patient expectations need to be examined to provide further insights into the determinants of pain and functional outcomes of total joint arthroplasties.

Acknowledgments

The authors express gratitude for the constructive comments by Dr. David H. Feeny.

References

[1] Liang MH, Cullen KE, Larson MG, et al. Cost-effectiveness of total joint arthroplasty in osteoarthritis. Arthritis Rheum 1986;29(8):937–43.

[2] Laupacis A, Bourne R, Rorabeck C, et al. Costs of elective total hip arthroplasty during the first year. Cemented versus noncemented. J Arthroplasty 1994;9(5):481–7.

[3] Chang RW, Pellisier JM, Hazen GB. A cost-effectiveness analysis of total hip arthroplasty for osteoarthritis of the hip. JAMA 1996;275(11):858–65.

[4] American Academy of Orthopaedic Surgeons. Primary total hip and total knee arthroplasty projections to 2030. Available at: http://www.aaos.org/wordhtml/pdfs_r/tjr.pdf. Accessed September 16, 2004.

[5] Katz BP, Freund DA, Heck DA, et al. Demographic variation in the rate of knee replacement: a multi-year analysis. Health Serv Res 1996;31(2):125–40.

[6] Wells VM, Hearn TC, McCaul KA, et al. Changing incidence of primary total hip arthroplasty and total knee arthroplasty for primary osteoarthritis. J Arthroplasty 2002;17(3): 267–73.

[7] Quam JP, Michet Jr CJ, Wilson MG, et al. Total knee arthroplasty: a population-based study. Mayo Clin Proc 1991;66(6):589–95.

[8] Madhok R, Lewallen DG, Wallrichs SL, et al. Trends in the utilization of primary total hip arthroplasty, 1969 through 1990: a population-based study in Olmsted County, Minnesota. Mayo Clin Proc 1993;68(1):11–8.

[9] Canadian Institute for Health Information. Canadian Joint Replacement Registry (CJRR) 2004 Report. Total Hip and Knee Replacements in Canada. Available at: http://secure.cihi.ca/cihiweb/dispPage.jsp?cw_page=PG_38_E&cw_topic=38&cw_rel=AR_30_E#full. Accessed September 16, 2004.

[10] Peterson MG, Hollenberg JP, Szatrowski TP, et al. Geographic variations in the rates of elective total hip and knee arthroplasties among Medicare beneficiaries in the United States. J Bone Joint Surg Am 1992;74(10):1530–9.

[11] Hawker GA, Wright JG, Coyte PC, et al. Differences between men and women in the rate of use of hip and knee arthroplasty. N Engl J Med 2000;342(14):1016–22.

[12] Mahomed NN, Barrett JA, Katz JN, et al. Rates and outcomes of primary and revision total hip replacement in the United States medicare population. J Bone Joint Surg Am 2003;85-A(1): 27–32.

[13] Hawker GA, Wright JG, Glazier RH, et al. The effect of education and income on need and willingness to undergo total joint arthroplasty. Arthritis Rheum 2002;46(12):3331–9.

[14] Dixon T, Shaw M, Ebrahim S, et al. Trends in hip and knee joint replacement: socioeconomic inequalities and projections of need. Ann Rheum Dis 2004;63(7):825–30.

[15] Seagroatt V, Tan HS, Goldacre M, et al. Elective total hip replacement: incidence, emergency readmission rate, and postoperative mortality. BMJ 1991;303(6815):1431–5.

[16] Dearborn JT, Harris WH. Postoperative mortality after total hip arthroplasty. An analysis of deaths after two thousand seven hundred and thirty-six procedures. J Bone Joint Surg Am 1998;80(9):1291–4.

[17] Paavolainen P, Pukkala E, Pulkkinen P, et al. Causes of death after total hip arthroplasty: a nationwide cohort study with 24,638 patients. J Arthroplasty 2002;17(3):274–81.

[18] Parvizi J, Sullivan TA, Trousdale RT, et al. Thirty-day mortality after total knee arthroplasty. J Bone Joint Surg Am 2001;83-A(8):1157–61.

[19] Laupacis A, Bourne R, Rorabeck C, et al. The effect of elective total hip replacement on health-related quality of life. J Bone Joint Surg Am 1993;75(11):1619–26.

[20] MacWilliam CH, Yood MU, Verner JJ, et al. Patient-related risk factors that predict poor outcome after total hip replacement. Health Serv Res 1996;31(5):623–38.

[21] Rissanen P, Aro S, Sintonen H, et al. Costs and cost-effectiveness in hip and knee replacements. A prospective study. Int J Technol Assess Health Care 1997;13(4):575–88.

[22] Borstlap M, Zant JL, Van Soesbergen M, et al. Effects of total hip replacement on quality of life in patients with osteoarthritis and in patients with rheumatoid arthritis. Clin Rheumatol 1994;13(1):45–50.

[23] Aarons H, Hall G, Hughes S, et al. Short-term recovery from hip and knee arthroplasty. J Bone Joint Surg Br 1996;78(4):555–8.

[24] Shields RK, Enloe LJ, Leo KC. Health related quality of life in patients with total hip or knee replacement. Arch Phys Med Rehabil 1999;80(5):572–9.

[25] Brander VA, Stulberg SD, Adams AD, et al. Predicting total knee replacement pain: a prospective, observational study. Clin Orthop 2003;416:27–36.

[26] Rissanen P, Aro S, Sintonen H, et al. Quality of life and functional ability in hip and knee replacements: a prospective study. Qual Life Res 1996;5(1):56–64.

[27] Kirwan JR, Currey HL, Freeman MA, et al. Overall long-term impact of total hip and knee joint replacement surgery on patients with osteoarthritis and rheumatoid arthritis. Br J Rheumatol 1994;33(4):357–60.

[28] Fitzgerald JD, Orav EJ, Lee TH, et al. Patient quality of life during the 12 months following joint replacement surgery. Arthritis Rheum 2004;51(1):100–9.

[29] Badley EM, Wagstaff S, Wood PH. Measures of functional ability (disability) in arthritis in relation to impairment of range of joint movement. Ann Rheum Dis 1984;43(4):563–9,

[30] Papagelopoulos PJ, Sim FH. Limited range of motion after total knee arthroplasty: etiology, treatment, and prognosis. Orthopedics 1997;20(11):1061–5.

[31] Roder C, Parvizi J, Eggli S, et al. Demographic factors affecting long-term outcome of total hip arthroplasty. Clin Orthop 2003;417:62–73.

[32] Miner AL, Lingard EA, Wright EA, et al. Knee range of motion after total knee arthroplasty: how important is this as an outcome measure? J Arthroplasty 2003;18(3):286–94.

[33] Bellamy N, Buchanan WW, Goldsmith CH, et al. Validation study of WOMAC: a health status instrument for measuring clinically-important patient-relevant outcomes following total hip or knee arthoplasty in osteoarthritis. J Orthopaed Rheumatol 1988;1:95–108.

[34] Bellamy N, Buchanan WW, Goldsmith CH, et al. Validation study of WOMAC: a health status instrument for measuring clinically important patient relevant outcomes to antirheumatic drug therapy in patients with osteoarthritis of the hip or knee. J Rheumatol 1988;15(12):1833–40.

[35] Lizaur A, Marco L, Cebrian R. Preoperative factors influencing the range of movement after total knee arthroplasty for severe osteoarthritis. J Bone Joint Surg Br 1997;79(4):626–9.

[36] Ritter MA, Harty LD, Davis KE, et al. Predicting range of motion after total knee arthroplasty: clustering, log-linear regression, and regression tree analysis. J Bone Joint Surg Am 2003; 85(7):1278–85.

[37] Harvey IA, Barry K, Kirby SP, et al. Factors affecting the range of movement of total knee arthroplasty. J Bone Joint Surg Br 1993;75(6):950–5.

[38] Ritter MA, Campbell ED. Effect of range of motion on the success of a total knee arthroplasty. J Arthroplasty 1987;2(2):95–7.

[39] Dalury DF, Jiranek W, Pierson J, et al. The long-term outcome of total knee patients with moderate loss of motion. J Knee Surg 2003;16(4):215–20.

[40] Milne S, Brosseau L, Robinson V, et al. Continuous passive motion following total knee arthroplasty. Cochrane Database Syst Rev 2003;2:CD004260.

[41] Beaupre LA, Davies DM, Jones CA, et al. Exercise combined with continuous passive motion or slider board therapy compared with exercise only: a randomized controlled trial of patients following total knee arthroplasty. Phys Ther 2001;81(4):1029–37.

[42] Chen B, Zimmerman JR, Soulen L, et al. Continuous passive motion after total knee arthroplasty: a prospective study. Am J Phys Med Rehabil 2000;79(5):421–6.

[43] MacDonald SJ, Bourne RB, Rorabeck CH, et al. Prospective randomized clinical trial of continuous passive motion after total knee arthroplasty. Clin Orthop 2000;380:30–5.

[44] Lau SK, Chiu KY. Use of continuous passive motion after total knee arthroplasty. J Arthroplasty 2001;16(3):336–9.

[45] Jones CA, Voaklander DC, Johnston DW, et al. Health related quality of life outcomes after total hip and knee arthroplasties in a community based population. J Rheumatol 2000; 27(7):1745–52.

[46] Fortin PR, Clarke AE, Joseph L, et al. Outcomes of total hip and knee replacement: preoperative functional status predicts outcomes at six months after surgery. Arthritis Rheum 1999;42(8):1722–8.

[47] March LM, Cross MJ, Lapsley H, et al. Outcomes after hip or knee replacement surgery for osteoarthritis. A prospective cohort study comparing patients' quality of life before and after surgery with age-related population norms. Med J Aust 1999;171(5):235–8.

[48] Hilding MB, Backbro B, Ryd L. Quality of life after knee arthroplasty. A randomized study of 3 designs in 42 patients, compared after 4 years. Acta Orthop Scand 1997;68(2):156–60.

[49] van Essen GJ, Chipchase LS, O'Connor D, et al. Primary total knee replacement: short-term outcomes in an Australian population. J Qual Clin Pract 1998;18(2):135–42.

[50] Hawker G, Wright J, Coyte P, et al. Health-related quality of life after knee replacement. J Bone Joint Surg Am 1998;80(2):163–73.

[51] Petrie K, Chamberlain K, Azariah R. The psychological impact of hip arthroplasty. Aust N Z J Surg 1994;64(2):115–7.

[52] Pitson D, Bhaskaran V, Bond H, et al. Effectiveness of knee replacement surgery in arthritis. Int J Nurs Stud 1994;31(1):49–56.

[53] McHorney CA, Ware Jr JE, Lu JF, et al. The MOS 36-item Short-Form Health Survey (SF-36): III. Tests of data quality, scaling assumptions, and reliability across diverse patient groups. Med Care 1994;32(1):40–66.

[54] Ware Jr JE, Sherbourne CD. The MOS 36-item short-form health survey (SF-36). I. Conceptual framework and item selection. Med Care 1992;30(6):473–83.

[55] Stewart AL, Hays RD, Ware Jr JE. The MOS short-form general health survey. Reliability and validity in a patient population. Med Care 1988;26(7):724–35.

[56] Sitzia J, Wood N. Patient satisfaction: a review of issues and concepts. Soc Sci Med 1997; 45(12):1829–43.

[57] Bullens PH, van Loon CJ, Waal Malefijt MC, et al. Patient satisfaction after total knee arthroplasty: a comparison between subjective and objective outcome assessments. J Arthroplasty 2001;16(6):740–7.

[58] Mancuso CA, Sculco TP, Salvati EA. Patients with poor preoperative functional status have high expectations of total hip arthroplasty. J Arthroplasty 2003;18(7):872–8.

[59] Dickstein R, Heffes Y, Shabtai EI, et al. Total knee arthroplasty in the elderly: patients' self-appraisal 6 and 12 months postoperatively. Gerontology 1998;44(4):204–10.

[60] Callahan CM, Drake BG, Heck DA, et al. Patient outcomes following tricompartmental total knee replacement. A meta-analysis. JAMA 1994;271(17):1349–57.

[61] Mancuso CA, Salvati EA, Johanson NA, et al. Patients' expectations and satisfaction with total hip arthroplasty. J Arthroplasty 1997;12(4):387–96.

[62] Lieberman JR, Dorey F, Shekelle P, et al. Differences between patients' and physicians' evaluations of outcome after total hip arthroplasty. J Bone Joint Surg Am 1996;78(6): 835–8.

[63] Nilsdotter AK, Petersson IF, Roos EM, et al. Predictors of patient relevant outcome after total hip replacement for osteoarthritis: a prospective study. Ann Rheum Dis 2003;62(10):923–30.

[64] Wright JG, Coyte P, Hawker G, et al. Variation in orthopedic surgeons' perceptions of the indications for and outcomes of knee replacement. CMAJ 1995;152(5):687–97.

[65] Braeken AM, Lochhaas-Gerlach JA, Gollish JD, et al. Determinants of 6–12 month postoperative functional status and pain after elective total hip replacement. Int J Qual Health Care 1997;9(6):413–8.

[66] Sharma L, Sinacore J, Daugherty C, et al. Prognostic factors for functional outcome of total knee replacement: a prospective study. J Gerontol A Biol Sci Med Sci 1996;51(4):M152–7.

[67] Anderson Jr FA, Hirsh J, White K, et al. Hip and Knee Registry Investigators. Temporal trends in prevention of venous thromboembolism following primary total hip or knee arthroplasty 1996–2001: findings from the Hip and Knee Registry. Chest 2003;24(6 Suppl):349S–56S.

[68] Mantilla CB, Horlocker TT, Schroeder DR, et al. Risk factors for clinically relevant pulmonary embolism and deep venous thrombosis in patients undergoing primary hip or knee arthroplasty. Anesthesiology 2003;99(3):552–60.

[69] Phillips CB, Barrett JA, Losina E, et al. Incidence rates of dislocation, pulmonary embolism, and deep infection during the first six months after elective total hip replacement. J Bone Joint Surg Am 2003;85-A(1):20–6.

[70] Gaine WJ, Ramamohan NA, Hussein NA, et al. Wound infection in hip and knee arthroplasty. J Bone Joint Surg Br 2000;82(4):561–5.

[71] Peersman G, Laskin R, Davis J, et al. Infection in total knee replacement: a retrospective review of 6489 total knee replacements. Clin Orthop 2001;392:15–23.

[72] Yuan L, Shih C. Dislocation after total hip arthroplasty. Arch Orthop Trauma Surg 1999; 119(5–6):263–6.

[73] Kreder HJ, Deyo RA, Koepsell T, et al. Relationship between the volume of total hip replacements performed by providers and the rates of postoperative complications in the state of Washington. J Bone Joint Surg Am 1997;79(4):485–94.

[74] Geerts WH, Heit JA, Clagett GP, et al. Prevention of venous thromboembolism. Chest 2001; 119(1 Suppl):132S–75S.

[75] Gillespie W, Murray D, Gregg PJ, et al. Risks and benefits of prophylaxis against venous thromboembolism in orthopaedic surgery. J Bone Joint Surg Br 2000;82(4):475–9.

[76] Walenkamp GHIM. Prevention of infection in orthopaedic surgery. In: Thorngren K-G, Soucacos PN, Horan F, Scott J, editors. European instructional course lectures. London: The British Editorial Society of Bone and Joint Surgery; 2001. p. 5–17.

[77] Xenos JS, Callaghan JJ, Heekin RD, et al. The porous-coated anatomic total hip prosthesis, inserted without cement. A prospective study with a minimum of ten years of follow-up. J Bone Joint Surg Am 1999;81(1):74–82.

[78] Engh Jr CA, Culpepper WJ, Engh CA. Long-term results of use of the anatomic medullary locking prosthesis in total hip arthroplasty. J Bone Joint Surg Am 1997;79(2):177–84.

[79] Hellman EJ, Capello WN, Feinberg JR. Omnifit cementless total hip arthroplasty. A 10-year average followup. Clin Orthop 1999;364:164–74.

[80] Heck DA, Robinson RL, Partridge CM, et al. Patient outcomes after knee replacement. Clin Orthop 1998;356:93–110.

[81] Rorabeck CH. Mechanisms of knee implant failure. Orthopedics 1995;18(9):915–8.

[82] Coyte PC, Hawker G, Croxford R, et al. Rates of revision knee replacement in Ontario, Canada. J Bone Joint Surg Am 1999;81(6):773–82.

[83] Mont MA, Booth Jr RE, Laskin RS, et al. The spectrum of prosthesis design for primary total knee arthroplasty. Instr Course Lect 2003;52:397–407.

[84] Mont MA, Hungerford DS. Proximally coated ingrowth prostheses. A review. Clin Orthop 1997;344:139–49.

[85] Geesink RG. Osteoconductive coatings for total joint arthroplasty. Clin Orthop 2002;395: 53–65.

[86] Rasquinha VJ, Ranawat CS. Durability of the cemented femoral stem in patients 60 to 80 years old. Clin Orthop 2004;419:115–23.

[87] Duffy GP, Berry DJ, Rand JA. Cement versus cementless fixation in total knee arthroplasty. Clin Orthop 1998;356:66–72.

[88] Heisel C, Silva M, Schmalzried TP. Bearing surface options for total hip replacement in young patients. Instr Course Lect 2004;53:49–65.

[89] Burnett RS, Bourne RB. Indications for patellar resurfacing in total knee arthroplasty. Instr Course Lect 2004;53:167–86.

[90] Clarke IC, Gustafson A. Clinical and hip simulator comparisons of ceramic-on-polyethylene and metal-on-polyethylene wear. Clin Orthop 2000;379:34–40.

[91] Schmalzried TP, Shepherd EF, Dorey FJ, et al. The John Charnley Award. Wear is a function of use, not time. Clin Orthop 2000;381:36–46.

[92] Brander VA, Malhotra S, Jet J, et al. Outcome of hip and knee arthroplasty in persons aged 80 years and older. Clin Orthop 1997;345:67–78.

[93] Jones CA, Voaklander DC, Johnston DW, et al. The effect of age on pain, function, and quality of life after total hip and knee arthroplasty. Arch Intern Med 2001;161(3):454–60.

[94] Malchau H, Herberts P, Eisler T, et al. The Swedish Total Hip Replacement Register. J Bone Joint Surg Am 2002;84-A(Suppl 2):2–20.

[95] Rand JA, Trousdale RT, Ilstrup DM, et al. Factors affecting the durability of primary total knee prostheses. J Bone Joint Surg Am 2003;85-A(2):259–65.

[96] Pedersen A, Johnsen S, Overgaard S, et al. Registration in the Danish hip arthroplasty registry: completeness of total hip arthroplasties and positive predictive value of registered diagnosis and postoperative complications. Acta Orthop Scand 2004;75(4):434–41.

[97] Lie SA, Havelin LI, Furnes ON, et al. Failure rates for 4762 revision total hip arthroplasties in the Norwegian Arthroplasty Register. J Bone Joint Surg Br 2004;86(4):504–9.

[98] Robertsson O, Knutson K, Lewold S, et al. The Swedish Knee Arthroplasty Register 1975–1997: an update with special emphasis on 41,223 knees operated on in 1988–1997. Acta Orthop Scand 2001;72(5):503–13.

[99] Jones CA, Voaklander DC, Suarez-Almazor ME. Determinants of function after total knee arthroplasty. Phys Ther 2003;83(8):696–706.

[100] Holtzman J, Saleh K, Kane R. Effect of baseline functional status and pain on outcomes of total hip arthroplasty. J Bone Joint Surg Am 2002;84-A(11):1942–8.

[101] Ackerman IN, Bennell KL. Does pre-operative physiotherapy improve outcomes from lower limb joint replacement surgery? A systematic review. Aust J Physiother 2004;50(1):25–30.

[102] Crowe J, Henderson J. Pre-arthroplasty rehabilitation is effective in reducing hospital stay. Can J Occup Ther 2003;70(2):88–96.

[103] Thomas KS, Muir KR, Doherty M, et al. Home based exercise programme for knee pain and knee osteoarthritis: randomised controlled trial. BMJ 2002;325(7367):752.

[104] Deyle GD, Henderson NE, Matekel RL, et al. Effectiveness of manual physical therapy and exercise in osteoarthritis of the knee. A randomized, controlled trial. Ann Intern Med 2000; 132(3):173–81.

[105] Ettinger Jr WH, Burns R, Messier SP, et al. A randomized trial comparing aerobic exercise and resistance exercise with a health education program in older adults with knee osteoarthritis. The Fitness Arthritis and Seniors Trial (FAST). JAMA 1997;277(1):25–31.

[106] Wang T, Ackland T, Hall S, et al. Functional recovery and timing of hospital discharge after primary total hip arthroplasty. Aust N Z J Surg 1998;68(8):580–3.

[107] Imamura K, Black N. Does comorbidity affect the outcome of surgery? Total hip replacement in the UK and Japan. Int J Qual Health Care 1998;10(2):113–23.

[108] Belmar CJ, Barth P, Lonner JH, et al. Total knee arthroplasty in patients 90 years of age and older. J Arthroplasty 1999;14(8):911–4.

[109] Guralnik JM. Assessing the impact of comorbidity in the older population. Ann Epidemiol 1996;6(5):376–80.

[110] Voaklander DC, Kelly KD, Jones CA, et al. Self report co-morbidity and health related quality of life—a comparison with record based co-morbidity measures. Soc Indic Res 2004;66(3): 213–28.

[111] Coyte PC, Hawker G, Croxford R, et al. Variation in rheumatologists' and family physicians' perceptions of the indications for and outcomes of knee replacement surgery. J Rheumatol 1996;23(4):730–8.

[112] Stern SH, Insall JN. Total knee arthroplasty in obese patients. J Bone Joint Surg Am 1990; 72(9):1400–4.

[113] Griffin FM, Scuderi GR, Insall JN, et al. Total knee arthroplasty in patients who were obese with 10 years followup. Clin Orthop 1998;356:28–33.

[114] McClung CD, Zahiri CA, Higa JK, et al. Relationship between body mass index and activity in hip or knee arthroplasty patients. J Orthop Res 2000;18(1):35–9.

[115] Jiganti JJ, Goldstein WM, Williams CS. A comparison of the perioperative morbidity in total joint arthroplasty in the obese and nonobese patient. Clin Orthop 1993;289:175–9.

[116] Winiarsky R, Barth P, Lotke P. Total knee arthroplasty in morbidly obese patients. J Bone Joint Surg Am 1998;80(12):1770–4.

[117] Smith BE, Askew MJ, Gradisar Jr IA, et al. The effect of patient weight on the functional outcome of total knee arthroplasty. Clin Orthop 1992;276:237–44.

[118] Chan CL, Villar RN. Obesity and quality of life after primary hip arthroplasty. J Bone Joint Surg Br 1996;78(1):78–81.

[119] Moseley JB, O'Malley K, Petersen NJ, et al. A controlled trial of arthroscopic surgery for osteoarthritis of the knee. N Engl J Med 2002;347(2):81–8.

ELSEVIER
SAUNDERS

CLINICS IN
GERIATRIC
MEDICINE

Clin Geriatr Med 21 (2005) 543–561

Rheumatic Diseases in the Elderly: Dealing with Rheumatic Pain in Extended Care Facilities

Bill H. McCarberg, MD

Chronic Pain Management Program, Kaiser Permanente, 732 North Broadway, Escondido, CA 92025, USA

The number of people 65 years or older in the United States is approximately 34 million, a number expected to increase to 70 million by the year 2030 [1]. Among the elder patient, pain is the most common symptom noted when consulting a physician [2], and a common source of this pain is rheumatic diseases. A study of 97 elderly patients in a long-term care environment found the most frequently reported sources of pain to be lower back pain (40%), arthritis (24%), previous fractures (14%), and neuropathies (11%) [3]. Other epidemiologic studies observed from 45% to 80% of residents have substantial pain from musculoskeletal origin that affected their functional status and quality of life [4]. In 325 patients randomly selected from 10 Los Angeles area nursing homes, arthritis accounted for 70% of the pain complaints [5]. Undertreatment of the pain has been reported to be as high as 85% in long-term care facilities [6].

Rheumatic diseases represent over 100 conditions. These diseases are disorders of connective tissue, especially the joints and related structures, characterized by inflammation, degeneration, or metabolic derangement. Osteoarthritis is the most common rheumatic disease seen in older individuals. More than 80% of people older than 75 have clinical osteoarthritis, and more than 80% over the age of 50 have radiologic evidence of osteoarthritis [7]. The pain resulting from rheumatic diseases is often unrecognized and untreated. Multiple reasons

E-mail address: bill.h.mccarberg@kp.org

0749-0690/05/$ – see front matter © 2005 Elsevier Inc. All rights reserved.
doi:10.1016/j.cger.2005.02.001
geriatric.theclinics.com

for this inadequate care have been cited, including patient fears and insufficient provider education. Treatment is also often withheld because of concerns about falling, diminished cognition, addiction, and constipation. The elderly patient may contribute to this problem by failing to report when pain is present. In one study, up to 56% of health symptoms are regularly underreported in our aging population [8].

Long-term care includes various residential settings where elderly and disabled persons may live. These facilities vary greatly in the amount of formal or informal health care they may provide. Along the continuum of long-term care, categories of these facilities may differ dramatically from state to state or region to region in the United States. Because of arbitrary distinctions and vast differences within these categories, it is not always easy to generalize information about these facilities. Most of what know about long-term health care facilities has come from data generated in nursing home and home care populations.

Twenty thousand nursing homes provide care for almost 2 million older persons in the United States. Nursing homes account for more than twice as many beds compared with acute care hospitals and more than three times as many facilities with residents who are typically poor and disabled. Medicaid is the largest payer for care in nursing homes and provides for more than 50% of nursing home reimbursement. About 45% of care is paid for out of the pockets of these residents. In some states, private pay lasts only a few months until all resources are exhausted and residents become eligible for Medicaid. The average length of stay in a nursing home is about 2 years, but a large number of individuals stay approximately 6 months, 20% stay for longer than 5 years, and 20% of discharges are secondary to death. The goals of nursing home care vary widely from short-term rehabilitation to short-term hospice care to long-term custodial care. It has been estimated that for every resident in a nursing home, there are three more similarly disabled persons living at home or other long-term care facility [9]. Depression, anxiety, decreased socialization, sleep disturbance, impaired ambulation, and increased health care use have all been found to be associated with the presence of pain in older people [10].

Rheumatic diseases and the pain related to these conditions increase in frequency with increasing age, but pain itself is not a normal part of aging and can aggravate age-related comorbidities. Deconditioning, gait disturbances, and falls result from poor pain management. The cognitively impaired elderly are even more at risk. In a study done by Won, 74% of a demented, elderly long-term care population suffered from inadequately treated pain [8]. Despite these patients being institutionalized and under the care of health professionals, the high prevalence of pain was overlooked, in part because identifying pain requires special assessment skills not used by many long-term care facilities.

The American Medical Directors Association advocates the proper evaluation and treatment of pain in our older population through the use of treatment guidelines [11] and concludes that "in the long-term care setting, the comfort and well-being of the individual patient must be paramount. This principle is the foundation for effective management of chronic pain. Neither resource constraints nor the perception of social disapproval... must ever be an excuse for inadequate pain control" [11].

Approach to pain

A different approach must be made when assessing and managing rheumatic diseases in elderly long-term care residents compared with younger patients. The spectrum of complaints, manifestations of distress, and differential diagnosis are often different in elderly persons. The implications for functional impairment are more important, and recovery from illness is often less dramatic and slower to occur. Elderly persons present with multiple medical problems, many of which are irreversible, and cure is rare. Despite this, relief of discomfort and disability modification can often be achieved. Without adequate awareness of subtlety of elderly patients' pain management, care is less than optimal. Aggressive testing or implementation of complicated treatment is less important than providing comfort and effective symptom management for many patients [12].

Incomplete medical records and unavailability of consultants often hamper initial assessment. Diagnostic laboratories, radiographs, or other resources common in ambulatory settings may not be available because of lack of convenient transportation. Testing or consultations disrupt the frail elderly's schedules, resulting in missed meals and missed medications.

Pain perception in elderly people

The experience of pain is dependent on a complex neural system incorporating excitatory and inhibitory mechanisms that exert differential effects depending on stimulus attributes and tissue integrity. It is widely believed that elderly persons do not experience pain with the same intensity as a younger population [8]. Aging is associated with widespread changes in the cellular and chemical substrates involved in the system designed to sense pain (nociception). The functional consequences of structural age-related changes are difficult to extrapolate given the highly integrated nature of pain processing, but some definite patterns have emerged from the literature. The threshold for pain is more likely to be increased in older people when stimuli are briefer and at peripheral cutaneous or visceral sites [13]. Decreased acuity for pain may place older people at a greater risk of injury. However, aging does not appear to be associated with substantive functional change over much of the pain stimulus-response curve [14]. Age-related increases in pain reports may be more apparent when stimuli are intense or persist for longer periods. The presence of sensitized pain fibers is a biologic benefit in the presence of injured tissues.

Sensitization is maladaptive when it does not resolve in concert with tissue healing. The slow resolution of peripheral sensitization of pain fibers in older people is of major clinical significance leading to prolonged pain states not seen in younger populations. The commonly held belief that older people are marginally insensitive to pain is not borne out in the literature. Under circumstances where pain is likely to persist, older people are especially vulnerable to the negative impacts of pain.

Pain assessment

Elderly persons in long-term care settings can present unique challenges to pain assessment because as many as 50% of the residents may have significant cognitive impairment of psychological illness. The high incidence of vision and hearing impairments also complicates communication and the assessment process [15]. Use of assessment scales in older persons often is inadequate, particularly in institutional settings [16]. Evaluation of pain intensity or severity is an essential component that guides treatment planning, and many investigators have examined the ability of older adults to use selected pain intensity rating scales to report their pain [17]. In a recent study of pain assessment in elderly persons by Herr et al [18], five pain scales were found to effectively discriminate different levels of pain sensation; however, the Verbal Descriptor Scale (VDS) (Fig. 1) was the most sensitive and reliable following experimentally induced thermal stimuli. The scale most preferred by elderly people to represent pain intensity was the Numeric Rating Scale (Fig. 2), followed by the VDS. Age did not impact failure rates.

Despite cognitive impairment, most elderly persons can provide meaningful and reliable information if given the time and consideration of a sensitive clinician [19]. A simple pain question requiring a yes or no answer is reliable in even most of those with severe cognitive impairment. Pain can wax and wane, making frequent assessments more valid than relying on patient memory. Behavioral observation and at times an analgesic medication trial may provide

VERBAL DESCRIPTOR SCALE

___ The most intense pain imaginable
___ Very severe pain
___ Severe pain
___ Moderate pain
___ Mild pain
___ Slight pain
___ No pain

Fig. 1. Verbal Descriptor Scale. (*From* Herr KA, Spratt K, Mobily PR, Rhichardson G. Pain intensity assessment in older adults: use of experimental pain to compare psychometric properties and usability of selected pain scales with younger adults. Clin J Pain July/August 2004;20(4):207–19; with permission.)

NUMERIC RATING SCALE

	20
	19
	18
	17
	16
	15
	14
	13
	12
	10
	9
	8
	7
	6
	5
	4
	3
	2
	1
	0

Fig. 2. Numeric Rating Scale. (*From* Herr KA, Spratt K, Mobily PR, Rhichardson G. Pain intensity assessment in older adults: use of experimental pain to compare psychometric properties and usability of selected pain scales with younger adults. Clin J Pain July/August 2004;20(4):207–19; with permission.)

the best information for caregivers in patients with severe cognitive impairment and those who are mute or comatose.

Nonpharmacologic approaches

Nondrug strategies used alone or in combination with appropriate analgesic medications should be an integral part of the treatment plan for most patients in pain. Many nursing homes provide substantial exercise, recreation, and rehabilitation resources for their residents [20]. The importance of physical activities cannot be overstated for these patients. Physical therapy aimed at improving flexibility, strength, and endurance can have substantial impact on the rheumatic diseases [21]. Most long-term residents have mobility deficits, deconditioning is endemic, and research supports appropriate exercise programs [22]. Patient education programs, cognitive-behavioral therapy, and stress management can all be practiced in long-term care facilities [23,24]. Long-acting heat can be used to reduce pain [25] in the form of Thermacare products. Cold [25] and transcutaneous electrical stimulation reduce pain in RA patients. Acu-

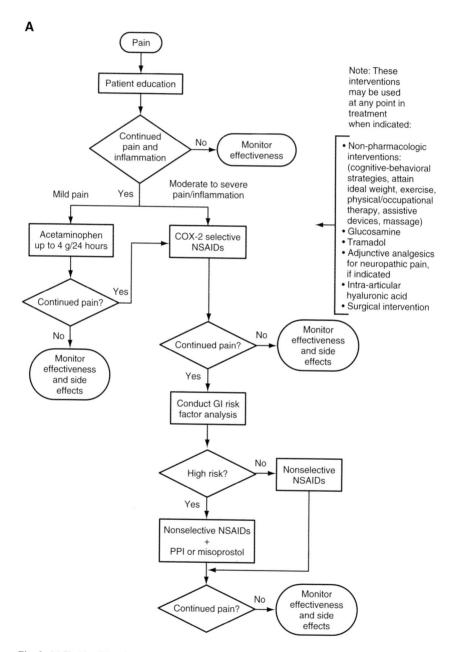

Fig. 3. (*A,B*) Algorithm for Management of Pain in Osteoarthritis. (*From* American Pain Society. Guideline for the management of osteoarthritis, rheumatoid arthritis, and juvenile chronic arthritis. 2nd ed. Glenview (IL): Author; 2002; with permission.)

B

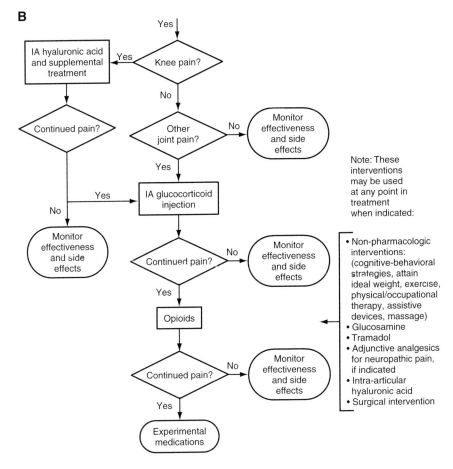

Fig. 3 (*continued*).

puncture and warmed pool exercises (Arthroswim), though often not available to long-term care patients, can also reduce pain. Surgical approaches to severely disabled patients should be considered early, before deconditioning becomes overwhelming [26]. This option is often not available or desired by many elderly people.

Pharmacologic options

Use of pharmaceuticals is often necessary to control pain in the elderly patient. It is always preferable to use evidence-based clinical practice guidelines that have specifically looked at the older patient in treating rheumatic diseases. These guidelines are often missing, and approaches need to be adapted from studies of younger populations and modified accordingly. No study to date has looked at

A

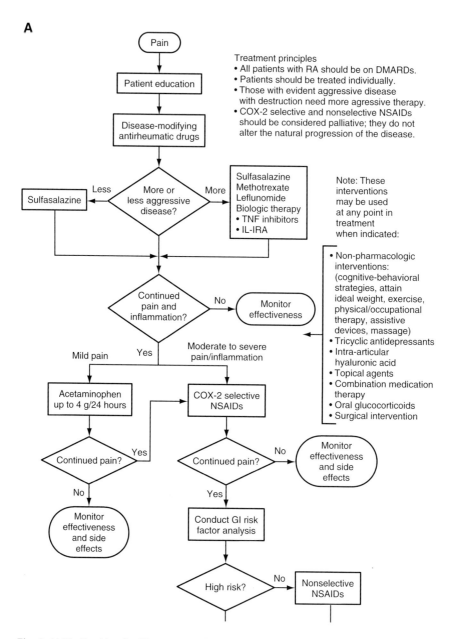

Fig. 4. (*A,B*) Algorithm for Management of Pain in Rheumatoid Arthritis. (*From* American Pain Society. Guideline for the management of osteoarthritis, rheumatoid arthritis, and juvenile chronic arthritis. 2nd ed. Glenview (IL): Author; 2002; with permission.)

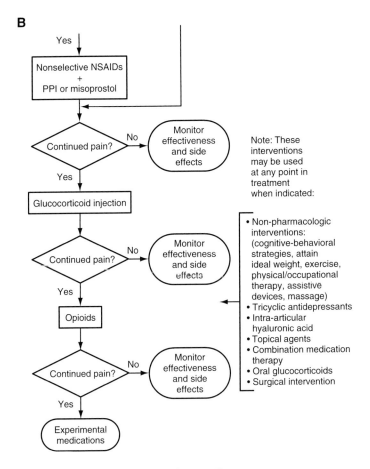

Fig. 4 (*continued*).

long-term use of any of the nonsteroidal agents in populations over the age of 85. Examples of a treatment algorithm for osteoarthritis are shown in Fig. 3, and rheumatoid arthritis in Fig. 4. Medication options to treat many rheumatic diseases are presented in Table 1, 2, and 3. These figures and tables have been reprinted from the newest evidence-based guidelines of the American Pain Society's *Guideline for the Management of Pain in Osteoarthritis, Rheumatoid Arthritis, and Juvenile Chronic Arthritis* [27]. The American College of Rheumatology has also published guidelines for the management of rheumatic diseases. Neither of these is specific to an older population. The American Geriatrics Society's (AGS) clinical guideline (*The Management of Persistent Pain in Older Persons*) addresses pain in the elderly patient; however, it does not concentrate solely the treatment of rheumatic disease.

The biological processes of aging alter most pharmacokinetic aspects of drug disposition and pharmacodynamic responses to pain-relieving drugs. Changing

Table 1
Dosages of acetaminophen and nonsteroidal antiinflammatory drugs (NSAIDs) used to treat people with osteoarthritis, rheumatoid arthritis, and juvenile chronic arthritis

Medication (trade name)	Usual 24-hour dose range (Adults)	Individual dosage and frequency (Adults) usual daily dose		Usual daily dose (Children) (mg/kg/24 hr)	FDA approved use
		Dosage	Frequency		
Acetaminophen (Anacin, Excedrin, Panadol, Tempra, Tylenol, others)	2–4 g	325–650 mg 650 mg–1 g	q 4 h qid	10–15mg/kg/q 4–6 h (maximum g/24 h)	RA, OA, AS, JCA, ST
Nonselective NSAIDs:					
Carboxylic acid derivatives (salicylic acid derivatives):					
Aspirin (acetylsalicylic acid)	2.4–6 g	600–1500 mg	qid	80–100 mg/kg/24 h/ + tid	RA, OA, AS, JCA, ST
Buffered aspirin (Acription, Bufferin, others)	2.4–6 g	600–1500 mg	qid	80–100 mg/kg/24 h/ + tid	RA, OA, AS, JCA, ST
Enteric-coated aspirin (multiple)	2.4–6 g	600–1500 mg	qid	80–100 mg/kg/24 h/ + tid	RA, OA, AS, JCA, ST
Choline magnesium trisalicylate (Tricosol, Trilisate)	1.5–3 g	500–1000 mg	tid	50–65 mg/kg/24 h + bid	RA, OA, pain, JCA
Diflunisal (Dolobid)	1–1.5 g	500–750 mg	bid		RA, OA, AS, JCA, ST
Salsalate (Disalcid)	1.5–3 g	750–1,500 mg	bid		RA, OA, AS, JCA, ST
Propionic acid derivatives:					
Fenoprofen (Nalfon)	1.2–2.4 g	300–600 mg	tid		RA, OA
Flurbiprofen (Ansaid)	100–200 mg	50–100 mg	bid		RA, OA, JCA
Ibuprofen (Advil, Motrin, others)	1.2–3.2 g (for pain) 2.4–3.2 g (for inflammation)	OTC: 200–400 mg Rx: 400, 600, 800 mg maximum: 3200 mg	qid tid–qid	30–50 mg/kg/24 h + tid (maximum 2.4g/24 h)	RA, OA
Ketoprofen (Orudis)	75–225 mg	25–75 mg	tid		RA, OA
Naproxen (Naporsyn, others)	500 mg–1 g	250, 375, 500 mg	bid	10–20 mg/kg/24 h + bid	RA, OA, JCA, ST
Naproxen sodium (Aleve, Anaprox)	550–1100 mg	275–550 mg	bid		RA, OA, ST
Acetic acid derivatives:					
Diclofenac[a] (N Arthrotec, Volaren, others)	150–200 mg	50 mg 75 mg	tid bid	1–4 mg/kg/24 h + bid	RA, OA, AS

Etodolac (Lodine)	400–1200 mg	200–300 mg maximum: 1200 mg	bid, tid, qid	15–20 mg/kg/24 h + bid	OA, pain
Indomethacin (Indocin, Indocin SR)	<200 mg	25–50 mg rarely >150 mg	tid or qid	2–3 mg/kg/24 h + bid (max 200 mg/24 hr)	RA, OA, G, AS, JCA
Sulindac (Clinoril)	300–400 mg	150, 200 mg	qd / bid	3–4 mg/kg/24 h + bid	RA, OA, AS, ST, G
Tolmetin[a] (Tolectin, Tolectin DS)	800–1800 mg	400, 600, 800 mg	tid	15–30 mg/kg/24 h + bid	RA, OA, AS, JCA
Fenamates (anthranilic acids):					
Meclofenamate (Meclomen)	50–400 mg	50–100 mg	tid or qid		RA, OA
Mefenamic acid (Ponstel)	1.0–2.0 g	250 mg	qid		RA, OA
Enolic acid derivatives:					
Meloxicam (Mobic)	7.5–15 mg	7.5 mg (OA) 15 mg (RA)	qd / qd		OA / Not approved
Phenylbutazone[b] (Butazolidin)	<600 mg	100 mg	tid up to 600 mg		Severe arthritis
Piroxicam (Feldene)	10–20 mg	10, 20 mg	qd	0.25–0.4 mg/kg/24 h qd	RA, OA
Naphthylalkanones:					
Nabumetone (Relafen)	1.0–1.5 g	500 mg	bid up to 1.5 g		RA, OA
COX-2 selective NSAIDs:					
Celecoxib (Celebrex)	200–400 mg	100, 200 mg 200 mg	q 12 h / qd		RA, OA, acute pain
Rofecoxib (VIOXX)	12.5–25 mg	12.5, 25 mg 50 mg	qd (chronic pain) / qd (acute pain)		OA / Acute pain
Valdecoxib (Bextra)	10 mg	10 mg	qd		RA, OA, acute pain

Abbreviations: AS, ankylosing spondylitis; G, gout; JCA, juvenile chronic arthritis; OA, osteoarthritis; RA, rheumatoid arthritis; ST, soft tissue injury.

[a] Long acting.

[b] Phenylbutazone has been withdrawn from commercial availability due to markedly decreased use. This is because of serious, potentially life-threatening toxicity (ie, blood dyscrasias). It is a potent and effective NSAID but has a higher incidence of minor (dyspepsia) and serious adverse events than most newer NSAIDs. It is only available in extemporaneously compounded dosage forms.

From American Pain Society. Guideline for the management of osteoarthritis, rheumatoid arthritis, and juvenile chronic arthritis. 2nd ed. Glenview (IL): Author; 2002.

Table 2
Disease-modifying antirheumatic drugs (DMARDs) and dosages

Medication (trade name)	Usual adult dosage	Usual pediatric dosage	Comments and special considerations
Azathioprine (Imuran)	PO: 50 mg up to 200 mg/24 h	PO: 2–3 mg/kg qd	Not associated with improved outcome as measured by radiograph
Cyclophosphamide (Cytoxan, Neosar, Pocytox)	PO or parenterally: 1–2 mg/kg	PO: 1–2 mg/kg q day or IV: 500–1000 mg/m^2 IV monthly	Experimental and highly toxic. Limited by associated leukemia, urinary tract cancers
Cyclosporine (Neoral, Sandimmune, Sang-cya)	3–5 mg/kg/24 h	PO: 3–5 mg/kg divided bid	Trough level between 100 and 200 mg. Use with caution in people with impaired renal or hepatic function, hypertension, and kidney dysfunction
D-penicillamine (Cuprimine, Depen)	PO: 75–125 mg to start, raising dose by 125 mg q 3 weeks to 750 mg	PO: 5–10 mg/kg q day Maximum daily dose = 750 mg	Rarely used because of toxicity
Etanercept (Enteril, Enbrel)	SQ: 25 mg 2x/week	SQ: 0.4 mg/kg 2x/week up to 25 mg	Soluble receptor to TNF-α. Use with caution in history of recurring infections
Hydroxychloroquine (Plaquenil)	PO: 200 mg bid to start then 200 mg qd	PO: <6.5 mg/kg qd	Retinal toxicity most important problem
Infliximab (Remicade)	IV: 3 mg/kg q 4A6 weeks up to 10 mg/kg	IV: 3A5 mg/kg (rounded up to nearest 100) q 8 weeks (maintenance)	(Monoclonalab to TNF-α) Use with caution in older adults
Intramuscular/Oral Gold Auranofin (Myochrysinc, Ridaura, Solganol)	IM: 10 mg q week, then 25 mg q week, then 50 mg q week; decrease to q mo. PO: 3–10 mg PO qd	IM: 0.5–1 mg/kg weekly Maximum weekly dose 50 mg	Risk of severe reactions; generally not used in children; heavy metal toxic reactions; diarrhea
Leflunomide (Arava)	PO: 100 mg qd × 3 days then 10 or 20 mg qd	PO: 0.5 mg/kg qd maximum 9 mg Too little data in children to specify dosage	Liver toxicity, rare
Methotrexate (Folex, Folex PFS, Mexate, Mexate-AQ, Rheumatrex)	PO, SQ, or IM: 7.5–15.0 mg q week up to 40 mg q week 1 g bid to qid	PO: 0.5–1.0 mg/kg q week 10–20 mg/m^2/week up to 1 mg/kg/week	Oral ulcers, liver, pulmonary, and bone marrow toxicity can occur. Teratogenic
Sulfasalazine (Alti-Sulfasalazine, Azullidine, PMS-Sulfasalazine, Salazopyrin)	PO: 1 g bid to qid bid up to 4 g/d	PO: 40–60 mg/kg divided bid	Sulfa allergy is contraindication. Enteric coated is better tolerated

Abbreviations: IM, intramuscularly; IV, intravenously; PO, orally; SQ, subcutaneously.
From American Pain Society. Guideline for the management of osteoarthritis, rheumatoid arthritis, and juvenile chronic arthritis. 2nd ed. Glenview (IL): Author; 2002.

Table 3
Usual starting doses for opioid analgesics in opioid naïve adults $\geq$ 50 kg body weight

Medication (Trade Name)	Usual Starting Oral Dose for Moderate to Severe Pain[a]	Special Considerations
Short-acting opioid agonists:		
Codeine	Not recommended because of adverse side effects common even at minimally effective analgesic doses.	Short-acting opioid agonist
Hydrocodone and acetaminophen[c] (Lorcel, Lortab, Vicodin)	5–10 mg qid hydrocodone[b]	Available only in combination with acetaminophen, aspirin, or ibuprofen
Hydrocodone and ibuprofen[c] (Vicoprofen)		More likely than most other opioids to cause side effects associated with histamine release
Hydrocodone and aspirin[c] (Lortab ASA)		
Hydromorphone[d] (Dilaudid, others)	2–3 mg qid	Short-acting opioid agonist
Meperidine (Demerol, others)	Not recommended because of potential CNS side effects.	Very short-acting opioid agonist. Risk of seizures when used for > 2 days
Morphine[d] (MSIR, Duramorph, Roxanol, others)	7.5–15 mg qid	Short-acting opioid agonist
Oxycodone (Roxicodone, Oxylr)	5–10 mg qid	Short-acting opioid agonist
Long-acting opioid agonists:		
Morphine, controlled-release (MS Contin, Oramorph SR) (Kadian)	30 mg q 12h 30 mg q 8h	Controlled-release opioid agonist
Oxycodone HydrochlorideAER (OxyContin)	10–20 mg q 12 h	Controlled-release opioid agonist. Tablets are to be swallowed whole and are not to be broken, chewed, or crushed. Taking broken, chewed, or crushed OxyContin leads to rapid release and absorption of a potentially fatal dose of oxycodone.
Fentanyl transdermal (Duragesic)	25 mcg (0.025mg)/h (one transdermal system for 72 h)	Controlled-release opioid agonist. Correct patch application procedure must be followed. Avoid direct exposure of application site to heat.

Caution: Recommended doses do not apply to adult patients with body weight less than 50 kg.

[a] Doses computed by using doses that are equianalgesic with dose of oxycodone shown to be effective in moderate to severe OA pain.

[b] This dosage is for hydrocodone only.

[c] Caution: These products contain aspirin, acetaminophen, or ibuprofen. Total daily doses of acetaminophen that exceed 6 gm may be associated with severe hepatic toxicity. Aspirin is contraindicated in children in the presence of lever or other viral disease, because of its association with Reye's syndrome.

[d] Caution: Recommended doses do not apply to patients with renal or hepatic insufficiency or other conditions affecting medication metabolism and kinetics.

From American Pain Society. Guideline for the management of osteoarthritis, rheumatoid arthritis, and juvenile chronic arthritis. 2nd ed. Glenview (IL): Author; 2002.

fat to muscle ratios alters drug distribution and changes in gastrointestinal motility lead to longer transit times. Renal function decreases resulting in drug accumulation as well as increases in drug metabolites. Comorbid conditions, such as congestive heart failure, diabetes, and hypertension—all associated with advanced age—complicate disease management and pain control in older patients. These myriad conditions, along with processes of senescence, lead to organ function impairment that influences pharmacokinetics. The additive influences of various pharmacologic interventions required for disease management in older patients further complicate clinical care.

Prescription drug use is often made more complex by the trend in United States society to use dietary supplements, herbal remedies, and a host of over-the-counter pharmaceuticals. Considerations of drug–drug and disease–drug interactions become more problematic. The risk to benefit assessment that is always made in treating diseases with medication becomes a delicate balancing act in the elderly arthritic patient. However, fear of potential harm must not overshadow the need for palliative pharmacotherapy, due to the high prevalence and overwhelming debilitating, life-altering nature of unabated persistent pain.

Pharmacotherapy is the mainstay of treatment to control pain in the older patient according to the AGS [28]. This statement is based on the aggregate literature that reveals a high prevalence of arthritis pain in the geriatric population. It is also evident that all drug therapies have potentially negative consequences. It is incumbent upon the prescribing practitioner to be cognizant of the potential risks associated with analgesic and pain-modulating therapies.

A key to success in the application of pharmacotherapy in geriatric arthritis pain is slow, careful titration of drugs with specific patient-centered endpoints. Anticipating and preventing adverse effects (eg, constipation, gastric upset, sedation, nausea, and cognitive disturbances) must also be considered. Patients who are experiencing severely debilitating pain require more rapid titration of medication for symptom control [29].

Drug regimens for the older patient should be simplified as much as possible, and regimens should be adjusted to meet individual needs and lifestyles [30]. Economic issues also play a role in pain management and should enter into the decision-making processes once sound principles of assessment and treatment have been followed. Clinicians should be aware of common economic barriers, including the lack of Medicare reimbursement for outpatient oral medications, limited formularies, and delays from mail-order pharmacies in some managed-care programs. Inner-city areas may not have pharmacies that are willing to carry certain analgesics [31].

Knowledge of each pain treatment drug's pharmacokinetic profile and relevant patient variables (eg, renal and hepatic function, concurrent medication use) allows for a reasoned approach to titration. This process may take 1 to 2 days for short half-life drugs in healthy patients and several days to a week with drugs having long half-lives or patients with diminished hepatic metabolism, impaired renal clearance [29].

Although pharmacotherapy is usually started after failure of nonpharmacologic options, for moderate to severe pain, efficacy is maximized when pharmacologic and nonpharmacologic treatments are employed together [32]. Combinations of drugs with different mechanisms of action may lead to improved outcomes as a result of therapeutic synergy, with less toxicity than can occur with higher doses of single drugs [33]. In rheumatoid arthritis, inflammation and erosions lead to significant damage of the joints. Pharmacotherapy with analgesics and anti-inflammatory agents is insufficient, and early introduction of disease-modifying antirheumatic drugs should be considered. In osteoarthritis where an inflammatory response is present, anti-inflammatories are the mainstay with analgesics if pain levels warrant multiple initial drug therapies.

Patients with mild to moderate arthritis pain may experience sufficient symptomatic relief with acetaminophen as recommended in the practice guidelines of the American Pain Society, the American College of Rheumatology, and the American Geriatric Society. The maximum recommended dosage for patients with normal renal and hepatic function, and in those with no history of alcohol abuse, is 4000 mg per day. This level may be reduced to 2000 mg per day with refinement of guidelines in the elder population. Hepatic or renal impairment requires dose reduction by 50% to 75% or an alternative form of therapy [27].

Nonselective nonsteroidal anti-inflammatory drugs (NSAIDs) are often used to treat the rheumatic diseases (see Table 1). Older patients, and especially those with multiple-system disease and the frail elderly, are at high risk for life-threatening gastrointestinal bleeding with chronic use of NSAIDs [34]. This risk is reduced with the concomitant administration of misoprostol or proton-pump inhibitors, but these pharmacologic additions are often not well tolerated by elderly patients [35].

When acetaminophen is not effective, safer alternatives to traditional NSAID therapy for patients who require daily chronic therapy are the cyclooxygenase-2 (COX-2) selective nonsteroidal anti-inflammatory drugs [36]. The COX-2 selective drugs offer reduced gastrointestinal morbidity compared with the nonselective NSAIDs and are devoid of antiplatelet effects. The COX-2 inhibitors are still new; one must stay vigilant to drug-drug interactions and postmarketing reports [37].

Contrary to previous thinking, it appears that in many cases, chronic low-dose opioid therapy for the pain of rheumatic diseases may have fewer life-threatening risks than does the long-term daily use of high-dose NSAIDs [38]. Over the past decade, largely as a result of observations derived from long-term opioid use in cancer pain patients, opioid analgesics for chronic arthritis have become increasingly more acceptable [39]. There are many different opioid analgesics and formulations from which to choose (see Table 3). Rational selection of opioid analgesics depends on several factors, including the pattern and intensity of the patient's pain, previous responses to opioid therapy, adherence to dosing regimens, routes of administration, convenience, and cost [40].

Propoxyphene is a weak opioid agonist that has been available for decades and is one of the most extensively prescribed analgesics in older patients [41]. Studies suggest that its efficacy is similar to that of aspirin or acetaminophen alone, but drug accumulation as well as ataxia or dizziness may add unnecessary morbidity. The current literature suggests that other analgesic strategies are more appropriate for patients with persistent mild to moderate pain, and the use of propoxyphene is discouraged [42]. Monitoring the side effects of opioid therapy should focus on neurologic, gastrointestinal, and cognitive effects. Serious side effects, such as impaired consciousness or respiratory depression, are rare.

Patients with borderline mobility capabilities and a propensity for falls must be monitored carefully for increasing gait and balance disturbances. Sustained-release opioid formulations are available for continuous treatment of moderate to severe pain. Chewing or crushing medications is common in the long-term care setting because of swallowing difficulty or the necessity of tube feeding. This practice destroys the controlled-release properties, causes rapid absorption of the entire dose, and may result in overdose.

Drug addiction is feared by patients, expected by providers, and has been reported in all age groups; however, the incidence of iatrogenic addiction in older patients with chronic arthritis appears to be negligible. Evidence from long-term studies of patients with stable disease states suggests that opioid tolerance (the need for more drugs to get the same therapeutic effect) is slow to develop [43]. Any dramatic change in a patient's dosing needs should prompt an evaluation of progression of the arthritic condition. Decisions regarding appropriateness of opioid therapy should be considered given known benefits and risks, similar to all other long-term care plans that have significant clinical implications.

Future areas for improving pain care

Improving pain management in long-term care facilities presents several unique barriers. Nursing homes are already highly burdened by local, state, and federal policies. Most of the care is delivered by nurse's aids with little or sometimes no formal medical education and high staff turnover rates. Monthly physician visits means that the doctor plays a minor role in directing resources and quality improvement in most facilities. The Joint Commission for Accreditation of Health Care Organizations as recently adopted pain management indicators in their review process; however, only about 5% of nursing homes are accredited by the commission. Yearly state licensure procedures or Medicaid and Medicare surveys do not have pain measures as quality indictors. Policies about use of heating pads, potent analgesic drugs, and use of outside services are being scrutinized more carefully to relieve unnecessary barriers. Substantial research with studies using long-term outcomes is critical in or to apply existing knowledge and technologies to this large segment of the health care industry.

Summary

Pain in elderly patients is often underreported, underdiagnosed, and under-treated. Increased understanding of the experience of pain in older persons, strategies for assessment, and appropriate use of pharmacologic and non-pharmacologic approaches is necessary to improve management of pain in this population. More valid and reliable pain measures are necessary as are new drugs with milder side effects. Nondrug strategies require further investigation for this highly disabled population. A pharmacologic regimen for the elderly patient suffering from a rheumatic disease must combine adequate analgesia with sufficient safety precautions, minimizing side effects. These regimens should also be simplified as much as possible. Long-acting medications are often best to provide longer durations of comfort and fewer doses for nurses or other caregivers to administer. In addition, any regimen must address the root cause of the pain as well as its severity, while taking into account comorbid conditions and concomitant medications.

Facilities must adopt contingency plans for pain management. These plans will prevent delays in pain care during medication changes or dosage adjustments. Institutional policies that limit activities should not be so rigid that they create barriers to pain control for most patients. As the need for health systems for frail elderly persons continues to grow, it is our most important obligation to provide comfort and effective pain control appropriate for these new settings.

References

[1] Centers for Disease Control and Prevention. Healthy aging: preventing disease and improving quality of life among older Americans. Atlanta (GA): CDC; 2001. Available at: www.cdc.gov/nccdphp/aag-aging.htm. Accessed January 7, 2002.

[2] Otis JAD, McGeeney B. Managing pain in the elderly. Clin Geriatr 2001;9:82–8.

[3] Ferrel BA, Ferrel BR, Osterweil D. Pain in the nursing home. J Am Geriatr Soc 1990;38: 409–14.

[4] Helm RD, Gibson SJ. Pain in older people. In: Crombie IK, Croft PR, Linton SJ, et al, editors. Epidemiology of pain. Seattle (WA): IASP Press; 1999. p. 103–12.

[5] Ferrel BA, Ferrel BR, Rivera L. Pain in cognitively impaired nursing home patients. J Pain Symptom Manage 1995;10:591–8.

[6] Mobily P, Herr K. Barriers to managing resident's pain. Contemp Longterm Care 1996;19: 60A–60B.

[7] Sharma L. Epidemiology of osteoarthritis. In: Moskowitz RW, Howell OS, Altman RD, et al, editors. Osteoarthritis: diagnosis and medical/surgical management. 3rd ed. Philadelphia: W.B. Saunders; 2001. p. 3–17.

[8] Won A, Lapane K, Gambassi G, et al. Correlates and management of nonmalignant pain in the nursing home. J Am Geriatr Soc 1999;47:936–42.

[9] Ouslander JG, Osterweil D, Morley J. Medical care in the nursing home. 2nd ed. New York: McGraw-Hill; 1997. p. 1–38.

[10] Parmelee PA, Katz IR, Lawton MP. The relation of pain to depression among institutionalized aged. J Geriatr 1991;46:15–21.

[11] American Medical Directors Association. Chronic pain management in the long-term care setting: clinical practice guideline. Columbia (MD): AMDA; 1999.

[12] Ferrell BA. Overview of aging and pain. In: Ferrell BA, Ferrell BR, editors. Pain in the elderly. Seattle (WA): IASP Press; 1996. p. 1–10.

[13] Birren JE, Schroots JF. History, concepts, and theory in the psychology of aging. In: Birren JE, Schaie KW, editors. Handbook of the psychology of aging. 4th ed. San Diego (CA): Academic Press; 1995. p. 3–23.

[14] Chakour M, Gibson SJ, Bradbeer M, Helme RD. The effect of age on A delta and C fibre thermal pain perception. Pain 1996;64:143–52.

[15] Ferrell BA. Pain evaluation and management in the nursing home. Ann Intern Med 1995; 123:681–7.

[16] Weissman DE, Matson S. Pain assessment and management in the long-term care setting. Theor Med Bioethics 1999;20:31–43.

[17] Weiner D, Peterson B, Ladd K, et al. Pain in nursing home residents: an exploration of prevalence, staff perspectives, and practical aspects of measurement. Clin J Pain 1999;15:92–101.

[18] Herr KA, Spratt K, Mobily PR, et al. Pain intensity assessment in older adults use of experimental pain to compare psychometric properties and usability of selected PAW scales with younger adults. Clin J Pain 2004;20(4):207–19.

[19] Ferrell BA, Ferrell BR, Rivera L. Pain in cognitively impaired nursing home residents. J Pain Symptom Manage 1995;10:591–8.

[20] Ouslander JG, Osterweil D, Morley J. Medical care in the nursing home. 2nd ed. New York: McGraw-Hill; 1997. p. 391–417.

[21] Gloth MJ, Matesi AM. Physical therapy and exercise in pain management. Clin Geriatr Med 2001;17:525–35.

[22] Simmons SF, Ferrell BA, Schnell JF. The effects of a controlled exercise trial on pain in nursing home residents. Clin J Pain 2002;18:380–5.

[23] Lorig K, Lubeck D, Kraines RG, Seleznick M, Holman HR. Outcomes of self-help education for patient with arthritis. Arthritis Rheum 1985;28:680–5.

[24] Keefe FJ, Bonk V. Psychosocial assessment of pain in patients having rheumatic arthritis pain: maintaining treatment gains. Arthritis Care Res 1999;25:81–103.

[25] Mihlovitz SL, Wolf SL. Thermal agents in rehabilitation. 2nd ed. Philadelphia (PA): Davis; 1990.

[26] Fortin PR, Clarke AE, Joseph L, et al. Outcomes of total hip and knee replacement: preoperative functional status predicts outcomes at six months after surgery. Arthritis Rheum 1999;42: 1722–8.

[27] American Pain Society. Guideline for the management of pain in osteoarthritis, rheumatoid arthritis, and juvenile chronic arthritis. 2nd ed. Glenview (IL): Author; 2002.

[28] American Geriatric Society Panel on Persistent Pain in Older Persons. The management of persistant pain in older adults. J Am Geriatr Soc 2002;50:S205–24.

[29] Grossberg GT, Sherman LK, Fine PG. Pain and behavioral disturbances in the cognitively impaired older adult: assessment and treatment issues. Annals of Long-Term Care 2000;8:22–4.

[30] Fine PG. Pain and aging: overcoming barriers to treatment and role of transdermal opioid therapy. Clin Geriatr 2000;8:28–36.

[31] Morrison RS, Wallenstein S, Natale DK, et al. "We don't carry that." A failure of pharmacies in predominantly nonwhite neighborhoods to stock opioid analgesics. N Engl J Med 2000;342: 1023–6.

[32] Gloth III FM. Pain management in older adults: prevention and treatment. J Am Geriatr Soc 2001;49:188–99.

[33] Mullican WS, Lacy JR. Tramadol/acetaminophen combination tablets and codeine/acetaminophen combination capsules for the management of chronic pain: a comparative trial. Clin Ther 2001;23:1429–45.

[34] Maclean CH. Quality indicators for the management of osteoarthritis in vulnerable elders. Ann Intern Med 2001;135:711–21.

[35] Graham DY, White RH, Moreland LW, et al. Duodenal and gastric ulcer prevention with misoprostol in arthritis patients taking NSAIDs. Misoprostol Study Group. Ann Intern Med 1993;119:257–62.

[36] Geba GP, Weaver AL, Polis AB, et al. Efficacy of rofecoxib, celecoxib, and acetaminophen in osteoarthritis of the knee: a randomized trial. JAMA 2002;287:64–71.

[37] Fine P. The role of rofecoxib, a COX-2-specific inhibitor, for the treatment of non-cancer pain: a review. J Pain 2002;3:272–83.

[38] Portenoy RK. Opiate therapy for chronic non-cancer pain. Can we get past the bias? Am Pain Soc Bull 1991;1:4–7.

[39] Portenoy RK. Opioid therapy for chronic non-malignant pain: current status. In: Fields HL, Libeskind JC, editors. Pharmacological approaches to the treatment of chronic pain. New concepts and critical issues: progress in pain research and management, vol. 11. Seattle (WA): IASP Press; 1994. p. 247–88.

[40] Hanks G, Cherny N. Opioid analgesic therapy. In: Doyle D, Hanks G, MacDonald N, editors. Oxford textbook of palliative medicine. 2nd ed. Oxford, United Kingdom: Oxford University Press; 1998. p. 331–55.

[41] Cramer GW, Galer BS, Mendelson MA, Thompson GD. A drug use evaluation of selected opioid and nonopioid analgesics in the nursing facility setting. J Am Geriatr Soc 2000;48:398–404.

[42] Leipzig RM, Cummings RG, Tinetti ME. Drugs and falls in older people: a systematic review and meta-analysis: II. Cardiac and analgesic drugs. J Am Geriatr Soc 1999;47:40–50.

[43] Portenoy RK. Opiod therapy for chronic non-malignant pain: current status. In: Fields H, Libeskind JC, editors. Progress in pain research and management. Seattle (WA): IASP Press; 1994. p. 247–88.

ELSEVIER
SAUNDERS

CLINICS IN
GERIATRIC
MEDICINE

Clin Geriatr Med 21 (2005) 563–576

Rheumatic Diseases in the Elderly: Assessing Chronic Pain

Susan L. Charette, MD*, Bruce A. Ferrell, MD

*Division of Geriatrics, University of California, Los Angeles, 10945 Le Conte Avenue, Suite 2339,
Los Angeles, CA 90095, USA*

Pain is a common yet frequently overlooked complaint among older patients. Population-based studies have estimated that the prevalence of pain may be as high as 25% to 50% in community-dwelling older persons and 45% to 80% in nursing home residents [1–5]. Unfortunately, many physicians and patients incorrectly view pain as an expected part of aging. Older patients frequently have multiple comorbid conditions, and their medical care is typically directed toward the management of the underlying disease processes. Little attention may be paid to the alleviation of associated symptoms such as pain. As a result, pain is a significant problem that frequently goes unrecognized and undertreated [5,6].

Pain must be accepted as a real and important issue for older patients. It can have multiple causes, variable presentations, and numerous meanings. Uncontrolled pain can negatively impact functional status, psychosocial well-being, and quality of life. The consequences of pain include impaired mobility, decreased socialization, depression, sleep disturbances, and increased health use and costs [2,7,8]. Pain may also negatively impact common geriatric conditions including gait impairment, falls, polypharmacy, cognitive dysfunction, and malnutrition [4]. Given this potential for negative consequences, it is recommended that older persons be assessed for pain on their initial presentation to any health care provider [1].

Effective pain management requires an accurate pain assessment. After a thorough initial assessment, ongoing reassessment is needed to ensure adequacy of the therapeutic plan, evaluate for new sources of pain, and monitor for side effects from the current treatment regimen. This article will review

---

* Corresponding author. Suite 420, 200 UCLA Medical Plaza, Los Angeles, California 90095.
  E-mail address: SCharette@mednet.ucla.edu (S.L. Charette).

0749-0690/05/$ – see front matter © 2005 Elsevier Inc. All rights reserved.
doi:10.1016/j.cger.2005.02.007

potential challenges and important pearls for the assessment of chronic pain in older patients.

What is pain? Definitions and descriptions

Before discussing assessment, a review of the common definitions and descriptions of pain is useful. Pain may be defined as an unpleasant sensory and emotional experience associated with actual or potential tissue damage, or described in terms of such damage [9]. Although pain often results from a physical insult, there are no reliable biologic markers for the presence or intensity of pain [10]. Ultimately, it is the patient's self-report that provides the most accurate and reliable evidence for the existence of pain [1,10–12].

Acute pain typically has a distinct onset, an obvious source, and a relatively short duration [10]. Acute pain may be self-limited or signify a serious condition that needs urgent attention. Patients may present with an acute physical response including signs such as an elevated heart rate, an elevated blood pressure, diaphoresis, and a mild increase in temperature. The intensity of acute pain usually correlates to the level of tissue damage, and typically disappears after the underlying cause has been treated.

Chronic pain is more difficult to define. It is characterized by a longer duration, and is usually associated with chronic medical conditions. Although chronic pain may lack distinct physiologic signs similar to acute pain, it is often associated with long-term changes in functional status and psychosocial well-being. Chronic pain is often defined arbitrarily as pain lasting longer than 3 to 6 months or beyond the time frame expected for healing [10]. For other conditions, the underlying disease and the associated chronic pain are synonymous with one another [10]. Common examples include fibromyalgia and osteoarthritis. Chronic pain may also present as recurrent attacks of acute pain, such as intermittent headaches and recurring mechanical low back pain. Given the range of processes that can produce chronic pain, it is essential to carefully diagnose the etiology and review the natural history of the associated pain syndrome with the patient.

Chronic pain may result from one or more physiologic mechanisms that perpetuate pain. Treatment plans specifically targeting the underlying pathophysiology are more likely to be effective. Chronic pain is typically generated by either a nociceptive or neuropathic mechanism. Nociceptive pain is the result of inflammation, traumatic injury, tissue destruction, or mechanical deformation that serves as a stimulus to a primary afferent sensory neuron [10]. Nociceptive pain can be visceral, derived from internal organs and viscera, or somatic, relating to muscle, soft tissue (ligaments, tendons), bones, joints or skin [13]. This type of pain is often described as a deep aching, throbbing, gnawing, or sore sensation, and examples include rheumatoid arthritis and polymyalgia rheumatica. Neuropathic pain results from nerve damage in either the central or peripheral nervous system [14]. Neuropathic pain is commonly experienced as burning, severe shooting pains, or persistent numbness or tingling. The diagnosis of neuropathic pain is often made by the presence of hyperalgesia (a stimulus that was previously only noxious now results in intense pain, eg, pinprick) or allodynia (stimulus that is typically not painful is now painful, eg, light touch). Common examples include postherpetic neuralgia and poststroke central pain. Typically nociceptive pain responds well to analgesics, while neuropathic pain may respond to nonanalgesic drugs such as antidepressants, anticonvulsants, or local anesthetics [10]. In addition to the pain descriptions provided by patients, the response to treatment or lack there of may be useful in determining the underlying type of pain.

Research over the last 2 decades suggests that chronic pain, whether nociceptive or neuropathic, can be perpetuated by remodeling within the spinal cord and brain. That is, after an event such as peripheral tissue injury or nerve injury, changes can occur in the central nervous system at the level of the spinal cord and thalamus, via physiologic, biochemical, cellular, and molecular mechanisms [15]. This neural plasticity, or ability for prolonged stimuli to induce changes in the central nervous system, is considered to be an important factor in the development of persistent pain after correction of the underlying pathology, and may lead to the development of hyperalgesia, allodynia, and the spread of pain to areas other than those involved with the initial pathology [16]. Animal studies have suggested that prolonged pain from a visceral source may also induce changes at the level of the dorsal column and thalamus, and that this neural plasticity may be a primary factor in chronic visceral pain [17]. Such changes in humans may help explain the persistence and intensity of pain observed with chronic conditions such as phantom limb pain, complex regional pain syndrome, and other neuropathic pain problems.

Barriers to effective pain assessment in older patients

The assessment of pain in older patients can be challenging. Social, cultural, and professional barriers have been documented that affect how patients, health care providers, and society perceive pain and the disabilities associated with it (Box 1). Misconceptions on the meaning, prevalence, and importance of pain are commonplace. Identifying the barriers that exist at both the patient and health provider level is an essential component of pain assessment and management.

There are a variety of patient-related barriers that make pain assessment difficult. Cognitive impairment is a common problem among older patients and can impede the assessment of pain. Cognitively impaired older people who retain communication skills are usually able to report experienced pain when asked; however, as their cognitive impairment advances, self-reports of pain decrease [18]. Other methods of pain assessment can be used in the cognitively impaired patient, and these will be discussed in a later section. Another common obstacle is sensory impairment. In particular, a majority of older patients experience some degree of vision and hearing impairment. These deficits may interfere with their ability to receive and provide information during a pain assessment [3].

Box 1. Barriers to pain assessment and management

Patient-related barriers

  Cognitive impairment
  Sensory impairment —vision and hearing
  Ageist attitudes
  Fear of the meaning of pain
  Fear of pain medication side effects
  Implications of tests and interventions
  Language issues
  Cultural background

Social and institutional barriers

  Stigma of chronic pain and physical disability
  Fear of addiction to pain medications
  Controlled substances laws
  Poor reimbursement

Health professional barriers

  Misconceptions and prejudice regarding pain
  Lack of adequate education in pain management

Unfortunately, ageist attitudes about pain are held by many older patients. The misconception that pain is a normal and expected part of aging is counterproductive to the evaluation and management of pain [5]. Additional patient-centered barriers include fears about the meaning of pain as well as the implications of tests and interventions. Some patients may fear that their pain represents a serious, underlying medical problem, and worry that divulging their pain to their physician will lead to tests, more pain, and an unfavorable diagnosis. Others may be concerned about the potential for drug interactions with their current medications and possible side effects. Often older patients have concerns about the cost of medications, including those for pain control. Yet other patients do not want to bother their health care provider or the staff at their residence, sometimes out of fear of reprisal [5,19]. Finally, language and cultural issues may present barriers to effective pain assessment. The language or wording employed by physicians may differ from that used by their older patients. Thus, older adults may deny "pain" but admit to having "discomfort" when questioned [11]. Cultural background can influence a patient's pain experience and his or her description of the pain, and these factors should be considered during the assessment [11].

Social and institutional factors also pose significant barriers to effective pain assessment. Patients frequently voice their unease about the potential for addiction to pain medications, and the media magnifies these concerns with stories of misuse and abuse among celebrities, for example. Other patients may choose not to report their pain due to fears about the implication of chronic pain and the potential stigma associated with the diagnosis of a disabling medical condition. In addition, the process of prescribing pain medications can be quite inconvenient due to restricted formularies by insurance companies, the need for special prescriptions for narcotic pain relievers, and constraints in pharmacy service availability, especially in the long-term care setting. Finally, labor-intensive pain assessment and management services receive poor reimbursement compared with other diagnoses, and this lack of adequate compensation may dissuade physicians and other health care professionals from addressing this common patient issue.

Barriers to the effective assessment of pain are common among the health care professionals who care for the elderly. Physicians and nurses may have misconceptions about pain like their patients. Research has shown that physicians underestimate pain in patients, whether they are cognitively intact or impaired, and elderly patients often receive inadequate analgesia [20,21]. Second, historically, physicians and nurses have received inadequate training in pain assessment and management. These health professionals typically lack an adequate background to perform an effective pain assessment, and one study showed that over one quarter of senior internal medicine residents felt inadequately prepared to manage pain [22]. Finally, patient care is often focused on active medical issues, and pain frequently falls to the bottom of the problem list. Multiple medical conditions may detract from the treatment of pain and often leave health care providers with inadequate time to address this symptom.

Recognizing these challenges is an important first step in the assessment and management of pain. Patients should be asked routinely about pain and reassured that their concerns are important and valid. Their questions about the meaning of pain, necessary tests, and side effects of medications need to be answered. For those who are unable to communicate or have significant cognitive impairment, the patient's family or primary decision maker should be included in the assessment and plan. Education and training of nurses and physicians in the evaluation of pain, particularly as it relates to older adults, is crucial. The next section will address effective means for pain assessment in older patients and pearls on how to overcome these barriers in clinical practice.

The assessment of chronic pain

Accurate pain assessment is the most critical component of effective pain management [10]. Initial assessment is essential to identify the underlying cause or causes, understand what modalities and medications have helped and those that have not or that have caused complications or side effects, and make optimal recommendations for an effective treatment plan [1]. In addition, the pain assessment should include an evaluation for acute pain that might indicate a new concurrent illness rather than an exacerbation of a chronic pain condition [1]. Reassessment after therapy has been initiated is essential to reevaluate the response to treatment, monitor for side effects, and determine if other sources of pain have developed. The pain assessment should uncover the sequence of events that led to the persistent pain complaint, and ultimately will establish the diagnosis, plan of care and likely prognosis [1]. This section will review the basics of pain assessment and other related issues including functional status, psychologic and social factors, assessment tools, and evaluation in the cognitively impaired.

History

The assessment of pain should begin with a thorough account of the patient's pain history and medical problems. Given that chronic pain is typically associated with an ongoing medical diagnosis, accurate history taking provides the necessary background to identify the probable source. Past medical and surgical history including reports of prior trauma or injury are especially valuable. An evaluation of the medication list and a review of systems provide important details that may be helpful in determining the diagnosis and developing a treatment plan. In addition, a psychosocial history, including alcohol consumption and illicit drug use, should be obtained as these factors may complicate the patient's pain experience and its management.

The pain history provides insight in the patient's pain experience. First, an evaluation of the pain characteristics should be pursued including features such as intensity, character, frequency (or pattern or both) location, duration, and precipitating and relieving factors [1]. Second, the patient should be asked about any recent event or activity that may be the source of the pain or have prompted an exacerbation or flare. Third, the patient should be asked questions about their use of analgesics and other therapies for his or her pain. This history should include current and previously used prescription medications, over-the-counter medications, and complementary or alternative remedies as well as their effectiveness and any experienced side effects [1]. In addition, inquiry regarding the use and helpfulness of other types of treatments such as physical therapy, chiropractic manipulation, massage, and acupuncture should be obtained. Finally, it is important to inquire about the patient's knowledge, attitudes, and beliefs regarding pain and its management [1]. In particular, pain may have different meanings for different people; some may view their pain as an "atonement for their sins" or "God's will," while others may believe that their symptoms are a sign that the end of life is near. An awareness of the patient's thoughts and ideas about pain is important, and may impact the expression of pain as well as treatment options and their effectiveness.

Most patients can report pain—all you have to do is ask them. This self-report provides the most accurate and reliable evidence for the existence of pain and its intensity [1,10–12]. It is imperative that physicians, nurses, other health care providers, as well as family and caregivers listen to patient's complaints of pain and take them seriously [1]. Even persons with mild to moderate cognitive impairment can answer simple questions about pain, and this information may helpful in completing the assessment and developing a management plan [7]. Older patients often use words other than "pain" to describe what they are feeling [10]. Many patients may not admit to having pain; however, they may use words such as "hurting," "aching," "soreness," or "discomfort" to characterize the sensation [1,21]. These words should be kept in mind and used when asking about pain. The history directs the physical examination and lays the groundwork for the management plan. Box 2 outlines some useful questions that may be

---

Box 2. Sample questions in a pain interview

1. How strong is your pain right now? What was the worst/ average pain over past week?
2. How many days over the past week have you been unable to do what you would like to do because of your pain?
3. Over the past week, how often has pain interfered with your ability of take care of yourself, for example, with bathing, eating, dressing, and going to the toilet?
4. Over the past week, how often has pain interfered with your ability to take care of your home-related chores, such as going grocery shopping, preparing meals, paying bills, and driving?
5. How often do you participate in pleasurable activities such as hobbies, socializing with friends, travel? Over the past week, how often has pain interfered with these activities?
6. How often do you do some type of exercise? Over the past week, how often has pain interfered with your ability to exercise?
7. How often does pain interfere with your ability to think clearly?
8. How often does pain interfere with your appetite? Have you lost weight?
9. How often does pain interfere with your sleep? How often over the past week?
10. Has pain interfered with your energy, mood, personality, or relationships with other people?
11. Over the past week, how often have you taken pain medication?
12. How would you rate your health at the present time?

From AGS Panel on Persistent Pain in Older Persons: The management of persistent pain in older persons. J Am Geriatr Soc 2002; 50:S205-24, with permission.

incorporated into a pain interview to help characterize a patient's pain and its impact on his or her life.

Physical examination

The physical examination is an integral component of the pain assessment. It builds upon the history, and should especially focus on potential pain sources and areas of concern identified during the history taking. The examination should include a careful evaluation of the location of reported pain and common sites for pain referral [1]. In particular, the musculoskeletal and nervous system should receive special attention, as they are the most frequent sources of pain [1]. The musculoskeletal examination should include an evaluation for trigger points of myofascial pain, tender points of fibromyalgia, inflammation, muscle spasm, deformities such as scoliosis, kyphosis, joint alignment, fracture, and gait disturbances [1,10]. In addition, joint range of motion and reproduction of aggravating movements may be useful to identify underlying physical impairment associated with pain and the need for rehabilitation [10]. Gait should be formally evaluated to see if it contributes to or is affected by the pain process; the timed "get up and go" test is an effective performance-based measure of functional status and gait [23]. The nervous system evaluation should search for evidence of weakness, hyperalgesia, hyperpathia, allodynia, numbness, paresthesia, and signs of autonomic neuropathies [1,10,11]. The physical examination may also give information on the status and contribution of other medical problems to the patient's pain. Health care providers who specialize in the evaluation and treatment of these systems, including physical therapists, physiatrists, rheumatologists, and neurologists, may be able to provide additional assistance with the physical diagnosis of the pain source as well as the treatment plan and should be considered for consultation [1].

Functional status

A patient's functional status may be adversely affected by pain, and the resulting functional losses may significantly impact one's quality of life and general well-being. Both the history and physical examination should address functional status to identify activity limitations and physical deficits caused by the underlying pain [5]. Impairments in functional status may range from difficulties in performing instrumental activities of daily living such as driving and house cleaning to an inability to perform basic activities of daily living such as bathing, transfers or toileting. Although many of the questions asked during the assessment may provide much of this information, validated functional status scales such as the Lawton Instrumental Activities of Daily Living Scale and the Katz Activities of Daily Living Scale may be incorporated into the assessment to address specific activities in an organized format [24,25]. Another way to elicit information about the impact of pain on a patient's function and behaviors is to ask the patient about his or her participation in activities such as hobbies, physical exercise, and socialization with family and friends [11]. One way to address these issues is to ask a question that addresses the global impact of the pain on one's life such as "How many days over the past 6 months have you been unable to do what you would like to do because of your pain"? [26]. The information on functional status obtained during the pain assessment should be incorporated into the goals of the treatment plan, and these should aim to maximize the patient's independence and enhance quality of life [10].

Psychologic and social assessment

Although pain can have a significant impact on physical function, its potential effect on the psychosocial well-being of older patients should not be overlooked. Depression is a common problem among older persons. Research has supported an association between pain and depressed mood in this patient population [8]. Many patients with chronic pain will experience concomitant depressive symptoms or anxiety [4]. The initial pain assessment should include an evaluation of psychologic function including mood, self-efficacy, pain coping skills, helplessness, and pain-related fears [1]. The Geriatric Depression Scale is a useful screening tool for depression and may be a useful adjunct during a comprehensive pain assessment [27]. Other validated instruments for the assessment of depression include the Hamilton Depression Rating Scale and the Cornell Scale for Depression in Dementia [28,29]. Counseling, supportive group therapy, biofeedback, or psychoactive medications may be indicated for patients with an underlying mood disorder, and they should be referred to these services [10].

An evaluation of the patient's social situation should be included as part of the initial pain assessment. Important issues include the patient's social support system, presence of caregivers, family relationships, work history, living arrangements, cultural environment, spirituality, and health care accessibility [1]. Cultural and social factors may influence a patient's experience with and expression of pain as well as his or her pain management choices and likelihood of compliance. Awareness of this background information during the initial assessment will be extremely useful for the development of the pain management plan and for reassessment.

Measurement of pain intensity and pain assessment scales

A variety of pain assessment scales have been designed for research and to assist health care practitioners in the evaluation of pain. There are multidimensional and unidimensional instruments for the assessment of pain. Multidimensional instruments have been developed to evaluate patients for multiple pain-related factors. These instruments typically ask questions from multiple domains including pain intensity, location, temporal effects, affective aspects, and functional status. The McGill Pain Questionnaire (MPQ), the Brief Pain Inventory (BPI), and the Geriatric Pain Measure are three validated multidimensional tools for the assessment of pain [30–32]. Although these instruments and others collect numerous important data points relevant to a person's pain experience, they are often long, time consuming, and difficult to score at the bedside, and it can be a challenge to implement such tools in the clinical setting [10].

Unidimensional instruments typically focus on one domain of the pain experience such as pain intensity. These tools take less time to administer and are more practical for use in a variety of clinical settings [10]. Pain intensity may be a primary factor that determines the impact of pain on a person's overall functioning and well-being, and it may be a useful endpoint for monitoring disease progression and the effectiveness of intervention strategies [11]. Many unidimensional pain intensity scales have been created to help quantify pain severity. Numeric rating scales have patients rate the intensity of their pain typically on a scale from 0 to 10. For example, the "Verbal 0–10 Scale" has patients rate their current pain on a scale from "0" or "no pain" to "10" or "the worst pain imaginable" [33,34]. Verbal descriptor scales (VDS) have patients identify the phrase or adjective that best quantifies the intensity of their pain such as "no pain," "mild pain," "moderate pain," "severe pain," "extreme pain," and "the most intense pain imaginable" [7,34]. A variation of the VDS is the pain thermometer that lists adjectives of pain from vertically from the bottom of the thermometer or "no pain" to the top of the thermometer or "pain as bad as it could be" [1,19]. Facial pain scales shows a series of progressively distressed facial expressions along a continuum and patients are asked to choose the face that reflects the intensity of their current pain [35]. The Visual Analog Scale consists of a 10-cm line denoted by "no pain" on the left end of the line and "most pain imaginable" on the right end of the line, and patients are asked to mark the intensity of their pain on the line [7,34]. Although the literature demonstrates fair to good reliability and validity for these instruments in the geriatric population, there are potential limitations to their use in patients with lower levels of education, deficits in vision and hearing, and moderate to ad-

Table 1
Table of pain assessment instruments

	Validity[a]	Reliability[a]	Subscales	Ease of use[b]	References
Multidimensional					
McGill pain questionnaire	++++	+++	5	+++	Melzack, 1975 [30]
Brief pain inventory	++++	+++	2	+	Daut et al, 1983 [31]
Geriatric pain measure	++++	+++	5	+	Ferrell et al, 2000 [32]
Unidimensional					
Verbal 0–10 scale	++++	++	N/A	+	Ferrell et al, 1995 [33]
Visual analog scale	++++	++	N/A	+++	Herr et al, 1993 [34]
Faces pain scale	++++	++	N/A	++	Herr et al, 1998 [35]
Present pain intensity	++++	+++	N/A	++	Melzack, 1975 [30]

[a] Relative strength of tool in authors' opinion: + = weak, ++++ = strong.
[b] Relative ease of use in authors' opinion: + = easy, ++++ = hard.

Box 3. Behavioral manifestations of pain in the cognitively impaired

Facial expressions

Slight frown; sad, frightened face
Grimacing, wrinkled forehead, closed or tightened eyes
Any distorted expression
Rapid blinking

Verbalizations, vocalizations

Sighing, moaning, groaning
Grunting, chanting, calling out
Noisy breathing
Asking for help
Verbally abusive

Body movements

Rigid, tense body posture, guarding
Fidgeting
Increased pacing, rocking
Restricted movement
Gait or mobility changes

Changes in interpersonal interactions

Aggressive, combative, resisting care
Decrease social interactions
Socially inappropriate, disruptive
Withdrawn

Changes in activity patterns or routines

Refusing food, appetite change
Increase in rest periods
Sleep, rest pattern changes
Sudden cessation of common routines
Increased wandering

Mental status changes

Crying or tears
Increased confusion
Irritability or distress

From AGS Panel on Persistent Pain in Older Persons: The management of persistent pain in older persons. J Am Geriatr Soc 2002;50:S205–24; with permission.

vanced cognitive impairment [11]. The pain reports of older patients, especially those with cognitive impairment, are influenced by "pain at the moment" so rather than using these scales to ask about recent or past pain experience, it is best to use them to evaluate current pain in the "here and now" [10]. Table 1 outlines examples of common multidimensional and unidimensional assessment tools described in this section.

Pain assessment in the cognitively impaired

Cognitive impairment is an important consideration in the assessment of pain in older patients. Although a potential barrier, research suggests that the self-report of pain from patients with mild to moderate cognitive impairment is reliable and valid [18,33]. Thus, the assessment of pain in those with early cognitive impairment should begin with the patient's self-report and a thorough history, as described earlier. Of the available pain intensity scales, the Pain Thermometer and the VDS are generally recommended for use in patients with mild to moderate cognitive impairment [11,34].

The evaluation of pain is more challenging in patients with severe cognitive impairment. Some individuals may be able to convey their needs through "yes" and "no" answers to simple questions [10]. However, for patients who are unable to make their needs known, the best method of pain assessment remains a subject of great debate. One area of research has focused on observational indicators of pain [11]. This type of assessment focuses on the behavioral manifestation of pain and potential indicators include nonverbal cues and behaviors, vocalizations, facial expressions, and changes in unusual behaviors (Box 3). The most reliable behavior may relate to guarding during examination or routine activities such as walking, morning care, and transfers [1]. In addition, an atypical behavior in a patient with severe dementia should trigger assessment for pain as a possible cause [1]. Family members, caregivers, and others who know the patient well may provide useful qualitative information about the patient's pain and changes in behavior; however, their quantitative assessment is often less reliable [10].

Summary

Pain is a unique experience for every person. An effective pain assessment sets the groundwork for optimal pain management. An understanding of the patient's personal pain history is essential, and should include detailed information on the pain complaint, prior treatments and their efficacy, functional status, and psychosocial well-being. Barriers exist at multiple levels and present considerable challenges to pain assessment in the elderly. A multifaceted approach that targets education, research, and public policy is needed if we are to break down these barriers. The training of physicians, nurses, and other health care professionals must include curricula on pain assessment and management in older patients. Continued research into the optimal tools and approaches to the evaluation and treatment of chronic pain is critical. In particular, further understanding of role of neural plasticity in chronic pain and the development of interventions to reduce or block the maladaptive response of the brain and spinal cord to injury are needed. Finally, it is imperative that our leaders in medicine, social institutions, and government recognize the prevalence and impact of chronic pain in the elderly. With the aging of the population, the importance and relevance of these issues will continue to grow in the future, and public policy must address the need for improvements in the evaluation and management of chronic pain in older patients.

References

[1] AGS Panel on Persistent Pain in Older Persons. The management of persistent pain in older persons. J Am Geriatr Soc 2002;50:S205–24.

[2] Helme RD, Gibson SJ. Pain in older people. In: Crombie IK, Croft PR, Linton SJ, LeResche L, Von Korff M, editors. Epidemiology of pain. Seattle: IASP Press; 1999. p. 103–12.

[3] Ferrell BA. Pain evaluation and management in the nursing home. Ann Intern Med 1995; 123(9):681–7.

[4] Ferrell BA. Pain management in elderly people. J Am Geriatr Soc 1991;39(1):64–73.

[5] Ferrell BA, Ferrell BR, Osterweil D. Pain in the nursing home. J Am Geriatr Soc 1990; 38(4):409–14.

[6] Bernabei R, Gambassi G, Lapane K, et al. Management of pain in elderly patients with cancer. SAGE Study Group. Systematic evaluation of geriatric drug use via epidemiology. JAMA 1998; 279(23):1877–82.

[7] Ferrell BA, Ferrell BR, Rivera L. Pain in cognitively impaired nursing home patients. J Pain Symptom Manage 1995;10(8):591–8.

[8] Parmelee PA, Katz IR, Lawton MP. The relation of pain to depression among institutionalized aged. J Gerontol 1991;46(1):P15–21.

[9] Merskey H, Lindblom V, Mumford JM, et al. Part III. Pain terms-a current list with definitions and notes on usage. In: Merskey H, Bogduk N, editors. Classification of chronic pain. 2nd edition. Seattle: IASP Press; 1994. p. 207–13.

[10] Ferrell BA. Pain. In: Osterweil D, Brummel-Smith K, Beck JC, editors. Comprehensive geriatric assessment. New York: McGraw-Hill; 2000. p. 381–97.

[11] Herr KA, Garand L. Assessment and measurement of pain in older adults. Clin Geriatr Med 2001;17(3):457–78.

[12] Turk DC, Melzack R. The measurement of pain and the assessment of people experiencing pain. In: Turk DC, Melzack R, editors. Handbook of pain assessment. New York: Guilford Press; 1992. p. 3–12.

[13] Myer RA, Campbell JN, Rija SN. Peripheral and neural mechanisms of nociception. In: Wall PD, Melzack R, editors. Textbook of pain. 3rd edition. New York: Churchill Livingstone; 1994. p. 13–44.

[14] Bennett GF. Neuropathic pain. In: Wall PD, Melzack R, editors. Textbook of pain. 3rd edition. New York: Churchill Livingstone; 1994. p. 201–24.

[15] Coderre TJ, Katz J, Vaccarino AL, et al. Contribution of central neuroplasticity to pathological pain: review of clinical and experimental evidence. Pain 1993;52(3):259–85.

[16] Marcus DA. Treatment of nonmalignant chronic pain. Am Fam Physician 2000;61(5):1331–8 [1345–6].

[17] Saab CY, Park YC, Al-Chaer ED. Thalamic modulation of visceral nociceptive processing in adult rats with neonatal colon irritation. Brain Res 2004;1008(2):186–92.

[18] Parmelee PA, Smith B, Katz IR. Pain complaints and cognitive status among elderly institution residents. J Am Geriatr Soc 1993;41(5):517–22.

[19] Herr KA, Mobily PR. Complexities of pain assessment in the elderly: clinical considerations. J Gerontol Nurs 1991;17(4):12–9.

[20] Morrison RS, Siu AL. A comparison of pain and its treatment in advanced dementia and cognitively intact patients with hip fracture. J Pain Symptom Manage 2000;19(4):240–8.

[21] Sengstaken EA, King SA. The problems of pain and its detection among geriatric nursing home residents. J Am Geriatr Soc 1993;41(5):541–4.

[22] Blumenthal D, Gokhale M, Campbell EG, et al. Preparedness for clinical practice: reports of graduating residents at academic health centers. JAMA 2001;286(9):1027–34.

[23] Mathias S, Nayak US, Isaacs B. Balance in elderly patients: the "get-up and go" test. Arch Phys Med Rehabil 1986;67(6):387–9.

[24] Katz S, Ford AB, Moskowitz RW, et al. Studies of illness in the aged. The index of activities of daily living: A standardized measure of biological and psychological function. JAMA 1963; 85:914–9.

[25] Lawton MP, Brody EM. Assessment of older people: Self-maintaining and instrumental activities of daily living. Gerontologist 1969;9(3):179–86.

[26] Von Korff M, Dworkin SF, Le Resche L, et al. An epidemiologic comparison of pain complaints. Pain 1988;32(2):173–83.

[27] Yesavage JA, Brink TL, Rose TL, et al. Development and validation of a geriatric depression screening scale: a preliminary report. J Psychiatry Res 1983;17(1):37–49.

[28] Hamilton M. A rating scale for depression. J Neurol Neursurg Psychiatry 1960;23:56–62.

[29] Alexopoulos GS, Abrams RC, Young RC, et al. Cornell scale for depression in dementia. Biol Psychiatry 1988;23(3):271–84.

[30] Melzack R. The McGill Pain Questionnaire: major properties and scoring methods. Pain 1975;1(3):277–99.

[31] Daut RL, Cleeland CS, Flanery RC. Development of the Wisconsin Brief Pain Questionnaire to assess pain in cancer and other diseases. Pain 1983;17(2):197–210.

[32] Ferrell BA, Stein WM, Beck JC. The Geriatric Pain Measure: validity, reliability and factor analysis. J Am Geriatr Soc 2000;48(12):1669–73.

[33] Ferrell BA. Pain in cognitively impaired nursing home residents. J Pain Symptom Manage 1995;10(8):591–8.

[34] Herr KA, Mobily PR. Comparison of selected pain assessment tools for use with the elderly. Appl Nurs Res 1993;6(1):39–46.

[35] Herr KA, Mobily PR, Kohout FJ, et al. Evaluation of the Faces Pain Scale for the use with the elderly. Clin J Pain 1998;14(1):29–38.

ELSEVIER
SAUNDERS

CLINICS IN
GERIATRIC
MEDICINE

Clin Geriatr Med 21 (2005) 577–588

Iatrogenic Rheumatic Syndromes in the Elderly

G. Andres Quiceno, MD, John J. Cush, MD*

Presbyterian Hospital of Dallas, 8200 Walnut Hill Lane, Dallas, TX 75231-4496, USA

More than 15% of all outpatient medical visits will be for musculoskeletal complaints, and up to 50% of outpatient evaluations will disclose a past or current musculoskeletal condition. The prevalence of these conditions often will rise in a geriatric population, where osteoarthritis, gout, pseudogout, rheumatoid arthritis, polymyalgia rheumatica, and infectious arthritis are commonly encountered. The onset of lupus, idiopathic inflammatory myositis, and sclerodermatous disorders is distinctly uncommon, and should question the diagnosis. The unusual occurrence of these rare disorders in the elderly should prompt consideration of drug-related (or iatrogenic) rheumatic disease.

In 1999, the Institute of Medicine reported that 7000 deaths in the United States each year could be attributed to medication-related errors, a magnitude greater than that from workplace injuries. Although such iatrogenic deaths are rare, daily medication-related adverse events are common, particularly in the elderly. The combination of aging, cumulative morbidities, and polypharmacy make the elderly a particularly susceptible target population for drug-related adverse events. In an aging population, it is not unusual for such iatrogenic events to masquerade as rheumatic disorders; alternatively, rheumatic complaints may presage overt drug toxicity. Although the osteoporotic effects of chronic corticosteroids or gastrotoxic effects of nonsteroidal antiinflammtory drugs are widely appreciated, drugs that may induce gout, lupus, vasculitis, arthralgia, or myopathy are often overlooked. This review will focus on several unusual rheumatic presentations that may be a consequence of pharmacotherapy in an elder patient.

---

* Corresponding author.
E-mail address: jackcush@texashealth.org (J.J. Cush).

0749-0690/05/$ – see front matter © 2005 Elsevier Inc. All rights reserved.
doi:10.1016/j.cger.2005.02.004   geriatric.theclinics.com

Statin-associated myopathy

"Statins" are a class of agents that act to decrease cholesterol production by inhibiting the HMG-CoA reductase and reducing the synthesis of mevalonate, an essential intermediary in the cholesterol biosytnetic pathway. These medications are primarily indicated in the management of elevated concentrations of low-density lipoprotein cholesterol (LDL-C). The use of these medications has grown considerably, owing to demonstrable reductions in cardiovascular events in patients with established coronary heart disease, mild to moderate elevations in LDL-C, as well as in healthy patients with elevated LDL-C values [1,2].

Statin therapy has been proven to generally be safe and well tolerated. It is estimated that over 11 million patients are currently taking statin therapy, and newly published guidelines suggest that up to 50 million Americans may be candidates for statin therapy. Although the benefit to risk ratio is favorable for most, potentially adverse effects (including statin-associated myopathy) need to be discussed in the context of the potential benefits [3].

Although definitions have varied among the investigators [4], the American College of Cardiology/American Heart Association/National Heart, Lung and Blood Institute has defined four myopathic syndromes related to statins (Table 1) [5]. The frequency of significant statin myopathy appears to be relatively low [6,7]. In clinical trials the dose-related prevalence of statin-related myalgia or weakness is generally less than 5%. Overt myopathy and rhabdomyolysis are rare events, with a reported incidence of rhabdomyolysis of 0.15 related deaths per 1 million prescriptions. Fatal rhabdomyolysis is rare, often emphasized, and potentially avoidable. Cerivastatin (Baycol) was voluntary withdrawn from the global market by the manufacturer in 2001 because it had a higher reported rate of rhabdomyolysis and fatalities at the highest recommended dose compared with other statins [1,3,8].

Risk factors associated with statin-associated myopathy

In general, statins are well tolerated and safe drugs. Postmarketing data report an overall adverse event frequency of $<0.5\%$ and a myotoxicity event rate of $<0.1\%$ [7,9]. All statins have been associated with myopathy, but some

Table 1
Myopathic syndromes related to statins

1. Statin myopathy	Any muscle complains associated to use of statin drugs.
2. Myalgia	Muscle complaints without elevation of serum CK levels.
3. Myositis	Muscle complaints with elevations of CK levels.
4. Rhabdomyolysis	CK levels > 10 times upper limit of normal associated with renal failure.

Abbreviation: CK, creatine kinase.
Adapted from Pasternak RC, et al. ACC/AHA/NIHLBI clinical advisory on the use and safety of statins. J Am Coll Cardiol 2000;40:567–72.

comorbidities and drugs may increase the risk of myopathy. Patients with a history of hypothyroidism, renal insufficiency, biliary obstruction, diabetes, recent trauma, perioperative periods, advanced age, or underlying myopathy are a greater risk. Also at risk are those receiving certain concomitant medications, including cyclosporine, fibrates, azole antifungals, and macrolide antibiotics, that inhibit specific cytochrome P450 (CYP-450) enzymes also involved in the metabolism of statins [4,10,11]. Hence, drug interactions, especially in older patients exposed to polypharmacy, account for many of the adverse events seen with the statins [12].

Lovastatin and simvastatin are administered in their prodrug form and are hydrolyzed in the active form in the liver, while pravastatin, atorvastatin, and fluvastatin are formulated in the open acid form [13]. The majority of the statins are highly bound to plasma proteins with minimal systemic exposure to the active drug [14]. Most of the statins are metabolized by the CYP-P450, specifically the 3A4 enzyme; exeptions are fluvastatin, which is metabolized via the cytochrome P450 2C9 enzyme, and pravastatin, which is enzymatically transformed in the liver and it does not use the CYP system [14]. Most of the drug interactions are the result of the inhibition or inductions of the CYP enzyme system (Table 2). Fluvastatin, atorvastatin, and pravastatin are hydrophilic, whereas cerivastatin, lovastatin, and simvastatin are lipophilic; lipophilic drugs appear to be more myotoxic (Table 2) [15]. Statins are also substrates for the P-Glycoprotein, a drug transporter in the small intestine that may influence their oral bioavailability [12]. The significance of this is seen when statins are combined with specific drugs, such as cyclosporine, which may augment the risk of myopathy or rhabdomyolysis because of a combined interference with the CYP P450 (CYP-3A4) and inhibition of P-Glycoprotein.

Pathogenesis of statin-associated myopathy

The mechanisms of action of statin-associated myopathy has not been completely elucidated. Proposed mechanisms have included (1) depletion of secondary intermediates, (2) induction of apoptosis, (3) alterations of the chloride

Table 2
Pharmacology of statins

Drug	Metabolized by	Distribution
Fluvastatin	P450 CYP 2C9	Hydrophilic
Rosuvastatin[a]	P450 CYP-2C9	Hydrophilic
Atorvastatin	P450 CYP-3A4	Hydrophilic
Lovastatin	P450 CYP-3A4	Lipophilic
Simvastatin	P450 CYP-3A4	Lipophilic
Cerivastatin	P450 CYP-3A4, CYP-2C8	Lipophilic
Pravastatin	Liver cytosol	Hydrophilic

Abbreviation: P450 CYP, cytochrome P 450 enzyme system.

[a] *From:* Mosby's Drug consult. Rosuvastatin, MD Consult; 2004.

channel conductance within the myocytes, (4) decreased cholesterol content of the muscle cell membranes causing membrane instability, (5) decrease in ubi-quinone, and (6) reduction in GPT binding proteins [1,2,12,16]. Oral sup-plementation with ubiquinone has not yielded clinical benefits. Biopsy studies have suggested a metabolic abnormality based on increase lipids stores, cytochrome-oxidase negative myofibers, ragged red fibers with variation in fiber diameter, and muscle necrosis and inflammation; all of these features are con-sistent with mitochondrial respiratory chain dysfunction [17–19]. Nonetheless, muscle biopsy findings are not specific for drug-induced damage, and may oc-cur in the absence of symptoms.

Management of statin-associated myopathy

Prevention is the best approach to avoid statin-associated myopathy. General recommendations include the use of the lowest effective dose to achieve the therapeutic goal and recognize the drugs interactions that increase the risk of myopathy [1].

Patients should be instructed to discontinue the statin and contact their physician if they develop myalgias, muscle weakness, or discoloration of the urine. Physicians should not ignore these complaints, even in the absence of increase creatine kinase (CK) [1]. Moreover, an asymptomatic elevated CK is not sufficient for to diagnose statin myopathy. Patients should be further evalu-ated in the setting of clinical or chemical abnormalities. Despite their differences in water solubility, there is no epidemiologic evidence that differentiates the risk of myotoxicity between statins [5].

Patients with symptomatic myalgias should be evaluated clinically and enzymatically, but may continue statin therapy if the symptoms are mild and tolerable. There are reports of improvement of the symptoms after switching to a different lipid-lowering agent. If symptoms are severe, the medication should be discontinued and a different class of lipid-lowering drug should be considered, such as niacin, bile sequestering salts, or ezetimibe [1,9].

Routine CK testing in asymptomatic patients are not recommended, but some physicians may choose to perform baseline CK levels to facilitate the evalua-tion of subsequent muscle complaints. In general, it is possible to continue the statin therapy in patients with asymptomatic mild elevations of the CK. However, marked elevations (levels greater than 5–10 times the upper limit of normal) should prompt cessation and evaluation. Discontinuation of statins should be considered before events that increase the risk of muscle injury (such as surgi-cal procedures) or unusual amounts of physical activity (Box 1).

There is no absolute contraindication to the combined use of a statin and an agent know to increase the risk of myopathy [1], as there may be circumstances wherein the benefit outweighs the risk [1].

Alternative therapies may be considered, as in the case of HIV or transplant patients who require the use of a statin or fibrates while receiving concomitant

---

Box 1. Recommendations for prescribing statin therapy

Check baseline renal, liver, and thyroid function tests before starting statins.

Consider drug interactions when prescribing statins.

Evaluate for risk factors for myopathy such as advance age, renal and liver impairment, diabetes with fatty liver, hypothyroidism, surgery, trauma, risk for ischemia-reperfusion, excessive alcohol intake, substance abuse, and heavy exercise.

Educate patients on the recognition of potential myopathic symptoms.

Instruct patient to discontinue the statin if they become ill or are to be admitted to the hospital.

Consider discontinuation of the statin with short-term use of macrolide antibiotics.

Check CK in all patients using statins who have symptoms of myopathy.

If CK levels are <5× ULN, repeat in 1 week.

If CK levels are >5× ULN, discontinue the agent and monitor CK levels.

Document the need of combination of lipid-lowering therapy and the lack of response to monotherapy.

When adding a statin for patients already receiving therapy with fibrates, initiate the lowest starting dose of statin.

Do not prescribe statin-fibrate combination therapy in patients with impaired liver or renal function (eg, creatinine level >2.0 mg/dL), concomitant cyclosporine or tacrolimus therapy, long-term macrolide antibiotic therapy, or azole antifungal therapy, advance age (>70 years), or known concomitant skeletal muscle pathologic conditions.

Abbreviations: CK, creatine kinase; ULN, upper limit of normal.
Adapted from Ballantyne CM, Corsine A, Davidson MH, et al. Risk of myopathy with statin therapy in high-risk patients. Arch Intern Med 2003;163:553–64.

---

treatment with protease inhibitors or cyclosporine. Ezetimibe is an inhibitor of intestinal cholesterol absorption that can be used with statins without the concomitant risk of myotoxicity [1].

In the presence of rhabdomyolysis, statins should be discontinued and treatment begins with aggressive hydration, mannitol diuresis, and alkalinization of the urine to avert renal damage [1].

Drug-induced lupus

Systemic Lupus Erythematosus (SLE) is an uncommon entity that typically affects young females. Less common is the occurrence of lupus-like manifestations resulting from a select group of drugs. Drug-induced lupus (DIL) typically affects elderly patients of both sexes, presumably because this population is exposed to a greater number of medications [20]. The classical presentation of DIL is a milder version of the idiopathic disorder, and is defined as the development of lupus-like symptoms, antinuclear antibody (ANA) positivity, and symptom resolution upon withdrawal of the offending drug. DIL also differs from SLE by having a different autoantibody profile (ie, fewer diverse autoantibodies and a predominance of only antihistone antibodies) and a more favorable outcome. However, several autoantibodies typically associated with idiopathic SLE have rarely been reported in DIL (eg, antiglobulin or Coombs antibody, lupus anticoagulant, and antiphospholipid antibodies) [21]. Although hemolytic anemias have rarely been ascribed to DIL, antiphospholipid syndrome (with thrombotic events or fetal loss) has not.

Historically, DIL was best described in patients receiving hydralazine, procainamide, methyldopa, and chlorpromazine. However, as the use of these agents has declined, the frequency of DIL appears to remains stable, owing to newer drugs that may also induce this syndrome. These newer drugs include quinidine, minocycline, carbemazepine, ticlodipine, and tumor necrosis factor inhibitors, such as infliximab, etanercept, and adalimumab. In general, DIL is an uncommon condition, with an estimated incidence of 30,000 cases per year in United States. However, the number of implicated medications appears to be increasing every year [22].

Clinical manifestations associated with drug-induced lupus

The diagnosis of DIL requires lupus specific findings, such as those that comprise the 11 classification criteria for lupus. However, most of these patients will present with less than four criteria (the usual requirement of a diagnosis of SLE) in the setting of ingesting a medication known to induce ANA positivity or frank DIL. It should be noted that the finding of ANA positivity alone is not sufficient to diagnose DIL, nor is it reasonable to discontinue any drug because of an asymptomatic ANA alone. For instance, up to 50% of those receiving higher doses of hydralazine will be ANA positive, but only 10% of these will develop DIL. The onset of DIL occurs months to years after drug initiation, and symptoms rapidly resolve discontinuation of the offending agent [23].

Articular complains are present in more than 80% of the people, with myalgias and arthralgias more common than arthritis. Constitutional symptoms, such as malaise, low-grade fever, and weight loss, are a frequent presenting symptom complex. Serositis (pleural effusion and pericarditis) and pneumonitis are classically found in procainamide-related DIL. Dermatologic manifestations, renal involvement, and neurologic symptoms are rare in classic DIL [23].

Table 3
Medications associated to drug-induced lupus

Definite	Probable	Possible
Procainamide	Hydantoins (phenytoin)	Estrogens
Hydralazine	Antithyroids (methimazole, propylthiouracil)	Penicillin
Methyl-dopa	Penicillamine	Gold salts
Quinidine	Lithium	Tetracycline
Chlorpromazine	Sulfasalazine	Reserpine
	Beta-blockers	Griseofulvin
	Carbamaepine	Para-aminosalicylic acid
	Minocycline	Atorvastatin
	Isoniazid	Simvastatin
	TNF inhibitors (etanercept, inflixmab, adalimumab)	Amiodarone
		Ticlopidine
		Terbinafine
		Interferons

Abbreviation: TFN, tumor necrosis factor.

Medications associated with DIL can be classified as *definitely, probably, and possibly* associated (Table 3). Classically, DIL has been associated with procainamide, hydralazine, methyldopa, quinidine, and chlorpromazine [24].

Other uncommon clinical manifestations reported with DIL include cutaneous vasculitis, pulmonary thromboembolism, pericardial tamponade, constrictive pericarditis, scleritis, lichen planus, stridor, granulocytopenia, and renal involvement [25–30].

Diagnostic tests in drug-induced lupus

DIL usually presents with clinical features of lupus with a positive ANA. In general, patients tend to have a high ANA titer (eg, > 1:1280), often in a diffuse or speckled pattern; such ANAs are directed toward deoxyribonucleoproteins (ie, histones). Antibodies against double-stranded DNA are not usually detected, and serum complement levels are usually normal. Hematologic findings such as leukopenia, lymphopenia, and Coombs-positive hemolytic anemia may be seen in DIL. Lupus anticoagulants and antiphospholipid antibodies are frequently found, but thrombosis and antiphospholipid syndrome are uncommon [31].

Antihistone antibodies are commonly found in DIL but they are also common in patients with idiopathic SLE; hence, they cannot distinguish between the two. They may be helpful in distinguishing between patients with symptoms that are secondary to DIL from asymptomatic patients with drug-induced ANA [32]. Nonetheless, antibodies against specific histone complexes have identified for procainamide and sulfasalazine (against H2A–H2B), hydralazine (H3–H2A), and quinidine (H1–H2B) [31,33,34].

Treatment

In general, DIL is a self-limited disease, with symptoms improving several weeks after discontinuation of the offending agent. Although symptoms tend to resolve quickly, the ANA and other serologic abnormalities may take up to 12 months to fully resolve.

Beyond drug cessation, the treatment of DIL is mainly symptomatic with the use of nonsteroidal anti-inflammatory drugs and occasionally corticosteroids in the setting of severe cytopenias or pleuropulmonary manifestations. Symptoms will seldom last for several months. Although such patients may benefit of treatment with antimalarials, this situation should raise concern for the onset of idiopathic SLE rather than DIL [24].

Gout

The incidence of gout rises with advancing age and higher serum uric acid levels. It is estimated that the prevalence of gout in the United States is between 2 and 5 million persons. The majority of patients with primary gout are men. Women rarely develop the disorder before menopause, as estrogen is thought to be uricosuric. Less than 15% of women have the onset of gout before menopause. Primary gout is often associated with obesity, hyperlipidemia, diabetes mellitus, hypertension, and atherosclerosis, conditions that are prevalent in the elderly. Secondary gout may be associated with alcoholism, myeloproliferative, and lymphoproliferative disorders and renal transplantation [35–37].

In most patients, gout is due to underexcretion rather than overproduction of uric acid. It is important to note that the onset or flare of secondary gout may be influenced by medications that either contribute to the body's total urate load (eg, cytotoxics) or impair renal excretion of urate (eg, diuretics, low-dose aspirin) (Table 4). Hence, the onset of gout or uncontrolled gout in the elderly should prompt a thorough reevaluation of medications that may contribute to hyperuricemia and the risk of gout or nephrolithiasis.

Table 4
Drugs that increase serum uric acid

Overproduction	Underexcretion
Ethanol	Ethanol
Cytotoxic drugs	Diuretics (loop, thiazide)
Warfarin	Low-dose salicylate
	Cyclosporine
	Ethambutol
	Pyrazinamide
	Levodopa
	Nicotinic acid

Colchicine and allopurinol

Allopurinol has rarely been implicated as a cause of vasculitis, which usually occurs in the setting of the observed acute allopurinol hypersensitivity syndrome. Such patients may manifest erythematous rashes, fever, eosinophilia, and severe exfoliative dermatitis (eg, toxic epidermal necrolysis), acute cutaneous or systemic vasculitis, hepatitis, and interstitial nephritis.

Colchicine is generally well tolerated and has no rheumatic consequences. However, both colchicine and allopurinol toxicity is markedly increased in the setting of renal insufficiency, such that these relatively inoccuous medications may lead to life-threading complications if used inappropriately or in the setting of renal insufficiency [37,38]. Some experts suggest that intravenous preparations of colchicine should never be used; they have been removed from clinical use in Great Britain and also in many academic centers in the United States. Fatalities have occurred with as little as 1 mg given intravenously. Severe colchicine toxicity may lead to skin necrosis, aplastic anemia, shock, disseminated intravascular coagulation, renal failure, myopathy, and rhabdomyolysis. Those at greatest risk include the elderly, those with renal failure, or those taking both oral and intravenously colchicines as well as concomitant therapy with statins, cyclosporine, or grapefruit juice.

Drug-induced arthralgia

Many drugs have been implicated in causing arthralgia. Less commonly tendinopathy and frank synovitis have been observed. Such cases are not examples of drug-induced lupus as they do not manifest lupus-specific features (or criteria). These events may be common, as in the case of interferons, or rare, as seen with beta-blockers. Nonetheless, the finding of unexplained and persistent articular or periarticular (ie, tendinitis) pains that coincide with the use of these medications may be sufficient reason to withdraw the drug. Although the time to resolution will depend on the pharmacokinetic properties of the agent,

Table 5
Drugs implicated in causing arthralgias

Class	Implicated agents
Anti-infectives	Quinolones, amphotericin, acyclovir, minocycline, BCG, vaccines
Biologic agents	Interferons, interleukin (IL)-2, IL-6, immunotoxins, tacrolimus, growth factors (G-CSF, erythropoietin)
Supplements	Excessive vitamin A, fluoride
Lipid-lowering	Statins, Fibrates (binding resins)
Cardiac	Quinidine, propranolol, acetabulol, nicardipine
Hormonal	raloxifene, tamoxifen, letrozole

Adapted from Cush JJ, Kavanaugh A, Stein MF. Gout. In: Cush JJ, Kavanaugh A, Stein MF, editors. Rheumatology: diagnosis and therapeutics. Philadelphia: Lippincott/Williams & Wilkins; 2005. p. 187–95.

Table 6
Drug-induced tight skin syndromes and vasculitis

Sclerodermatous disorders	Vasculitis
Bleomycin	Allopurinol
Docetaxel	Amphetamines
Pentazocine	Cocaine
Carbidopa	Hydrochlorthiazide
L-Tryptophan	Penicillamine
Organic solvent exposure	Propylthiouracil
Rapeseed oil	Trimethoprim-sulfamethoxazole
Vinyl chloride	Montelukast
	Cytarabine
	Hepatitis B vaccine
	TNF inhibitors (infliximab, etanercept, adalimumab)

most patients will require an observation period of several days or weeks to determine if there is improvement off drug. Implicated agents are listed in Table 5.

Vasculitis and scleroderma

The unlikely occurrence of certain forms of vasculitis, scleroderma, or
myositis in the elderly should prompt the clinician to consider that the disorder
may be secondary to infection, neoplasia (ie, a paraneoplastic phenomena), or
related to medications. Although the last is quite rare, case reports continue to be
reported that implicate a variety of agents as the cause of these uncommon
immune-mediated disorders. Table 6 details some of the reported associations
[39,40]. These drug-related events are usually not as severe as the idiopathic
disorders, and tend to be more limited in the extent of tissue involvement. The
etiology of most of these events is unknown. In most cases drug cessation is an
effective means to improvement or resolution.

Acknowledgments

J.J.C. is an investigator, lecturer, and consultant for Abbott, Amgen, Aventis,
Centocor, Wyeth.

References

[1] Thompson PD, Clarkson P, Kara RH. Statin associated myopathy. JAMA 2003;289(13):
     1681–90.
[2] Jamal SM, Eisenberg MJ, Chrsitopoulos S. Rhabdomyolysis associated with hydroxymethyl-
     glutaryl-coenzyme A reductase inhibitors. Am Heart J 2004;147(6):956–65.
[3] Ballantyne CM, Corsine A, Davidson MH, et al. Risk of myopathy with statin therapy in high-
     risk patients. Arch Intern Med 2003;163:553–64.

[4] Daugird AJ, Crowell K. Do statins cause myopathy? J Fam Pract 2003;52(12):973–6.

[5] Pasternak RC, Smith SC, Bairey-Merz CN, et al. ACC/AHA/NIHLBI clinical advisory on the use and safety of statins. J Am Coll Cardiol 2000;40:567–72.

[6] Mantel-Teeuwise AK, et al. Myopathy due to statin/fibrate use in the Netherlands. Ann Pharmacother 2002;36(12):1957–60.

[7] Gaist D, et al. Lipid-lowering drugs and risk of myopathy: a population-based follow-up study. Epidemiology 2001;12(5):565–9.

[8] Prieto JC. Safety profile of statins. Rev Med Chil 2001;129(11):1237–40.

[9] Evans M, Rees A. Effects of HMG-CoA reductase inhibitors on skeletal muscle: are all the statins the same? Drug Saf 2002;25(9):649–63.

[10] Borrego FJ, et al. Rhabdomyolisis and acute renal failure secondary to statins. Nefrologia 2001; 21(3):309–13.

[11] Reineveld JC, et al. Differen effects of 3-hydroxy-3methylgluaryl-coenzyme A reductase inhibitors on the development of myopathy in young rats. Pediatr Res 1996;39(6):1028–35.

[12] Williams D, Feeley J. Pharmacokinetic-pharmacodynamic drug interactions with HMG-CoA reductase inhibitors. Clin Pharmacokinet 2002;41(5):343–70.

[13] Slater EE, et al. Mechanism of action and biological profile of HMG CoA reductase inhibitors. Drugs 1998;36(Suppl 3):72–82.

[14] Corsini A, et al. New insights into the pharmacodynamic and pharmacokinetic properties of statins. Pharmachol Ther 1999;84:413–28.

[15] Paoiletti R, et al. Pharmacological interactions of statins. Atheroscler Suppl 2002;3(1):35–40.

[16] Matzno S, Tazuya-Murayama K, Tanaka H, et al. Evaluation of the synergistic adverse effects of concomitant therapy with statins and fibrates on rhabdomyolysis. J Pharm Pharmacol 2003; 55(6):795–802.

[17] Phillips PS, Hass RH, Bannykhs S, et al. Statin-associated myopathy with normal creatinine kinase levels. Ann Intern Med 2002;137(7):581–5.

[18] Farne JA. Statin and myotoxicity. Curr Atheroscler Rep 2003;5(2):96–100.

[19] Carvalho AA, et al. Statin and fibrate associated myopathy: study of eight patients. Arq Neuropsiquiatr 2004;62(2A):257–61.

[20] Calkins E, Vladutiu A. Drug induced lupus. Musculoskeletal disorders. In: Duthie EH, Katz P, editors. Practice of geriatrics. 3rd ed. Philadelphia: WB Saunders; 1998. p. 430.

[21] Olsen NJ. Drug-induced autoimmunity. Baillieres Best Pract Res Clin Rheumatol 2004;18(5): 677–88.

[22] Blazes DL, Martin GJ. Drug-induced lupus erythematosus secondary to nafcillin: the first reported case. Rheumatol Int 2004;24(4):242–3.

[23] Buyon JP. Drug-related Lupus. Primer on the rheumatic diseases. 12th ed. Atlanta (GA): The Arthritis Foundation; 2001. p. 345.

[24] Ferri FF. Systemic Lupus Erythematosus. In: Ferri FF, editor. Practical guide to the care of the medical patient. 6th ed. St. Louis: Mosby, Inc.; 2004. p. 810–1.

[25] Cohen MG, Prowse MV. Drug-induced rheumatic syndromes. Diagnosis, clinical features and management. Med Toxicol Adverse Drug Exp 1989;4(3):199–218.

[26] Asherson RA, Zulman J, et al. Pulmonary thromboembolism associated with procainamide induced lupus syndrome and anticardiolipin antibodies. Ann Rheum Dis 1989;48(3):232–5.

[27] Turgeon PW, Slamovits TL. Scleritis as the presenting manifestation of procainamide-induced lupus. Ophthalmology 1989;96(1):68–71.

[28] Sherertz EF. Lichen planus following procainamide-induced lupus erythematosus. Cutis 1988; 42(1):51–3.

[29] Maxwell D, Silver R. Laryngeal manifestations of drug induced lupus. J Rheumatol 1987;14(2): 375–7.

[30] Wing SS, Fantus IG. Adverse immunological effects of antithyroid drugs. CMAJ 1987;136(2): 12–7.

[31] Cush JJ, Kavanaugh AF. Drug-induced lupus. In: Cush JJ, Kavanaugh AF, editors. Rheumatology diagnosis and therapeutics. Baltimore (MD): Williams & Wilkins; 1999. p. 193–7.

[32] Epstein A, Barland P. The diagnostic value of antihistone antibodies in drug-induced lupus erythematosus. Arthritis Rheum 1985;28(2):158–62.

[33] Bray VJ, West SG, Schultz KT, et al. Antihistone antibody profile in sufasalazine induced lupus. J Rheumatol 1994;21(11):2157–8.

[34] Rubin RL. Etiology and mechanism of drug-induced lupus. Curr Opin Rheumatol 1999;11(5): 357–63.

[35] Kim KY, Ralph Schumacher H, Hunsche E, et al. A literature review of the epidemiology and treatment of acute gout. Clin Ther 2003;25:1593–617.

[36] Rott KT, Agudelo CA. Gout. JAMA 2003;289:2857–60.

[37] Cush JJ, Kavanaugh A, Stein MF. Gout. In: Cush JJ, Kavanaugh A, Stein MF, editors. Rheumatology: diagnosis and therapeutics. Philadelphia: Lippincott Williams & Wilkins; 2005. p. 187–95.

[38] Boomershine KH. Colchicine-induced rhabdomyolysis. Ann Pharmacother 2002;36(5):824–6.

[39] ten Holder SM, Joy MS, Falk RJ. Cutaneous and systemic manifestations of drug-induced vasculitis. Ann Pharmacother 2002;36(1):130–47.

[40] Doyle MK, Cuellar ML. Drug-induced vasculitis. Expert Opin Drug Saf 2003;2(4):401–9.

ELSEVIER
SAUNDERS

CLINICS IN
GERIATRIC
MEDICINE

Clin Geriatr Med 21 (2005) 589–601

New Developments in Osteoarthritis

Christopher W. Wu, MD, Kenneth C. Kalunian, MD*

*Center of Innovative Therapies at the University of San Diego at California,
9320 Campus Point Drive, Suite 225, La Jolla, CA 92037-0943, USA*

The prior notion of osteoarthritis (OA) as a bland disease related to aging and "wear and tear" of the joint has given way to views of a dynamic system with multiple pathogenic contributors. Traditional views of articular cartilage failure have centered on a variety of genetic, metabolic, and biochemical factors. Recent work has elucidated the importance of local factors as well as crystals and inflammation in contributing to disease progression. The new paradigm of OA considers it a heterogenous disease with numerous factors leading to its pathologic hallmark of cartilage loss and the clinical manifestation of joint pain with movement. Conceptualizing OA as phenotypic subsets related to a primary abnormality allows more targeted investigation into disease pathophysiology and treatment. Of course, it must be recognized that this distinction is somewhat artificial, and disease expression is almost certainly a summation of different, interrelated components.

Better appreciation of the chondrocyte and its phenotypic alteration in OA has provided mechanistic explanations for the contribution of repetitive injury and aging to the disease. The advances in our understanding of OA have led to a treatment that emphasizes reduction of joint vulnerability and load. Pharmacologic therapy in the twenty-first century has added cyclooxygenase-2 specific (Cox-2) inhibitors, glucosamine-chondroitin, and viscosupplementation to the standard armamentarium. Clinical trials are currently underway for a number of potential disease modifying agents that may significantly change the treatment approach for OA. With the possibility of disease-modifying OA drugs (DMOADs), the necessity for instruments sensitive to change in clinical trials has become very apparent. Advances in the fields of magnetic resonance imaging

---

* Corresponding author. 9320 Campus Point Drive, #227, La Jolla, CA 92037.
  E-mail address: kkalunian@ucsd.edu (K.C. Kalunian).

doi:10.1016/j.cger.2005.02.008

(MRI) and ultrasound (US) have made these modalities useful tools in the research arena and in the clinics as well.

Epidemiology

Although OA does not invariably lead to disability in those who have clinical signs of joint damage, its impact is enormous. OA disables about 10% of people who are older than 60 years of age, compromises the quality of life of more than 20 million Americans, and its economic impact in the United States is greater than $60 billion dollars a year [1]. OA is second only to ischemic heart disease as a cause of work disability in men over age 50 years [2].

The prevalence of OA in all joints increases with age [1]. In some populations, more than 75% of the people over age 65 years have OA that involves one or more joints [3]. Epidemiologic studies further suggest that there are clear sex-specific differences [4,5]. Before 50 years of age, the prevalence of OA in most joints is higher in men than in women. After about age 50 years, women are more often affected with hand, foot, and knee OA than men. Of course, the growing elderly population in addition to the obesity epidemic implies that OA will assume an even greater societal impact in the near future.

Pathogenesis

OA pathology is characterized by cartilage destruction with subsequent joint space loss, osteophye formation, and subchondral sclerosis. Most experts believe that the initiating insult occurs against hyaline cartilage with subsequent eburnation and osteophyte formation. Recent data, however, has questioned this fundamental notion. Rogers et al [6] have proposed that primary OA may be a systemic disease of bone. Based upon fossil examinations of 563 skeletons from an archaeologic site in England, they demonstrated a strong association between "classic OA" and widespread eburnation of bone and osteophyte formations, as well as widespread formation of enthesophytes. This group concluded that the most likely explanation for these associations is that OA represents a disease primarily dependent on a systemic bony response to mechanical stress. In an accompanying editorial, Felson and Neogi [7] cite several limitations of the study (difficult in distinguishing osteophytes and enthesophytes from fossils, the age of the subjects, and the possibility that subjects had concomitant rheumatic disorders); nevertheless, these findings provide a rationale for further investigation into a concept that would radically change the approach to OA management.

The pathogenesis of OA progression likely revolves around a complex interplay of numerous factors. The major contributors include chondrocyte regulation of the extracellular matrix, genetic influences, local mechanical factors, and inflammation. We believe that although these factors clearly influence one another, individual patients have a predominant pathogenic contributor, thus having a specific OA phenotype. This classification, albeit somewhat artificial, allows more specific targeting for disease subsets.

Chondrocyte biology

Chondrocytes comprise the sole cellular component of hyaline cartilage, and the balance between the expressions of anabolic versus catabolic factors is the common pathway for cartilage degradation. For example, OA cartilage from animals with experimental arthritis and patients with OA are hyporesponsive to IGF-1 [8,9], a major growth cytokine. It has also been proposed that upon stimulation with pro-inflammatory cytokines, OA chondrocytes express inducible nitric oxide synthase and Cox-2, leading to products that induce chondrocyte apoptosis. The role of matrix metalloproteinases (MMPs) and tissue inhibitors of MMPs have also received a great deal of attention. Disappointedly, pharmacologic interventions to alter the balance of these factors have not lead to clinical improvement. Chondrocytes are clearly sensitive to mechanical forces and alteration in their production of matrix components is influenced by extrinsic load [10,11]. Differences in responses to repetitive loading of cultured chondrocytes from healthy and osteoarthritic cartilage have been noted. In response to repetitive loading, OA chondrocytes demonstrated an increase in aggrecan mRNA transcription and a decrease in MMP-3 transcription compared with normal cartilage [12].

Genetic contributions

Genetic factors are implicated in the development of OA via the results of conventional twin and nontwin sibling, population, and modern molecular studies [13,14]. Genetic factors may have more influence on the expression of some subsets of OA than in others [14]. Classic twin studies have shown that the influence of genetic factors is between 39% and 65% in radiographic OA of the hand and knee in women, about 60% in OA of the hip, and about 70% in OA of the spine. Taken together, these estimates suggest a heritability of OA of 50% or more [15]. Potential genetic abnormalities that predispose to OA include structural defects in collagen and alterations in cartilage or bone metabolism [14]. These defects may influence the effect of additional risk factors, such as obesity, on the development of OA.

Proposed candidate OA genes include the collagen genes that encode for type II collagen. Using linkage analysis, for example, two reports on three unrelated families showed coinheritance of generalized OA with specific alleles of a type II pro-collagen gene (COL2A1) on chromosome 12 [16,17]. This allele has been found to have a single base mutation that was noted in all affected members of a family, but in none of the unaffected or unrelated individuals [18]. In addition, linkage between COL2A1 and OA has been demonstrated in several families [19,20] in a large population-based study [21].

The genetic nature of primary generalized OA may be heterogeneous and mutations in genes other than COL2A1 may be responsible. The role of mutations in genes encoding minor collagen types and extracellular matrix protein such as aggrecan, decorin, and the link protein, therefore, needs to be investigated.

Biomechanical factors

Local mechanical factors such as malalignment, laxity, and a reduction in proprioceptive activity may play a role in the development and progression of knee OA [22]. Muscle strength, once thought to have a prominent role in OA progression, may in fact be significantly influenced by joint laxity [23]. It is felt that the summation of these local factors in addition to systemic susceptibility factors lead to intrinsic joint vulnerability, and when compounded with load (ie, obesity, injury), leads to disease expression.

Sharma et al [24] have recently demonstrated the contribution of knee alignment to OA disease progression. In their study, varus alignment at baseline was associated with a fourfold increase in the odds of medial progression (odds ratio 4.09; confidence interval [CI], 2.20–7.62). Similar increased risks for lateral progression were found in patients with baseline valgus deformities. Malalignment most likely increases local stresses in the joint, thereby causing OA progression [25].

Significant contributions, albeit to a lesser degree than alignment, have been found for joint laxity and proprioception. Joint laxity, as defined by abnormal rotation or displacement of the tibia, results in large displacements at the articular surface and increased sheer stress. Proprioception refers to position sense of the joint as it relates to coordinated movement. Alterations in proprioception lead to decreased coordination of movement, and ultimately increases in joint load. Three-year data from the Mechanical Factors in Arthritis of the Knee study suggested that each $3°$ increment in ligamentous laxity was associated with an increase of about 1.5-fold in the odds of a poorer outcome [26]. Proprioception inaccuracy modestly increased the likelihood of a poor functional outcome in this study.

Inflammation (crystals, cytokines)

Recent evidence over the past decade has implicated synovial inflammation as a central component of OA pathogenesis. Histologic evidence of severe inflammation, heightened levels of pro-inflammatory cytokines in OA chondrocytes, and elevated levels of biomarkers related to synovitis all support the notion that inflammation is a key player in cartilage destruction. The use of US and MRI in clinical trials of patients with knee OA have shown synovial thickening and effusions in 50% to 73% of patients studied [27,28]. Haynes et al [29] performed histologic grading for 104 patients with knee OA who had undergone total joint replacement or arthroscopy. Their study showed that, in this population of late stage OA, 31% (32 of 104) of tissue samples had severe inflammation; thickened intimal lining and associated lymphoid aggregates were often observed. Further immunohistochemical analysis of knee OA synovium has shown abundance of T-cell infiltrates and large cellular aggregates with immune activation markers [30]. The T cells from these samples revealed a Th1 phenotype, thus providing further evidence of a pro-inflammatory state in this disease.

An important question of ongoing debate is the etiology of inflammation in OA. Multiple factors have been proposed in triggering synovial inflammation, including crystals [31], immune complex formation [32], or chards of articular cartilage [33]. The inflammatory phenotype of some cases of OA is presumed to lead to heightened levels of IL-1 and tumor necrosis factor-alpha, which result in increases of chondrocyte MMP expression, inhibiting synthesis of proteoglycan and collagen, and upregulation of nitric oxide and prostaglandin E2 production. This leads to a balance that favors degradative forces acting upon the extracellular matrix as well as chondrocyte apoptosis.

Radiography

Plain film radiography has been the main diagnostic modailty for assessing the severity and progression of OA. As clinical trials are underway to examine DMOADs, the utility of plain radiography to detect structural changes in relatively short periods of time have come in to question. In fact, NEGMA convened an ad hoc advisory board in early 2002 to specifically address this issue. It was the conclusion of the board that "none of the protocols discussed could be endorsed for use in a DMOAD trial at the present time" [34].

The prospect of DMOADS has served as an impetus for the investigation of more sensitive techniques for the diagnosis and staging of OA. Two of the most promising imaging modalities are US and MRI. Most of this data is derived from studies examining knee OA as well as studies in rheumatoid arthritis patients. The development of high-frequency transducers have made US a practical and viable modality for studying joints. US allows assessment of synovial inflammation, identification of tendon and ligament integrity, and with the use of power doppler, vascularity can be quantified [35]. US has also been reported to be more sensitive for visualizing bone erosions in the finger joints than conventional radiography and is comparable to MRI [36]. Cartilage defects, specifically femoral condylar cartilage, can be clearly shown with US [37]. We and other researchers have used US to look for signs of synovitis in knee OA. This technique has been validated with arthroscopy as the "gold standard" [38]. Although this is a very exciting technique in OA, its applicability to OA other than the knee has not been clearly studied.

MRI has also shown great promise as a noninvasive means of assessing OA. It provides superb soft tissue contrast, multiplanar and volumetric capabilities, superior inplane resolution, and sensitivity to early pathologic changes [39]. Abnormalities of articular cartilage appear as alterations in signal intensity, morphology, or both. Although results of accuracy, sensitivity, and specificity in the detection of cartilage surface irregularities have varied widely among different studies [40], very early lesions appear to be detected by this method. Addition of gadolinium, either by intra-articular (IA) or intravenous infusion, further increases the ability of MRI to detect small defects in the cartilage integrity [41]. The advent of ultrashort echo time pulse sequences has even further improved upon the limit of clinical detectability, and holds great promise for future use [42]. In clinical practice, the current primary role of MRI in OA is to rule out concomitant or alternative sources of knee pain, such as mechanical abnormalities, osteonecrosis, and Paget's disease. Felson et al [43,44] have reported that bone marrow edema in OA significantly correlates with pain and is indicative of a poor prognosis. Although perhaps having a limited role in clinical use, sensitivity to change and the noninvasive nature have made MRI an exciting tool in clinical studies assessing DMOADs. Ayral et al [45] have completed a 1-year study of MRI to detect knee OA progression in comparison to plain radiographs and arthroscopy. Using a unique scoring method, they found that MRI assessment of cartilage was even more responsive than arthroscopy.

Biomarkers

The promise of biomarkers has yet to be fulfilled in OA. Type II collagen, cartilage oligomeric matrix protein, hyaluronan, and aggrecan have been some of the many biomarkers investigated. Although numerous clinical studies have suggested that specific or combinations of biomarkers can have predictive value in terms of disease presence and severity, the wide variability in these values limits use for individual patients.

Treatment

Treatment for OA should be separated into three different categories: nonpharmacologic, pharmacologic, and surgical. Interest in nonpharmacologic treatment has heightened given our improved understanding of local factors and their influences on OA progression. Weight loss, physical therapy to strengthen related musculature, and an exercise program should be a part of the treatment plan for most patients with OA of the knee and hip. In patients with unicompartmental knee OA, braces have been shown to significantly reduce pain and improve function [46]. Less cumbersome and a more practical alternative is use of a neoprene sleeve. Although no clear randomized, controlled trials exist to support its use, this orthotic likely reduces symptoms by decreasing joint laxity and increasing proprioception. Additionally, lateral wedge inserts with subtalar strapping for patients with varus deformity has been shown to improve alignment as well as functional and pain scores compared with traditional inserts [47].

Pharmacologic treatment for OA is targeted toward symptomatic relief. The current algorithm uses analgesics (ie, acetaminophen), nonsteroidal anti-inflammatory drugs (NSAIDs), IA steroid injections, and viscosupplementation. Other proposed therapies include colchicine, topical NSAIDs, arthroscopic irrigation, and acupuncture. Several authors [48–50] have debated whether acetaminophen or NSAIDs should be first-line therapy in treating OA. In clinical practice, this distinction is probably overstated. Acetaminophen and NSAIDs have additive analgesic effects and are generally well tolerated in combination. We propose, however, that patients with an inflammatory phenotype of OA should have NSAIDs as part of their pharmacologic therapy.

New therapies for OA over the last decade have included Cox-2 inhibitors, glucosamine/chondroitin, and viscosupplementation. The Cox-2 specific inhibitor rofecoxib was withdrawn from the market in September 2004 following results of the APPROVe (Adenomatous Polyp Prevention of Vioxx) trial showing significant associations with cardiovascular (CV) morbidity/mortality. A recent meta-analysis examining 18 randomized controlled trials and 11 observational trials further support this association [51]. Subsequent studies have suggested that both celecoxib and valdecoxib, the remaining Food and Drug Administration-approved Cox-2 inhibitors, may have concerning CV and cerebrovascular risk profiles. Thus, the increased risk for adverse CV outcomes may be a class-wide effect, due to inhibition of prostaglandin I2 without any disruption of thromboxane A2 [52].

One of the more intriguing medications for OA is the nutraceutical, glucosamine/chondroitin. Supplementation with chondroitin sulfate, a major component of aggrecan, and glucosamine sulfate, a normal constituent of glycosaminoglycans, is thought to shift cartilage metabolism to a positive balance. Although most of the studies have examined the compounds individually, the data is fairly convincing for their effects in symptomatic relief (glucosamine at 1500 mg/d, chondroitin at 800 mg/d) [53–55]. Symptom relief of these nutraceuticals has generally been thought to be similar to that of naproxen. It is worth mentioning that despite the numerous different preparations of glucosamine, 75% of the studies in a Cochrane review evaluated exclusively the prescription medicine manufactured by Rotta Pharmaceutical Company (a glucosamine sulfate preparation that is approved as a prescription drug for OA in the European Union countries) [53]. A study to determine the actual content of glucosamine and chondroitin in several products in the marketplace found between 0% and 115% deviation from the labeled amount [54], suggesting that there may be variable efficacy seen with the different available products.

A question of great debate and interest is the role of glucosamine/chondroitin in structural modification. A 2003 meta-analysis was performed to address this question and included 15 randomized, double-blinded, placebo-controlled trials that assessed either glucosamine or chondroitin on structure modification of knee or hip OA [55]. This analysis concluded that there was highly significant evidence ($P < 0.001$) that glucosamine had a positive effect in reducing joint space narrowing (JSN). Through their calculations, the potential minimal JSN difference between placebo and active allocated drug groups would be 0.27 mm (95% CI, 0.13–0.41 mm) after 3 years of daily administration of 1500 mg of glucosamine [55]. Fewer studies have been performed examining the potential for structural modification of chondroitin, and thus no conclusions have been drawn to this regard. Despite this seemingly convincing data, one major criticism of these studies has been reliability of JSN as a surrogate for structural modification. Improved knee extension as a result of decreased pain could be the explanation for the decreased JSN, independent of any true structural modifying effects. As a consequence of these questions, National Institute of Health studies are underway to more definitively answer this question using MRI to measure cartilage volume.

The 2000 recommendations by the American College of Rheumatology include IA hyaluronic acid (HA) for use in the treatment of OA patients at risk for gastrointestinal side effects [56]. However, a meta-analysis in 2003 pooled the results of 22 trials comparing HA injections to IA placebo injections and concluded that HA injections were only minimally superior to the IA saline injections [57]. The largest study randomly assigned 495 patients with OA of the knee to one of three treatment groups; some received a series of five weekly IA injections of HA, the others received oral naproxen or a placebo for 26 weeks [58]. The group that completed the series of injections had greater improvement in knee pain than the placebo group (difference 8.8 mm on a 100-mm scale) 26 weeks after beginning treatment. However, there was no statistically significant difference between those who received injections compared with the naproxen group. In addition, a reanalysis of the data from this trial on an intention to treat basis suggested that there was no difference between HA and placebo groups at either 12 or 26 weeks of treatment [59]. In the meta-analysis there were three groups that used high molecular weight HA; two of these trials showed a dramatic effect size, while the third study showed almost no benefit. Although several mechanistic concepts may explain the greater efficacy of this particular formulation, the dichotomous nature of the three trials suggests that further, more rigorous studies need to be conducted. Given the dearth of treatment options and minimal risks associated with IA HA, this is probably a reasonable option for patients who do not respond to other agents.

Colchicine is a treatment option in patients with inflammatory OA who have symptoms that are unresponsive to nonpharmacologic interventions and NSAIDs. The basis for the use of colchicine in inflammatory OA that is refractory to NSAIDs or IA corticosteroids is that the majority of such patients have evidence of calcium pyrophosphate dihydrate crystals [60]. Inflammation is attenuated by colchicine via microcrystal-induced tyrosine phosphorylation [61]. Das et al [62] performed a randomized controlled trial using colchicine in 39 patients with OA of the knee. All patients included in the study had at least two of the following four clinical signs of inflammation: warmth over the joint area, joint margin tenderness, synovial effusion, and soft tissue swelling around the knee. Patients were given an IA steroid injection at baseline and were maintained on piroxicam in addition to colchicine 0.5 mg twice a day or placebo. At 16 and 20 weeks the groups receiving colchicine had more significant improvement in pain as reported by patients using visual analog scales and the modified Western Ontario and

McMasters osteoarthritis Index (WOMAC). Whether or not colchicine's effect on these outcomes was related to modulation of inflammation, however, cannot be answered by this study.

A topical preparation of diclofenac (diclofenac epolamine) is effective for pain relief in patients with knee OA but is not currently available in the United States. Its efficacy was illustrated in a study that randomly assigned 103 patients to a diclofenac or placebo-containing skin patch [63]. Self-reported knee pain decreased significantly more in the group receiving diclofenac than the placebo patch. The efficacy of topical NSAIDs, however, appears to be of relatively short duration. A 2004 meta-analysis included 13 trials involving almost 2000 patients who were randomly assigned to treatment with a topical NSAID, oral NSAID, or placebo [64]. There was evidence of significant short-term (1 to 2 weeks) efficacy for pain relief and functional improvement when topical NSAIDs were compared with placebo but the effect was not apparent at 3 to 4 weeks. Topical NSAIDs were generally inferior to oral NSAIDs, although the topical route was safer than oral use.

Acupuncture, a technique in existence for thousands of years, has gained renewed interest as a treatment for OA. A multicenter, 26-week National Institute of Health-funded randomized controlled trial found acupuncture to be effective as adjunctive therapy for reducing pain and improving function in patients with knee OA [65]. This study of 570 patients randomized patients to traditional Chinese acupuncture and sham acupuncture. Follow-up at 26 weeks demonstrated significant improvements in WOMAC pain and function outcomes (traditional Chinese acupuncture pain—3.79, function—2.42 versus sham acupuncture pain—2.92, function—9.87, $P = 0.003$ and 0.009, respectively). Another randomized controlled study by Vas et al [66] also showed positive results for acupuncture. Given this data, the small potential for adverse effects from acupuncture, and the dearth of other treatment options, acupuncture should be considered in the OA armamentarium.

Enthusiasm for the role of arthroscopic irrigation with or without debridement in knee OA severely declined following the results of two studies showing no benefit over a sham control group [67,68]. However, an American College of Rheumatology-sponsored study of 90 patients was able to demonstrate a significant response to arthroscopic irrigation in the subset of patients who had evidence of calcium pyrophosphate crystals at IA examination [69]. The patients with crystals had significant benefits after 1 year postirrigation in a patient report of pain by the visual analog scale and in WOMAC scores. Based on the results of this study, we believe that patients with knee OA who exhibit inflammatory characteristics should be considered for arthroscopic irrigation after other noninvasive measures have failed.

Surgery should be considered in patients with severe symptomatic OA who have failed to respond to medical management and who have marked limitations in performing activities of daily living. Surgical options include total joint arthroplasty, unicompartmental arthroplasty, patellofemoral arthroplasty, osteotomy, and chondrocyte grafting. Improvements in materials used in the surgeries and methods of properly aligning the prosthetics have led to longer durability of the replacements [70].

Summary

OA has been a frustrating disease for both the patient and the physician. Its current impact on society is tremendous, and rivals that of ischemic heart disease in many regards. As the baby boomers reach late adulthood and the obesity epidemic rages on, OA will assume an even greater impact on society. The current OA armamentarium only reduces pain and perhaps improves function, and has no impact on the disease incidence or progression. Thus, the challenge for researchers to develop DMOADs becomes an issue of paramount importance. Several advances in our understanding of OA pathophysiology have provided a glimpse of optimism that disease modification is a real possibility. Appreciation of the local factors involved in OA progression as well as the inflammatory nature in a subset of patients has led to different treatment strategies based on predominant phenotype. Further understanding of the initiating events in cartilage destruction, the relationship between the different pathologic influences, and the role of the chondrocyte in maintaining extracellular matrix homeostasis will be necessary to reveal potential targets of therapy.

References

[1] Buckwalter J, Saltzman C, Brown T. The impact of osteoarthritis. Clin Orthop 2004;427S: S6–15.
[2] Lawrence RC, Helmick CG, Arnett FC, et al. Estimates of the prevalence of arthritis and selected musculoskeletal disorders in the United States. Arthritis Rheum 1998;41:778–99.
[3] Felson DT. The epidemiology of osteoarthritis: prevalence and risk factors. In: Kuettner KE, Goldberg VM, editors. Osteoarthritic disorders. Rosemont (IL): American Academy of Orthopedic Surgeons; 1995. p. 13–24.
[4] Cunningham LS, Kelsey JL. Epidemiology of musculoskeletal impairments and associated disability. Am J Public Health 1984;74:574–9.
[5] Felson DT, Naimark A, Anderson J, et al. The prevalence of Knee osteoarthritis in the elderly. The Framingham Osteoarthritis Study. Arthritis Rheum 1987;30:914–8.
[6] Rogers J, Shepstone L, Dieppe P. Is osteoarthritis a systemic disorder of bone? Arthritis Rhuem 2004;50:452–7.
[7] Felson D, Neogi T. Editorial: osteoarthritis: is it a disease of cartilage or bone? Arthritis Rheum 2004;50:341–4.
[8] Morales TI. The role and content of endogenous insulin-like growth factor-binding proteins in bovine articular cartilage. Arch Biochem Biophys 1997;343:164–72.
[9] Tardif G, Reboul P, Pelletier J-P, et al. Normal expression of type 1 insulin-like growth factor receptor by human osteoarthritic chondrocytes with increased expression and synthesis of insulin-like growth factor binding proteins. Arthritis Rheum 1996;39:968–78.
[10] Urban JP. The chondrocyte: a cell under pressure. Br J Rheumatol 1994;33:901–8.
[11] Sah RL, Kim YJ, Doong JY, et al. Biosynthetic response of cartilage explants to dynamic compression. J Orthop Res 1989;7:619–36.

[12] Millward-Sadler SJ, Wright MO, Davies LW, et al. Mechanotransduction via integrins and interleukin-4 results in altered aggrecan and matrix metalloproteinase 3 gene expression in normal, but not osteoarthritic, human articular chondrocytes. Arthritis Rheum 2000;43:2091–9.

[13] Wordsworth P. Genes and arthritis. Br Med Bull 1995;51:249.

[14] Holderbaum D, Haqqi TM, Moskowits RW. Genetics and osteoarthritis: exposing the iceberg. Arthritis Rheum 1999;42:397.

[15] Spector T, MacGregor A. Risk factors for osteoarthritis: genetics. Osteoarthritis Cartilage 2004; 12:S39–44.

[16] Palotie A, Vaisanen P, Ott J, et al. Predisposition to familial osteoarthritis linked to type II collagen gene. Lancet 1989;1:924.

[17] Knowlton RG, Katzenstein PL, Moscovitz RW, et al. Genetic linkage of a polymorphism in the type II procollagen gene (Col 2A1) to primary osteoarthritis associated with mild chondro-dysplasia. N Engl J Med 1990;322:526.

[18] Ala-Kokko L, Baldwin CT, Moskowitz RW, et al. Single base mutation in the type II procollagen gene (COL2A1) as a cause of primary osteoarthritis associated with a mild chondrodysplasia. Proc Natl Acad Sci USA 1990;87:6565.

[19] Hull R, Pope FM. Osteoarthritis and cartilage collagen genes. Lancet 1989;1:1337.

[20] Vikkula M, Palotie A, Ritvaniemi P, et al. Early onset osteoarthritis linked to the type II procollagen gene: detailed clinical phenotype and further analysis of the gene. Arthritis Rheum 1993;36:401.

[21] Uitterlinden AG, Burger H, van Duijn CM, et al. Adjacent genes, for COL2A1 and the vitamin D receptor, are associated with separate features of radiographic osteoarthritis of the knee. Arthritis Rheum 2000;43:1456.

[22] Sharma L. The role of proprioceptive deficits, ligamentous laxity, and malalignment in development and progression of knee osteoarthritis. J Rheum 2004;31S70:87–92.

[23] Sharma L, Hayes K, Fleosn D, et al. Does laxity alter the relationship between strength and physical function in knee osteoarthritis? Arthritis Rheum 1999;42:25–32.

[24] Sharma L, Song J, Felson D, et al. The role of knee alignment in disease progression and functional decline in knee osteoarthritis. JAMA 2001;286:188–95.

[25] Felson DT. Risk factors of osteoarthritis. Clin Orthop 2004;427:S16–21.

[26] Sharma L, Cahue S, Song J, et al. Physical functioning over three years in knee osteoarthritis: role of psychosocial, local, mechanical and neuromuscular factors. Arthritis Rheum 2003;48: 3359–70.

[27] Karim Z, Wakefield R, Quinn M, et al. Validation and reproducibility of US in detection of synovitis in the knee. Arthritis Rheum 2004;50(2):387–94.

[28] Tarhan S, Unlu Z, Gotkan C. MRI and US evaluation of the patients with knee arthritis: a comparative study. Clin Rheumatol 2003;22:181–8.

[29] Haywood L, McWilliams D, Pearson C, et al. Inflammation and angiogenesis in osteoarthritis. Arthritis Rheum 2003;48(8):2173–7.

[30] Haynes M, Hume E, Smith J. Phenotypic characterization of inflammatory cells from OA synovium and synovial fluids. Clin Immunol 2002;105(3):315–25.

[31] Concoff A, Kalunian K. What is the relationship between crystals and OA? Curr Opin Rheum 1999;11(5):436–42.

[32] Kato T, Xiang Y, Nakamura H, et al. Neoantigens in osteoarthritic cartilage. Curr Opin Rheumatol 2004;16:604–8.

[33] Nalbant S, Martinez J, Kitummuaypong T, et al. Synovial fluid features and their relations to osteoarthritis severity: new findings from sequential analysis. OA Cartilage 2003;11:50–4.

[34] Brandt K, Mazzuca S, Conrozier T, et al. Which is the best radiographic protocol for a clini-cal trial of a structure modifying drug in patients with knee osteoarthritis? J Rheum 2002;29: 1308–20.

[35] Ostergaard M, Szkudlarek M. Imaging in rheumatoid arthritis—why MRI and ultrasonography can no longer be ignored. Scand J Rheumatol 2003;32:63–73.

[36] Wakefield R, Gibbon W, Conhaghan P et al. The value of sonogrpahy in the detection of bone erosions in patients with rheumatoid arthritis. Arthritis Rheum 2000;43:2762–70.

[37] Grassi W, Lamanna G, Farina A, et al. Sonographic imaging of normal and osteoarthritic cartilage. Semin Arthritis Rheum 1999;28:398–403.

[38] Karim Z, Wakefield RJ, Quinn M, et al. Validation and reproducibility of ultrasonography in the detection of synovitis in the knee. Arthritis Rheum 2004;50:387–94.

[39] Waldschmidt J, Braunstein E, Buckwalter K. Magnetic resonance imaging in osteoarthritis. Rheum Dis Clin N Am 1999;25:451–65.

[40] Hodler J, Resnick D. Current status of imaging of articular cartilage. Skeletal Radiol 1996;25: 703–9.

[41] Gylys-Mroin VM, Hayek PC, Satoris DJ, et al. Articular cartilage defects: detectability in cadaver knee with MRI. AJR 1987;148:1153–7.

[42] Gatehouse PD, Bydder GM. Magnetic resonance imaging of short T2 components in tissue. Clin Radiol 2003;58:1–19.

[43] Felson DT, McLaughlin S, Goggins J, et al. Bone marrow edema and its relation to progressive knee osteoarthritis. Ann Intern Med 2003;139:330–6.

[44] Felson DT, Chaisson CE, Hill CL, et al. The association of bone marrow lesions with pain in knee OA. Ann Intern Med 2001;134:541–9.

[45] Pessis E, Drape JL, Ravaud P, et al. Assessment of progression in knee osteoarthritis: results of a 1 year study comparing arthroscopy and MRI. Osteoarthritis Cartilage 2003;11(5):361–9.

[46] Draper ER, Cable JM, Sanchez-Ballester J, et al. Improvement in function after valgus bracing of the knee. An analysis of gait symmetry. J Bone Joint Surg Br 2000;82(7):1001–5.

[47] Toda Y, Tsukimura N. A six-month followup of a randomized trial comparing the efficacy of a lateral-wedge insole with subtalar strapping and anin-shoe lateral-wedge insole in patients with varus deformity osteoarthrits of the knee. Arthritis Rheum 2004;50(10):3129–36.

[48] Bradley J, Brandt K, Katz B, et al. Treatment of OA: relationship of clinical features of joint inflammation to the response to a NSAID or pure analgesic. J Rheum 1992;19:1950–4.

[49] Pincus T, Koch G, Sokka T, et al. A randomized, double-blind, crossover clinical trial of diclofenac versus acetaminophen in patients with osteoarthritis of the hip or knee. Arthritis Rheum 2001;44(7):1587–98.

[50] Brandt K, Bradley J. Should the initial drug used to treat osteoarthritis pain be a nonsteroidal anti-inflammatory drug? J Rheum 2001;28:467–73.

[51] Juni P, Nartey L, Reichenbach S, et al. Risk of cardiovascular events and rofecoxib: cumulative meta-analysis. Lancet 2004;364:2021–9.

[52] Fitzgerald G. Coxibs and cardiovascular disease. N Engl J Med 2004;351:1709–11.

[53] Townheed T. Current status of glucosamine therapy in osteoarthritis. Arthritis Rheum 2003; 49:601–4.

[54] Adebowale AO, Cox DS, Liang Z, et al. Analysis of glucosamine and chondroiten sulfate content in marketed products and the caco-2 permeability of chondroitin sulfate raw materials. J Am Nutraceutical Assoc 2000;3:37–44.

[55] Richy F, Bruyere O, Ethgen O, et al. Structural and symptomatic efficacy of glucosamine and chondroitin in knee osteoarthritis. Arch Intern Med 2003;163:1514–22.

[56] Recommendations for the medical management of osteoarthritis of the hip and knee: 2000 update. American College of Rheumatology Subcommittee on Osteoarthritis Guidelines. Arthritis Rheum 2000;43:1905–15.

[57] Lo G, LaValley M, McAlindon T, et al. Intra-articular hyaluronic acid in treatment of knee osteoarthritis. JAMA 2003;290:3115–21.

[58] Altman RD, Moskowitz R. Intra-articular sodium hyauronate in the treatment of patients with osteoarthritis of the knee: a randomized, double-blind, placebo controlled clinical trial. J Rheumatol 1998;25:2203.

[59] Felson DT, Anderson JJ. Hyaluronate sodium injections for osteoarthritis: hope, hype and hard truths. Arch Inten Med 2002;162:245.

[60] Klashman DJ, Moreland LW, Ike RW, et al. Occult presence of CPPD crystals in patients undergoing arthroscopic knee irrigation for refractory pain related to osteoarthritis [abstract]. Arthritis Rheum 1994;37:S240.

[61] Roberge C, Gaundry M, Medicis R, et al. Crystal-induced neutrophil activation. IV Specific inhibition of tyrosine phosphorylation by colchicine. J Clin Invest 1993;92:1722.

[62] Das S, Mishra K, Ramakrshnan S, et al. A randomized controlled trial to evaluate the slow-acting symptom modifying effects of a regimen containing colchicines in a subset of patients with OA of the knee. OA Cartilage 2002;10:247–52.

[63] Bruhlmann P, Michel BA. Topical diclofenac patch in patients with knee osteoarthritis: a randomized, double-blind, controlled clinical trial. Clin Exp Rheumatol 2003;21:193.

[64] Lin J, Zhang W, Jones A, et al. Efficacy of topical non-steroidal anti-inflammatory drugs in the treatment of osteoarthritis: meta-analysis of randomised controlled trials. BMJ 2004;329:324.

[65] Hochberg M, Lixing L, Bausell B, et al. Traditional Chinese acupuncture is effective as adjunctive therapy in patients with osteoarthritis of the knee [abstract]. Arthritis Rheum 2004; 50:S644.

[66] Vas J, Mendex C, Perea-Milla E, et al. Acupuncture as a complementary therapy to the pharmacological treatment of osteoarthritis of the knee: randomized controlled trial. BMJ 2004; 329:1216–21.

[67] Bradley JD, Heilman DK, Katz BP, et al. Tidal irrigation as treatment for knee osteoarthritis: a sham-controlled, randomized, double-blinded evaluation. Arthritis Rheum 2002;46:100.

[68] Moseley JB, O'Malley K, Petersen NJ, et al. A controlled trial of arthroscopic surgery for osteoarthritis of the knee. N Engl J Med 2002;347:81.

[69] Kalunian KC, Moreland LW, Klashman DJ, et al. Visually-guided irrigation in patients with early knee osteoarthritis: a multicenter randomized, controlled trial. Osteoarthritis Cartilage 2000; 8:412.

[70] Schurman DJ, Smith RC. Osteoarthritis: current treatment and future prospects for surgical, medical, and biologic intervention. Clin Orthop 2004;427(Suppl):S183–9.

ELSEVIER
SAUNDERS

Clin Geriatr Med 21 (2005) 603–629

CLINICS IN
GERIATRIC
MEDICINE

Osteoporosis

Lee S. Simon, MD

*Harvard Medical School, Beth Isreal Deaconess Hospital, 330 Brookline Avenue,
Boston, MA 02215, USA*

Bone is a complex organ. It contains an organic matrix that serves as scaffolding—mineral as calcium distributed in a pattern which provides structure and serves as an ion reservoir for the body. Within this complex tissue reside specialized bone cells, including osteoblasts, osteocytes, and osteoclasts. There are other cells in contact with the inner or endosteal surface of bone, including monocytes, macrophages, and fibroblasts, all of which modulate the activities of the osteoblasts and osteoclasts [1,2]. The organic matrix of bone consists predominantly of type I collagen (about 95% of the organic matrix is this type of collagen) [3]. The primary structure of the type I collagen in bone is similar to that of type I collagen in skin; however, bone type I collagen contains certain secondary posttranslational modifications distinguishing it chemically from that collagen found in skin [4,5].

Bone is a dynamic organ and remodels itself throughout life. This process involves removal or resorption of bone from one surface of bone and the subsequent deposition of new bone on another nearby surface. These two specific actions, bone resorption and formation, are performed by the specialized bone cells, and these events are tightly coupled in time and space. Factors that participate in modulating these processes include systemic hormones and local paracrine factors as well as gravity, physical activity, and weight bearing [1,2].

The specialized cells that perform remodeling include the osteoblasts and the osteoclasts. The osteoblasts are the cells that form bone. They synthesize the organic matrix and subsequently perform the actions leading to mineralization. The organic matrix synthesized by osteoblasts includes other proteins in addition to type I collagen. There are also noncollagenous proteins within the organic structure [3]. These include osteocalcin (also known as bone-GLA protein or BGP) [6]. Osteocalcin contains γ-carboxyglutamic acid and is a vitamin K-dependent protein. The other noncollagenous proteins include osteonectin, thrombospondin, and other sialyted and phosphorylated proteins [3,6–11]. These

doi:10.1016/j.cger.2005.02.002
geriatric.theclinics.com

proteins probably have important roles in chemotaxis and cell adherence. Their synthesis is controlled by serum levels of hormones, such as parathyroid hormone (PTH) and 1,25 dihydroxy vitamin D $(1,25(OH)_2D)$ [3,7].

The osteoclasts are the bone resorbing cells. Structurally they are polarized cells, multinucleated and characterized by their large size. The cell's basolateral membrane is closely apposed to the bone marrow and maintains sodium pumps and a bicarbonate/chloride exchanger [12]. The opposite cellular membrane in contact with mineralized bone contains contractile proteins such as actin. The peripheral edge of the cell in contact with the bone surface forms a "sealing zone." The cell attaches to the matrix osteopontin through an $av\beta3$ integrin (vitronectin) receptor that seals off a compartment [13–16] that is sub-osteoclastic. In this interface between the osteoclast and bone, bone resorption takes place (Howships lacunae). The plasma membrane is invaginated in this area and forms the typical ruffled border of the cell. Osteoclasts are derived from the same stem cells as monocyte/macrophages [13,17]. Macrophages also participate in the process of bone resorption through phagocytosis of residual debris and by producing cytokines. These cytokines have been demonstrated to participate in increased osteoclast recruitment, differentiation, and function [18–22].

Systemic hormones and local factors regulate the recruitment, replication, and function of the osteoblasts and the osteoclasts. Hormones act on cells directly or indirectly by altering the synthesis, activation, and receptor binding of locally active factors or regulating availability or activity of specific binding proteins modulating the effects of these factors. Locally produced factors include growth factors, cytokines, and prostaglandins and leukotrienes [18,23,24].

Parathyroid hormone is one of the systemic hormones with important effects on bone cell function. It stimulates bone resorption by increasing osteoclast activity; however, no PTH receptors have been demonstrated on these cells. Specific PTH receptors have been identified on cells of the osteoblast lineage or stromal cells. PTH stimulates these cells to produce soluble factors that communicate with and stimulate the osteoclasts to increase bone resorption including a substance termed RANK ligand [23,25,26]. This important molecule interacts with transcription factors that serve to increase osteoblastic development; it is inhibited by another soluble factor, osteoprotegerin. PTH also directly inhibits ostoblastic mediated synthesis of collagen. However, it has been shown that it will also stimulate the local production of insulin-like growth factor (IGF) I, which has the paradoxical effect of increasing matrix synthesis [27]. The inhibitory effects on synthesis of collagen matrix are observed after continuous exposure to the hormone, but intermittent exposure leads to the stimulation of new matrix synthesis [28]. These opposite actions of PTH are mediated through a single receptor coupled to different regulatory (G) proteins.

Calcitonin is another important hormone with specific effects on bone cells. It inhibits osteoclastic bone resorption directly through high-affinity receptors on osteoclasts. There is little evidence to suggest that calcitonin has an effect on osteoblastic function [29,30].

The remodeling process in the adult skeleton is a dynamic process, continuous throughout life to a greater or lesser degree. It is required to maintain the strength of bone and occurs on all bone surfaces, including the periosteal, haversian, cortical, and endosteal surfaces [1,2,23,24,31–34]. Once the bone mass has reached adult proportions, which is probably genetically predetermined, it remains constant with equal rates of bone formation and resorption. This equilibrium is achieved through coupling of packets of interacting cells called "remodeling units" [24,32–34]. Peak bone mass is reached by men and women about in the middle of the third decade of life. A plateau period then ensues during which there is a constant turnover of bone formation, which approximates bone resorption. Following this plateau phase there begins, in men and women, a period of net bone loss equivalent to about 0.3% to 0.5% per year. Beginning with the decrease in estrogen associated with the menopause, women accelerate this net bone loss about 10-fold for approximately 5 to 7 years.

Osteoporosis

Osteoporosis is a heterogeneous group of abnormal processes characterized biologically by the net loss of bone, which results in a decrease in total mineralized bone without a decrease in the ratio of bone mineral to the organic matrix such as seen in osteomalacia [35–41]. Thus there is a decrease in the overall amount of bone. By histomorphometric analysis, the size of the osteoid seams is normal, but there is a decrease in the thickness of the cortex and a decrease in the number and size of the trabeculae in cancellous bone. The trabecular plates have increased perforations, and there is a decrease in trabecular connectivity [41–44]. Trabecular connectivity is probably an important determinant of the extent that bone may be compressible and thus absorb energy, suggesting that connectivity is an important determinant of the tensile strength of bone. Ultimately, osteoporosis leads to bone with less tensile strength and significantly more susceptibility to fracture with less force. At some point, the amount of bone available for mechanical support falls below a certain threshold (the "fracture threshold") and the patient may sustain a fracture. It is important to remember that there is no absolute fracture threshold for a population of patients; rather, it is different for each individual. The bone loss affects cortical and trabecular bone, with trabecular bone loss more predominant in typical postmenopausal osteoporosis.

Pathophysiology

Peak bone mass is achieved by men and women in the middle of the third decade of life. After a plateau period, during which there is a constant turnover of bone formation approximately equal to bone resorption, there begins a period of net bone loss equivalent to about 0.3% to 0.5% per year. Beginning with menopause, women sustain an accelerated period of bone loss, which may increase 10-fold, so that for approximately 5 to 7 years they may lose bone at the rate of 3% to 5% per year [35–41]. This same issue of constant bone loss affects men and women over the age of 70. Whereas accelerated bone loss is the dominant effect in postmenopausal osteoporosis, it is likely that a decrease in synthesis of new bone with either stable or accelerated bone loss is the main problem in the older age group in men and women both.

Though the osteoblasts and osteoclasts are under the control of systemic hormones and cytokines as well as other local factors, such as parathyroid hormone (PTH), calcitonin, estrogen, and 1,25-dihydroxyvitamin D_3 [1,25-$(OH)_2D_3$] (see references [19,21,22,25–27,45–47]), estrogen deficiency is a significant cause of accelerated bone loss (see references [20–22,46,47]). Estrogen deficiency is described to affect circulating levels of specific cytokines, such as IL-1, tumor necrosis factor-α (TNF-α), granulocyte-macrophage colony stimulating factor (GM-CSF), and IL-6 [46,47]. With the progressive loss of estrogen, levels of these cytokines rise and enhance bone resorption by increasing the recruitment, differentiation, and activation of osteoclast cells [46–61]. Calcitonin levels are decreased in women compared with men; however, calcitonin deficiency has not been shown to play a role in age-related osteoporosis (see references [35–37,49,62–66]). This increase in activity of cytokines leads to the generation of transcription factors, which lead to increased osteoclastic recruitment and development. The mediator of this activity is RANKL, generated from osteoblasts and other cells, including of the immune system leading to increased bone resorption.

Other factors also affect bone mass (see references [35–37,49,62,67–85]). Physical activity tends to increase bone mass, whereas immobilization leads to increased bone loss. Obesity is associated with higher bone mass. Typical patients with osteoporosis tend to be thin and possess less muscle mass (see references [48,78,86,87]). Low dietary intake of calcium, phosphorous, and vitamin D are associated with age-related bone loss. The body's acid-base balance is also important; for example, the alkalization of the blood with bicarbonate has been shown to retard bone loss [85]. Late menarche and early menopause, caffeine ingestion, alcohol use and cigarette smoking are also important ingredients determining decreased bone mass (see references [48,71,72,79, 86–90]). Race and sex also influence bone mass. Blacks and Hispanics have higher bone mass than Caucasians and Asians, and men have higher bone mass than women [83,84,87]. Genetic factors are probably the most important of these in defining an increased risk of the development of osteoporosis. A family history of fractures in postmenopausal women probably predicts future problems (see references [48,78,91,92]). Some investigators have also demonstrated a correlation with abnormal receptors for vitamin D in some families with osteoporosis in multiple generations [93]. Unfortunately, this seems to be evident in some portions of the world but not in others, and is probably only an important problem in a small number of patients. However, other types of genetic abnormalities may explain the expression of an osteoporosis phenotype in certain families [48,91,92].

Specific abnormalities in genetic and hormonal factors appear to be important to define two clinical subtypes of age-related osteoporosis (see references [35–37,67,68]). Type I osteoporosis occurs in hypogonadal women or men. Postmenopausal women, women with premature oligo- or amenorrhea (due to anorexia nervosa or obsessive exercise programs), and men after castration or associated with testosterone deficiencies develop net bone loss directly related to the loss of gonadal function (see references [35–37,70–72]). As described, the loss of estrogen leads to increased serum levels of cytokines, which is thought to lead to increased recruitment and responsiveness of osteoclast precursors in trabecular bone, resulting in increased bone resorption [46,47]. As a result, these patients present with fractures of the skeleton where trabecular bone is predominant, such as the distal forearm and vertebral bodies.

Type II osteoporosis, on the other hand, is associated with the normal aging process and is seen in men and women typically after the age of 60 to 70 (see references [35–37,67,68,94]). Normal aging is associated with a progressive decline in the supply of osteoblasts and a decrease in their activity, but not primarily with an increase in osteoclast activity [33,42–44]. However, there remains a net loss of bone, but this time due to decreased formation and not necessarily due to increased resorption. Fractures of cortical bone, such as in the femur, femoral neck, proximal tibia, and pelvis, are more common in this group.

Other pathological circumstances leading to abnormalities of bone metabolism that increase the risk of bone loss include those patients with increased endogenous production of glucocorticoids or those with inflammatory diseases, regardless of whether they are treated with exogenous glucocorticoids. The pathogenesis of glucocorticoid-induced osteoporosis is complex, but is probably due to several induced abnormalities, including changes in gonadal hormone secretion, an induced decrease in calcium absorption, and an increase urinary calcium excretion as well as the direct effects of glucocorticoids on bone cells [45,95–98]. Glucocorticoids have been shown to decrease pituitary gonadotrophin secretion and suppress adrenal androgen production. These powerful anti-inflammatory drugs also decrease intestinal calcium absorption even with normal serum levels of calcitriol. In addition, the other skeletal effects of glucocorticoids include inhibition of osteoblast function, increased sensitivity of the cells to the effects of parathyroid hormone, and possibly transiently increased osteoclast activity. However, long-term use of glucocorticoids decreases osteoclast recruitment and cellular activity. Glucocorticoids also inhibit the generation of osteoprotegerin, a factor that inhibits RANK ligand. Thus, by decreasing inhibition of the inhibitor for RANK ligand there is increased generation of osteoclastic precursors and the generation of more osteoclasts. Bone loss with glucocorticoid therapy is most marked in trabecular bone and appears to be related to the dose and duration of glucocorticoid therapy and can be rapid. A significant amount of this bone loss is due to glucocorticoid-induced secondary changes in calcium balance and can be blunted by adequate use of calcium supplementation and vitamin D repletion concomitantly with the anti-inflammatory therapy [99–102]. The use of certain diuretics, such as thiazide derivatives, has been shown to decrease the hypercalciuria associated with the use of glucocorticoids [103]. Furthermore, it has been shown that the use of bisphosphonates is clearly beneficial and appropriate when starting systemic glucocorticoid therapy. Those patients with systemic inflammatory diseases are already at increased risk for bone loss, and the use of glucocorticoids to control the inflammation in these clinical circumstances enhances the problem.

Not everyone with low bone mass will fracture. The quantity of bone is measurable as the bone density and is predictive of future fracture; however, without a bone biopsy it is hard to define the quality of bone. The quality of bone, which partially reflects the extent of its connectivity, is also an important component of bone strength. Patient awareness of the potential risks associated with falling down is also important (see references [48,80–82,101]). Many elderly people are at risk for falling as a result of poor coordination, poor vision, muscle weakness, confusion, and the use of hypnotics or other medications that alter the sensorium. Because they are at a higher risk of falling they are also at an increased risk of sustaining a fracture. It has been shown that the use of hip pads by elderly nursing home occupants can reduce the incidence of hip fracture when patients fall.

Differential diagnosis

Osteoporosis can occur as a primary disorder or as a disorder associated with various diseases. Primary osteoporosis is a disease of the elderly, particularly among older women, with most cases occurring in the sixth and later decades of life. This form of osteoporosis is sometimes referred to as "involutional" osteoporosis.

Secondary osteoporosis is a series of abnormalities and diseases that may manifest with effects in bone. Those disease states associated with osteoporosis include endocrine disorders, systemic inflammatory diseases, bone mineral and metabolic defects, and other chronic illnesses. Some endocrine diseases that commonly effect bone include hyperthyroidism (due to primary thyroid disease or excessive supplemental thyroxine), hyperadrenocortism (primary or iatrogenic), and hyperparathyroidism. Some examples of systemic inflammatory diseases associated with osteoporosis include inflammatory bowel disease, rheumatoid arthritis, and systemic lupus erythematosus [37,62]. Osteoporosis may also result from therapeutic interventions, such as with methotrexate drug therapy (decreased osteoblast function), heparin (increased osteoclast activity at doses higher than 15,000 units in 24 h), glucocorticoids at or higher than 7.5 mg/d, or the use of anticonvulsants (which effect vitamin D metabolism and calcium absorption) (see references [45,48,94–96,99,104–106]). Other diseases commonly associated with an increased incidence of osteoporosis include diabetes mellitus, chronic obstructive pulmonary disease, and alcoholism [86–90].

Clinical manifestations

The clinical features of osteoporosis are bone fracture, pain, and deformity. Many patients are surprised to discover they have surreptitiously lost height due to previous asymptomatic vertebral fractures. Pain is the most common of symptoms. The axial skeleton is the most commonly involved area, with fractures occurring frequently in the mid thoracic, lower thoracic, and lumbar spine vertebrae. Spontaneous high thoracic or cervical fractures associated with minimal trauma should raise the suspicion of a malignancy. Osteoporotic fractures are typically sudden in onset and may be caused by a fall, sudden movement, lifting, jumping, or even with innocent traumatic events, such as a cough. Pain may be severe and typically localized to the site of fracture but can radiate to the abdomen or flanks. Activities that increase vertebral pain include valsalva maneuver, bending, or prolonged sitting or standing. Factors that decrease pain include lying on one's side with knees and hips flexed and arising from the lateral position rather than upright from the supine position. Generalized bone pain is rare and should raise the possibility of other diseases, such as metastatic cancer or osteomalacia.

Pain from an acute fracture usually subsides in a few weeks, and it is typically gone in 3 months. Persistent nagging back pain may continue for years even in the absence of new fracture because of the mechanical changes resulting from the fracture. Classic sciatica or pain characteristic of nerve root impingement is unusual in osteoporosis. Most patients with an osteoporosis related fracture sustain further fractures within the first few years [48,67,107]. Femoral neck fractures occur mainly in people over 65 years of age and increase in incidence as patients age [36,37]. Once a patient fractures a hip, there is a significant increased risk of death within 1 year [69]. This increased mortality is typically the result of complications of the fracture or reparative surgery; however, hip fractures are often sustained by patients who are chronically debilitated for other reasons.

Physical examination typically demonstrates tenderness to palpation over an area of fracture, spinal deformity, loss of height, and, over time, development of a lax abdominal musculature with a protuberant abdomen. Progressive anterior vertebral compression produces an exaggerated kyphosis of the thoracic spine, which leads to a characteristic deformity called a "dowager's hump."

Laboratory and radiologic features

Histomorphometry remains the gold standard for determining the state of bone turnover and diagnosing disease, unfortunately, the method is invasive requiring transiliac bone biopsies obtained with a trefine that has an internal diameter of 7 to 8 mm [43,108,109]. With tissue fixation, the samples are not demineralized, are embedded into plastic, and then thin sections are cut by microtome. Tetracycline labeling may be used as an in vivo marker to determine the rate of bone formation [110,111]. In normal adults, about 1 pmole of bone is deposited daily within active areas of remodeling [110,111]. Although it is a technique providing an enormous amount of information, it is not commonly used in clinical practice because of its invasiveness.

There are now methods to approximate the extent of bone turnover without relying on radiocalcium kinetics or direct measurement by bone biopsy. Biochemical markers can be measured in blood or urine, which define either markers of osteoblastic or osteoclastic function, the amount of new collagen or noncollagenous proteins synthesized, the extent of activity of osteoblasts, or the amount of bone collagen that has been resorbed [112–132]. The degree of elevation of indices of resorption and formation reflects the extent or severity of the abnormal bone turnover. Unfortunately, these markers of bone turnover have not yet been determined to reflect bone mass, quality of bone, or predict risk for fracture alone.

The biochemical markers for new synthesis, which may be clinically useful, include serum alkaline phosphatase, bone specific alkaline phosphatase, type I procollagen carboxyterminal peptide, and osteocalcin (see references [112–114, 116–118,123,132]). As a result of bone resorption, several of the collagen breakdown products are excreted in the urine. These include peptides containing hydroxyproline, hydroxylysine, and glycosylated hydroxylysine that are present in all type I collagens of all sources, or the 3hydroxy-pyridinium crosslink compounds that are unique to bone type I collagen (see references [112,114,116, 119–130,132]).

Elevated levels of serum alkaline phosphatase activity reflect increased activity of the osteoblasts [128]. The available bone specific serum alkaline phosphatase assays have not yet been proven to add more information except in patients with concomitant liver disease [128]. Measurement of bone-specific alkaline phosphatase is more accurate then fractionation of total serum alkaline phosphatase. Another possible marker for bone synthesis includes serum osteocalcin measurements. Osteocalcin contains γ-carboxyglutamic acid, which is a vitamin K-dependent protein, is 49 amino acids, represents about 20% of the noncollagenous component of the organic bone matrix, and undergoes variable processing that can lead to multiple possible immunoreactive peptides circulating in serum, which might profoundly confound the results of some assays. It appears to be a marker associated with osteoblast function, is deposited within the matrix, and thus may be variably released with resorption. There is some evidence that it might be associated with the process of mineralization. This marker appears to be substantially less useful than serum alkaline phosphatase for osteoblast activity and has unpredictable changes associated with it in Paget's disease (see references [112–114,116,123,132]). In patients suffering from even mild chronic renal failure, the clearance of this peptide is significantly affected.

Serum levels of the type I procollagen carboxyterminal extension peptide have been shown to be highly correlated with trebecular bone formation as determined by histomorphometry [123]. This is particularly true in those patients with osteoporosis whose net loss of bone is associated with increased bone formation, but, unfortunately, their extent of bone resorption is more than their bone formation. It is not as predictive of changes in new bone synthesis in patients with low bone formation. This is probably due to the lack of specificity of this measurement. This assay measures new collagen synthesis from all collagenous tissues, not just bone. At low levels of new bone synthesis, new collagen synthesis in other tissues is probably at a higher rate, which then serves to confound the usefulness of the assay.

Typically, the urinary markers of resorption or osteoclast activity include the hydroxyproline-containing peptides or pyridinium cross-linked peptides, which serve as rapid predictors of changes in osteoclastic activity. The levels of the urinary resorption peptides may fall within hours of exposure to an antiresorptive agent [123] The newer pyridinium crosslink markers are remarkably reproducible and are predominantly directly related to bone collagen resorption particularly in active disease states (see references [112,119,120,126,127,129,131,132]). Although the extent of absolute values of the individual markers varies when compared one to another, their net change after baseline seems to be useful to monitor therapeutic intervention and responsiveness [129].

There have recently been data evaluating the usefulness of the various available urinary pyridinium markers, either the free deoxypyridinuim (Dpd), the N-terminal telopeptide, or C-terminal telopeptide pyridinium peptide. Cummings et al [133] demonstrated that in 410 women 67 years of age or older who were not prescribed hormone replacement therapy, those patients with higher urinary concentrations of the free Dpd marker within the higher quartiles had a higher risk for fracture and were correlated with lower bone density. More directly, a study of 7598 women, 75 years of age or older and followed for 22 months, sustained 109 hip fractures. High urinary levels of the free Dpd and the C-terminal telopeptide pyridinium peptides were correlated with lower bone mass at the hip and more hip fractures [134]. These two studies suggest what is obvious. The patients with high levels of the urinary markers for bone resorption have lower bone densities as determined by densitometry. Low bone mass is associated with an increased risk for fracture. Gannero et al [134] have demonstrated that the relative risk for a hip fracture in elderly women was increased if the patients had low bone mass as determined by standard bone densitometric techniques and high levels of the urinary markers for resorption [femoral neck BMD standard deviation (SD) less than 2.5 = odds ratio (OR) for future hip fracture of 2.7, femoral neck BMD SD less than 2.5 and either elevated levels of the C-terminal telopeptide pyridinium peptide or the free Dpd peptide had an increased risk for future hip fracture of OR, 4.7 and 4.1]. Thus, it is possible with the newer improved assays of urinary pyridinium crosslinks in development that these urinary peptide markers may be useful to predict future fracture risk. Those presently available have been approved for diagnostic use in the United States.

Measurements of skeletal mass

Standard radiologic measurements allow for the definition of skeletal architecture. However, the typical radiograph reveals only a semiquantitative assessment of skeletal mass [135]. In specific epidemiologic studies, the cortex of a specific bone, typically the midshaft of the second metacarpal, is accurately measured using radiogrametry [136]. Although inexpensive and available, this technique provides little information about trebecular bone, which is the most metabolically active, and as noted, the area of bone most involved in post-menopausal osteoporosis. Instead, methods have been developed for quantization of cortical and trabecular bone mass as well as potential risk for fracture [137–145].

Single-photon densitometry is performed using an iodine [125] absorptiometric technique during which a radiation source with a fixed detector is directed over a bone or bones. This method is best to determine the mineral density of the distal radius. This area is predominantly cortical bone with some trebecular bone, which is considered to be less metabolically active than the trebecular bone found in the vertebral bodies or the femoral neck [137,143,144]. Age-related disease in men and women can be approximated by this measurement; however, as a single photon source, the amount of soft tissue can confound the results.

Dual-photon absorptiometry (DPA) (see references [137,138,143–145]), dual energy x-ray absorptiometry (DXA) [137,142–145], and quantitative computed tomography (QCT) (see references [139,143,145–148]) are used to accurately and reproducibly assess the mineral content of the vertebrae and femoral neck. DPA uses two separate photon energies obtained from a gadolinium [153] source that allows for distinction between the mineral content of bone and soft tissues. Short-term precision is between 1% and 2% [143]. DXA uses x-rays of two separate energies to analyze the distinctions between the mineral content of bone and the density of adjacent soft tissues. DXA is used to examine different skeletal sites and in addition to bone density can provide an estimate of total skeletal mineral. Short-term precision of this technique is between 0.5% and 1.2% [143–145]. QCT is the most expensive technology with a slightly higher dose of radiation per study. As noted, in patients with estrogen-deficient or glucocorticoid-induced osteoporosis, trabecular bone is lost more rapidly than cortical bone. QCT of the forearm or vertebrae is preferred in this setting because QCT is able to measure trabecular bone apart from the surrounding bony cortex. Spinal DXA in the lateral projection is used and appears to be nearly equivalent to spinal QCT. Spinal DXA in the anterior-posterior projection lacks sensitivity because the posterior elements of the spine, which are composed of cortical bone, are included in the measurement. In addition, many patients with osteoporosis are older and may have complicating osteoarthritis of the spine leading to hypertrophic boney changes that can alter the approximation of bone density. For these patients, measurement of the bone mineral density at the hip may be more accurate. For other patients, the most sensitive bone density measurements are made in cortical bone. In these clinical settings, measurement of the shaft of the radius, which is composed entirely of cortical bone, can be measured equally well by DXA, DPA, and pQCT (peripheral QCT). The method used depends on time, cost, and the clinical question being asked. In general, DXA is cheaper, faster, and more reproducible than DPA. There is increasing data that demonstrates that ultrasound of the calcaneous may be as predictive of risk for trebecular bone fracture as a spinal DXA [141].

Presently, DXA has become the measurement of choice for osteoporosis, and by using population standards, osteoporosis is defined in a patient with a bone density measurement of the spine that is 2.5 or greater standard deviations from the mean of the standard 35-year-old population in the appropriate gender (T score). Osteopenia is defined as a bone density between 1.0 and 2.5 standard deviations below the bone density of a standard 35-year-old population that is gender appropriate (T score). Thus, patients do not have to sustain a fracture to be diagnosed with this insidious problem. In addition, the Z score provides similar information regarding a patient's BMD as it relates to age matched controls. Therefore, with this calculation, it is possible to screen for superimposed causes of accelerated bone loss [149].

DXA is used for bone mineral screening because it identifies individuals whose osteoporosis is sufficiently severe that it places them at increased risk for fracture. There is an exponential correlation between the fall in BMD and the rise in fracture risk. For approximately every 1 SD fall in bone mass as measured by a bone densitometer there is a twofold rise in risk for fracture [147]. Perimenopausal and postmenopausal women are at particular risk for osteoporosis (see references [35–44,143,150]). Patients with osteoporotic vertebral compression fractures also develop chronic pain syndromes, which can be hard to diagnose [40,150,151]. Most of these patients suffer from osteoarthritis as well as degenerative disc disease. Some investigators are using single-photon emission computed tomography bone scintigraphy (SPECT) to help differentiate acute vertebral compression fractures from other causes of back pain, such as osteoarthritis [152,153].

Diagnosis

The diagnosis of osteoporosis in a postmenopausal woman or older individual who presents with pain and a vertebral compression fracture is uncomplicated; however, before a pathologic fracture occurs the diagnosis of osteoporosis can be more difficult. As noted, radiograph changes are insensitive to early changes of osteoporosis, and clinical symptoms of pain are typically lacking. Additionally, there are no characteristic laboratory abnormalities associated with osteoporosis. The serum calcium, phosphate, and alkaline phosphatase are usually normal for age and sex. There may be hypercalciuria, and urinary hydroxyproline or hydroxypyridinium excretion may be elevated indicative of increased bone resorption, but not invariably, and therefore these are not yet clinically useful screening tests for diagnosis. The biochemical markers presently available to determine the extent of bone resorption, such as the hydroxypyridinium (pyridinoline) urinary markers represented by assays for the free pyridinoline peptides (Dpd), the n-terminal telopeptides of type I collagen, and the c-terminal telopeptides of type I collagen, have been useful to determine those patients who are in a state of high bone resorption, as well as to define the response to specific therapy but have not yet been shown to be useful as a screen for diagnosis or to predict fracture risk [101,112,116]. Markers of new bone formation have not been shown to be useful as a measure for osteoblast function in these patients [112,116,123].

Before the diagnosis of osteoporosis is assigned to a patient with risk factors for osteoporosis or a screening radiograph consistent with osteoporosis, it is prudent to exclude other diseases that are associated with osteoporosis. In addition to establishing that there is a normal hematocrit, white blood cell count, platelet count, and erythrocyte sedimentation rate along with normal serum chemistries, renal function, and liver tests, other laboratory tests that are useful in excluding diseases associated with osteoporosis include serum calcium, serum phosphorous, serum alkaline phosphatase, 24-hour urine calcium/creatinine clearance, plasma 25-$(OH)D_3$, and 1,25-$(OH)_2D_3$ levels. Elevated serum calcium suggests either carcinomatous skeletal metastases or hyperparathyroidism. Hypophosphatemia is usually present in osteomalacia, although in some circumstances the serum phosphorous levels may be normal; typically, the serum calcium is normal. Low 25-$(OH)D_3$ serum levels suggest hypovitaminosis D from either inadequate dietary sources, including states of malabsorption or low levels of exposure to sunlight. In the Northeastern part of the United States, it is not unusual for older, homebound people to become depleted of their vitamin D stores over the long winter. Urinary calcium excretion is usually normal or may be elevated in osteoporosis. Normal levels of urinary calcium essentially exclude hypovitaminosis D as a result of intestinal malabsorption but do not rule out a renal calcium or phosphate-leak syndrome. Concentrations of serum 1,25-$(OH)_2D_3$ should be normal in premenopausal patients with adequate renal function. However, serum 25-$(OH)D_3$ and 1,25-$(OH)_2D_3$ levels have been shown to be lower in elderly patients with osteoporotic hip fracture [76,77]. Serum parathyroid hormone may be elevated in states of secondary hyperparathyroidism as found in some patients with glucocorticoid-induced bone loss.

Management

The fundamental management goals for patients with osteoporosis are to prevent fractures, decrease pain when present, and maintain function. The drugs available today decrease the risk for further bone loss and reduce the risk of bone fracture when combined with nonpharmaceutical measures. Studies have shown that women with multiple risk factors and low bone density are at high risk for fracture, and that this risk can be reduced by maintaining body weight, walking for exercise, avoiding long-acting benzodiazepines, minimizing caffeine intake, and treating impaired visual function (see references [42,48, 101,143,154]). It is important to educate patients about the risks of falling [42,101].

The first step to good therapeutic choices is an appropriate diagnosis. As noted, it is not difficult to diagnose a patient who has pain resulting from a vertebral compression fracture. The goal is to diagnose the patient with osteoporosis before they have sustained enough bone loss to be at risk for a fracture. Patients should be identified early who are at risk for future fracture based on their family history and other known risk factors. These patients should undergo a bone densitometry test to determine their bone mass as it relates to an age-matched cohort (Z score) and determines the T score. If the resultant BMD has a standard deviation of 1 or greater, then serious consideration needs to be given to close follow-up and potential therapy.

Once a patient has fractured, therapeutic interventions to decrease the pain include local physical measures, such as warm, moist packs to decrease muscle spasm or occasional cold compresses, gentle physical therapy, appropriate bed rest, and pharmacologic interventions, such as simple analgesics, nonsteroidal anti-inflammatory drugs, muscle relaxants when appropriate, and even the use of calcitonin for its acute analgesic effects.

The pharmacologic treatment strategies for the prevention and treatment of type I and type II osteoporosis include medications that decrease osteoclast-induced bone resorption (antiresorptive therapy) even though increased osteoclastic resorption likely does not play a key role in age-related disease affecting men and women 60 to 70. Therefore, in clinical states associated with decreased osteoblastic activity, an improved bone turnover balance can be restored by decreasing the resorption of bone by drug therapy while new bone formation is decreased naturally due to the aging of the osteoblast lineage of cells. There is also therapy available to increase bone mass by stimulating new osteoblastic activity using parathyroid hormone.

Antiresorptive drugs include calcium and vitamin D supplementation, hormone replacement therapy (HRT), such as estrogen supplementation in women, calcitonin either as parenteral therapy or as an inhaled product, and bisphosphonate therapy. Treatment aimed at stimulating osteoblasts and new bone formation includes sodium fluoride, androgens, and intermittent parenteral parathyroid hormone therapy. Because type II osteoporosis is related to decreased osteoblastic activity, drugs to stimulate osteoblast function would be preferable. Unfortunately, there are significant problems with several of the anabolic therapies, including the potential for virilization and hepatic toxicity because of androgens, or the potential for increased bone pain or the development of bone of poor quality associated with fluoride treatment. PTH treatment has been shown to be successful; however, combination therapy with bisphosphonates and PTH has been a problem [101,102].

Calcium, vitamin D, and calcitriol

Calcium supplementation of the normal diet increases bone mass in adolescents and reduces bone loss associated with advancing age (see references [40,102,107,154–159]). Calcium supplements should be given to all patients with low calcium intake (less than 400 mg/d), postmenopausal women, the elderly, and patients treated with glucocorticoids. Calcium supplements when given alone to women with established osteoporosis have shown variable results in reducing fracture risk in controlled trials [155,157,159]. Recommended total calcium intakes for white women (diet and supplementation) include 1000mg/day for adults, 1500 mg/d for postmenopausal women and women with known osteoporosis, and 1200 mg/d for adolescents [42,160–163].

Relative vitamin D deficiency, like calcium deficiency, is a problem in postmenopausal women, the elderly, and institutionalized people who do not have enough access to the sun. Serum 25-OH vitamin D_3 and 1,25-$(OH)_2$vitamin D_3 levels are variable and thus not useful as clinical diagnostic tools except in patients with a history compatible with malabsorption; therefore, empiric treatment with vitamin D supplements is preferred [160–166]. Some studies have shown that vitamin D_3 plus calcium appears to reduce the risk of hip and other nonvertebral fractures by as much as 43% in elderly institutionalized women [164]. Calcitriol therapy, though safe, requires careful monitoring of serum and urine calcium levels to avoid hypercalcemia and significant hypercalciuria.

Estrogen

Estrogen deficiency is now well established as a major cause of bone loss in postmenopausal women [167]. In young women with amenorrhea or ovulatory disturbances, cyclic medroxyprogesterone has been demonstrated to increase bone density, further demonstrating the central role that female sex hormones play in osteoporosis [168]. Estrogen replacement therapy is associated with increased bone mass, decreased urinary biochemical resorption markers, and reduced fracture rate in many studies [169–172]. Therapeutic regimens that include estrogen are more effective in protecting against osteoporosis than those that contain calcium alone (see references [101,154,155,163,173–187]). Estrogen replacement appears to be most effective at maintaining bone mass when begun soon after menopause and continued. This is due to the accelerated period of bone loss during the early postmenopause during which women may lose bone mass at the rate of up to 3% to 5% per year for approximately 5 to 7 years. Unfortunately, estrogen therapy has significant risks [188–192]. Unopposed estrogen therapy is associated with an increased incidence of uterine cancer, and there is also an increased cumulative risk for breast cancer in women who are treated with estrogen, which may be important in women with a family history of the disease. Furthermore, recent data has demonstrated that use of HRT is associated with an increased risk for acute myocardial infarction and stroke. Thus the use of HRT has been relegated to only short-term use at low dose for those few patients with significant perimenopausal symptoms.

However, there is continued use of the estrogen-like drugs or SERMs. Raloxifene is a commonly used drug for women with postmenopausal osteoporosis, but it does not have preventative effects on perimenopausal symptoms. It has been shown that raloxifene (60 mg/d) decreases the risk of vertebral fracture by 30%. Whether use of this agent prevents the development of breast cancer or heart disease is still not known [193].

Calcitonin

Salmon calcitonin inhibits bone resorption by decreasing osteoclast function by binding to high-affinity receptors [194–197]. Calcitonin is available in the United States as a subcutaneous injection and as an intranasal spray (200 U) for the treatment of osteoporosis [197–206]. In one study it has been shown to be effective in increasing bone mineral content in patients with normal or high bone turnover. Femoral bone mineral content decreased in that study, however, and there was no analysis of the effect of calcitonin on fracture rate [207]. Patients were treated in the standard fashion with calcium (500 to 1000 mg/d) and calcitonin 50 U SQ every other day for 2 years. Common side effects of calcitonin therapy included nausea and flushing, but these were seldom severe enough to warrant discontinuation of therapy. Calcitonin therapy is also hampered by cost and the inconvenience of injections. Though nasal salmon calcitonin appears to reduce spinal bone loss in early postmenopausal woman, it has not been shown to have any effect on the peripheral skeleton [198,199]. There is some evidence that calcitonin has analgesic effects, probably mediated centrally [208].

Bisphosphonates

The bisphosphonates are synthetic analogs of pyrophosphate, a naturally occurring substance that inhibits bone mineralization. The bisphosphonates have been shown to inhibit bone resorption by inhibiting the action of osteoclasts [193,209–220]. These compounds once absorbed orally or by intravenous injection are bound tightly to hydroxyapatite crystals. During the process of bone resorption, the bisphosphonates bound to the hydroxyapatite crystal are released, are taken up by osteoclasts, and inhibit the bone-resorbing function of these cells. Bone surfaces once coated with bisphosphonates also are less able to bind and activate osteoclasts that subsequently arrive.

The bisphosphonates clinically available for the treatment of osteoporosis include etidronate, alendronate, and risedronate. Another choice, pamidronate, is available as a parenteral drug to treat hypercalcemia of malignancy. Some studies have shown that etidronate given in cyclical fashion (400 mg for 2 weeks every 3 months) along with calcium supplementation (500 mg/d) increased spinal bone density by 4% and reduced the rate of new fracture by 50% to 75% when compared with placebo. Unfortunately, there has been conflicting evidence regarding change in the vertebral fracture rate, and possible protective effects of etidronate on fracture rates in nonvertebral sites were not demonstrated.

Treatment with the next generation of bisphosphonates, such as alendronate or risedronate, has led to decreased fracture rates with years of continuous therapy at vertebral and nonvertebral sites, such as the hip and forearm, with no effect on mineralization. There is some evidence that bone mass continues to improve as measured by densitometry with continuation of these drugs. Other bisphosphonates, such as pamidronate, tiludronate, zolandronate, and ibandronate, are or soon will be available.

Although bisphosphonate therapy has been shown to be of benefit in specific patient populations, there are some risks with these drugs. The complicated intermittent therapy regimen with etidronate was developed because of drug-induced inhibition of mineralization. The intermittent dose decreases that effect. In addition, all bisphosphonates are poorly bioavailable and thus should be taken on an empty stomach to ensure some absorption. For alendronate and residronate, there are further important issues. The major noted toxicity in most clinical studies and in practice has been esophageal irritation. To reduce this effect, a bisphosphonate should be taken fasting first thing in the morning, on an empty stomach, with 8 ounces of water, and the patient should remain upright for 30 to 45 minutes before eating.

Sodium fluoride

Sodium fluoride therapy increases trabecular bone mass, but may at the same time decrease cortical bone mass even in the presence of adequate calcium supplementation [221–223]. Though patients receiving sodium fluoride might improve bone mass with a lower dose, confirmation of a benefit from sodium fluoride is lacking. A study employing a new formulation of sodium fluoride has demonstrated better results. When slow release sodium fluoride was used there were similar improvements in BMD at all sites without any one site containing cortical bone losing its content [221]. Although, sodium fluoride therapy clearly increases bone density and increases the activity of osteoblasts, some investigators continue to be concerned about the quality rather than quantity of the bone that is formed.

Parathyroid hormone

Traditional therapies for osteoporosis have been aimed at inhibiting bone resorption. Therapies that target increased osteoblast activity, replacing lost bone by increasing new bone formation, are now available. Various forms of parathyroid hormone therapy have been considered for years. One treatment available now is the use of the synthetic (1–34) amino acid fragment of PTH with or without 1,25 (OH)$_2$ D [224–232]. Small daily doses of PTH have been shown to stimulate bone formation in osteoporotic patients without increasing bone resorption or causing hypercalcemia. The accumulated evidence shows that there may be large increases in bone density over short periods of time correlated with decreased fracture risk of about 65% after 21 months of treatment. The use of this powerful anabolic therapy when combined with bisphosphonates is still controversial [230].

Androgens

Because androgen deficiency likely plays an important role in age-associated bone loss, androgen replacement might stimulate osteoblasts to produce new bone. Androgens have been shown to decrease urinary calcium excretion, increase muscle mass (thereby improving strength and perhaps stability), and perhaps provide an improved sense of well-being [233]. Stanozolol and nandrolone augment bone mass in postmenopausal women, but at the expense of lowering serum HDL concentrations [233,234]. Other concerns include the potential for virulization, alteration in blood lipid levels, which might increase risk for heart disease, and increased risk for hypertension. These concerns, along with the risk of hepatotoxicity when androgens are used for more than 3 months, have limited the usefulness of this form of therapy.

The male patient with osteoporosis presents a unique problem. As in the case of the female hypogonadal patient, the male patient will also benefit from repleting calcium, ensuring adequate vitamin D intake, an appropriate exercise regimen, and the use of antiresorptive agents if applicable. If the patient is hypogonadal, the use of testosterone by injection or patch is appropriate [101].

Strontium ranelate

A new agent, strontium ranelate, with a novel mechanism of action acting on bone resorption to reduce the rate of bone growth (as do bisphosphonates) and on bone formation to promote the growth of new bone (as does the parathyroid hormone) has recently been approved for osteoporosis in Europe [235,236]. The recommended dose is 2 g daily. The drug comes in the form of granules to be taken as a suspension in a glass of water. Given the slow absorption, it should be taken at bedtime, preferably at least 2 hours after eating. Food, milk and derivatives, and medicinal products containing calcium may reduce bioavailability by 60% to 70%, so should be avoided for at least 2 hours. Sontium ranelate is reported to reduce the risk of vertebral fractures by 49% after a year, and by 41% over the 3 years of the study. Side effects include an increased frequency of nausea, diarrhea, and headache in the first few months of treatment, not usually requiring withdrawal of treatment, and an excess of venous thromboembolism.

In summary, effective therapies are available for the older patient with osteoporosis. The approach is critical to ensure an optimal quality of life in these individuals who suffer a disease that clearly is treatable.

References

[1] Rodan GA. Introduction to bone biology. Bone 1992;13:S3.
[2] Robey PG. The biochemistry of bone. Endocrinol Metab Clin North Am 1989;18:859.
[3] Heinegard D, Hultenby K, Oldberg A, et al. Macromolecules in bone matrix. Connect Tissue Res 1989;21:3.
[4] Bork P. The modular architecture of vertebrate collagens. FEBS Lett 1992;307:49.
[5] Krane SM, Simon LS. Organic matrix defects in metabolic and related bone diseases. In: Veis A, editor. The chemistry and biology of mineralized connective tissues. New York: Elsevier Science; 1981. p. 185.
[6] Brown JP, Delmas PD, Malaval L, et al. Serum bone GLA-protein: a specific marker of bone formation in postmenopausal osteoporosis. In Proceedings of the Copenhagen International Symposium on Osteoporosis. Department of Clinical Chemistry, Glostrop Hospital, Denmark; 1984.
[7] Lian JB, Coutts M, Canalis E. Studies of hormonal regulation of osteocalcin synthesis in cultured fetal rat calvariae. J Biol Chem 1985;260.8706.
[8] Triffitt JT. Plasma proteins present in human cortical bone: enrichment of the α_2HS-glycoprotein. Calcif Tissue Res 1976;22:27.
[9] Ashton BA, Smith R. Plasma α_2HS-glycoprotein concentrations in Paget's disease of bone: its possible significance. Clin Sci 1980;58:435.
[10] Franzen A, Heinegard D. Isolation and characterization of two sialoproteins present only in bone calcified matrix. Biochem J 1985;232:715.
[11] Sage EH, Bornstein P. Extracellular proteins that modulate cell-matrix interactions, SPARC, tenascin, and thrombospondin. J Biol Chem 1991;266:14831.
[12] Baron R. Polarity and membrane transport in osteoclasts. Connect Tissue Res 1988;20:109.
[13] Suda T, Takahashi N, Martin TJ. Modulation of osteoclast differentiation. Endocr Rev 1992; 13:66.
[14] Aubin JE. Osteoclast adhesion and resorption: the role of podosomes. J Bone Miner Res 1992;7:365.
[15] Blair HC, Teitelbaum SL, Ghiselli R, et al. Osteoclast bone resorption by a polarized vacuolar proton pump. Science 1989;245:855.
[16] Chatterjee D, Chakraborty M, Leit M. Sensitivity to vanadate and isoforms of subunits A and B distinguish the osteoclast proton pump from other vacuolar H^+ ATPases. Proc Natl Acad Sci USA 1992;89:6257.
[17] Jones SJ, Hogg NM, Shapiro IM, et al. Cells with Fc receptors in the cell layer next to osteoblasts and osteoclasts in bone. Metab Bone Dis Relat Res 1981;2:357.
[18] Canalis E, McCarthy TL, Centrella M. Growth factors and cytokines in bone cell metabolism. Annu Rev Med 1991;42:17.
[19] Gravallese EM, Galson DL, Goldring SR, Auron PE. The role of TNF-receptor family members and other TRAF-dependent receptors in bone resorption. Arthritis Res 2001;3:6–12.
[20] Jilka RL, Hangoc G, Girasole G. Increased osteoclast development after estrogen loss: mediation by interleukin-6. Science 1992;257:88.
[21] Roodman GD, Kurihara N, Ohsaki Y, et al. Interleukin 6: a potential autocrine/paracrine factor in Paget's disease of bone. J Clin Invest 1992;89:46.
[22] Passeri G, Girasole G, Knutson S, et al. Interleukin-11 (IL-11): a new cytokine with

osteoclastogenic and bone resorptive properties and a critical role in PTH and 1,25(OH)$_2$D$_3$-induced osteoclast development. J Bone Miner Res 1992;7:S110.

[23] Raisz LG, Kream BE. Regulation of bone formation. N Engl J Med 1983;309:29.

[24] Parfitt AM. Surface specific bone remodeling in health and disease. In: Kleerekopper M, Krane SM, editors. Clinical disorders of bone and mineral metabolism. New York: Mary Ann Liebert; 1989. p. 7.

[25] Chambers TJ, McSheehy PMJ, Thomson BM, et al. The effect of calcium-regulating hormones and prostaglandins on bone resorption by osteoclasts disaggregated from neonatal rabbit bones. Endocrinology 1985;60:234.

[26] Mundy GR, Shapiro JL, Bandelin JG, et al. Direct stimulation of bone resorption by thyroid hormones. J Clin Invest 1976;58:529.

[27] McCarthy TL, Centrella M, Canalis E. Regulatory effects on insulin-like growth factor I and II on bone collagen synthesis in rat calvarial cultures. Endocrinology 1989;124:301.

[28] Hock JM, Fonseca J. Anabolic effect of human synthetic parathyroid hormone-(1–34) depends on growth hormone. Endocrinology 1990;127:1804.

[29] Lin H, Harris TL, Flannery MS, et al. Expression cloning of an adenylate cyclase-coupled calcitonin receptor. Science 1991;254:1022.

[30] Gorn A, Lin HY, Yamin M, et al. Cloning, characterization, and expression of a human calcitonin receptor from an ovarian carcinoma cell line. J Clin Invest 1992;90:1726.

[31] Johnson LC. The kinetics of skeletal remodeling. A further consideration of the theoretical biology of bone. Birth Defects 1966;2:66.

[32] Frost HM. Bone remodeling and its relationship to metabolic bone diseases. Springfield (IL): Charles C. Thomas; 1973.

[33] Parfitt AM. The coupling of bone formation: a critical analysis of the concept and of its relevance to the pathogenesis of osteoporosis. Metab Bone Dis Relat Res 1982;4:1.

[34] Parfitt AM, Kleerehoper M. Diagnostic value of bone histomorphometry and comparison on histologic measurements and biochemical indices of bone remodeling. In: Christiansen C, Arnaud CD, Nordin BEC, et al, editors. Proceedings of the Copenhagen International Symposium on Osteoporosis, Aalborg Stiftsbogtrykkeri, Denmark, 1984. p. 111.

[35] Riggs BL, Melton III LJ. Involutional osteoporosis. N Engl J Med 1986;314:1676.

[36] Riggs BL, Melton III LJ. Evidence for two distinct syndromes of involutional osteoporosis. Am J Med 1983;75:899.

[37] Melton III LJ, Riggs BL. Further characterization of the heterogeneity of the osteoporotic syndromes. In: Kleerekoper M, Krane SM, editors. Clinical disorders of bone and mineral metabolism. New York: Mary Ann Liebert; 1989. p. 145.

[38] Marcus R, Kosek J, Pfefferbaum A, et al. Age-related loss of trabecular bone in premenopausal women. A biopsy study. Calcif Tissue Int 1983;35:406.

[39] Avioli LV, Lindsay R. The female osteoporotic syndrome(s). In: Avioli LV, Krane SM, editors. Metabolic bone disease and clinical related disorders. Philadelphia: W.B. Saunders; 1990. p. 397.

[40] Nagant de Deuxchaisnes C. The pathogenesis and treatment of involutional osteoporosis. In: Dixon AStJ, Russell RGG, Stamp TCB, editors. Osteoporosis, a multi-disciplinary problem. Royal Society of Medicine International Congress and Symposium Series No. 55. London: Academic Press; 1983. p. 291.

[41] Parfitt AM, Shih M-S, Rao DS, et al. Relationship between bone formation rate and osteoblast surface in aging and osteoporosis: evidence for impaired osteoblast recruitment in pathogenesis. J Bone Miner Res 1992;7(Suppl 1):S116.

[42] Riggs BL, Melton LJ. The prevention and treatment of osteoporosis. N Engl J Med 1992; 327:620.

[43] Parfitt AM. Bone remodeling: relationship to the amount and structure of bone, and the pathogenesis and prevention of fractures. In: Riggs BL, Melton III LJ, editors. Osteoporosis: etiology, diagnosis, and management. New York: Raven Press; 1988. p. 45.

[44] Parfitt AM, Mathews CHE, Villanueva AR, et al. Relationships between surface, volume, and thickness of iliac trabecular bone in aging and in osteoporosis: implications for the microanatomic and cellular mechanisms of bone loss. J Clin Invest 1983;72:1396.

[45] Lukert BP, Raisz LG. Glucocorticoid-induced osteoporosis: pathogenesis and management. Ann Intern Med 1990;112:352–64.

[46] Stavros CM, Jilka RL. Bone marrow, cytokines, and bone remodeling: emerging insights into the pathophysiology of osteoporosis. N Engl J Med 1995;332:305–11.

[47] Hurwitz MC. Cytokines and estrogen in bone: anti-osteoporotic effects. Science 1993; 260.623.

[48] Cummings SR, Nevitt MC, et al. Risk factors for hip fracture in white women. N Engl J Med 1995;332:767–73.

[49] Bauer DC, Browner WS, Cauley JA, et al. Factors associated with appendicular bone mass in older women. Ann Int Med 1993;118:657–65.

[50] Prince RL, Smith M, Dick IM, et al. Prevention of postmenopausal osteoporosis. N Engl J Med 1991;325:1189.

[51] Pacifici R. Is there a causal role for IL-1 in postmenopausal bone loss? Calcif Tissue Int 1992;50:295.

[52] Jilka RL, Hangoc G, Girasole G, et al. Increased osteoclast development after estrogen loss: mediation of interleukin-6. Science 1992;257:88.

[53] Girasole G, Jilka RL, Passeri G, et al. 17β-Estradiol inhibits interleukin-6 production by bone marrow-derived stromal cells and osteoblasts in vitro: a potential mechanism for the antiosteoporotic effect of estrogens. J Clin Invest 1992;89:883.

[54] Chaudhary LR, Spelsberg TC, Riggs BL. Production of various cytokines by normal human osteoblast-like cells in response to interleukin-1β and tumor necrosis factor-α: lack of regulation by 17β-Estradiol. Endocrinology 1992;130:2528.

[55] Rickard D, Russel G, Gowen M. Oestradiol inhibits the release of tumor necrosis factor but not interleukin 6 from adult human osteoblasts in vitro. Osteoporos Int 1992;2:94.

[56] Keeting PE, Rifas L, Harris SA, et al. Evidence for interleukin-1β production by cultured normal human osteoblast-like cells. J Bone Miner Res 1991;6:827.

[57] Oursler MJ, Cortese C, Keeting P, et al. Modulation of transforming growth factor-β production in normal human osteoblast-like cells by 17β-estradiol and parathyroid hormone. Endocrinology 1991;129:3313.

[58] Mbalaviele G, Orcel P, Bouizar Z, et al. Transforming growth factor-β enhances calcitonin-induced cyclic AMP production and the number of calcitonin receptors in long-term cultures of human umbilical cord blood monocytes in the presence of 1,25- dihydroxycholecalciferol. J Cell Physiol 1992;152:486.

[59] Schneider HG, Michelangeli VP, Frampton RJ, et al. Transforming growth factor-β modulates receptor binding of calciotropic hormones and G protein-mediated adenylate cyclase responses in osteoblast-like cells. Endocrinology 1992;131:1383.

[60] Knappe V, Raue F, Pfeilschifter J, et al. Tumor necrosis factor-alpha inhibits the stimulatory effect of the parathyroid hormone-related protein on cyclic AMP formation in osteoblast-like cells via protein kinase-C + blind E. Biochem Biophys Res Commun 1992;182:341.

[61] Takahashi N, Udagawa N, Akatsu T, et al. Role of colony-stimulating factors in osteoclast development. J Bone Miner Res 1991;6:977.

[62] Melton LJ, Cummings SR, Johnston CC. Heterogeneity of age-related fractures: implications for epidemiology. Bone Miner 1987;2:321.

[63] Stevenson JC, Hillyard CJ, MacIntyre I, et al. A physiological role for calcitonin: protection of the maternal skeleton. Lancet 1979;2:769.

[64] Deftos LJ, Weissman MH, Williams GW, et al. Influence of age and sex on plasma calcitonin in human beings. N Engl J Med 1980;302:1351.

[65] Taggart HM, Chestnut III CH, Ivey JL, et al. Deficient calcitonin response to calcium stimulation in postmenopausal osteoporosis? Lancet 1982;1:475.

[66] Tiegs RD, Body JJ, Barta JM, et al. Secretion and metabolism of monomeric human calcitonin: effects of age, sex, and thyroid damage. J Bone Miner Res 1986;1:339.

[67] Melton LJ, Wahner HW, Richelson LS, et al. Osteoporosis and the risk of hip fracture. Am J Epidemiol 1986;124:154.

[68] Whyte MP, Bergfeld MA, Murphy WA, et al. Postmenopausal osteoporosis: a heterogeneous

disorder as assessed by histomorphometric analysis of iliac crest bone from untreated patients. Am J Med 1982;72:193.

[69] Cummings SR, Rubin SM, Black D. The future of hip fractures in the United States: numbers, costs, and potential effects of postmenopausal estrogen. Clin Orthop 1990;252:163.

[70] Finklestein JS, Neer RM, Biller BMK, et al. Osteopenia in men with a history of delayed puberty. N Engl J Med 1992;326:600.

[71] Prior JC, Vigna YM, Schechter MT, et al. Spinal bone loss and ovulatory disturbances. N Engl J Med 1990;323:1221.

[72] Klibanski A, Neer RM, Beitins IZ, et al. Decreased bone density in hyperprolactinemic women. N Engl J Med 1980;303:1511.

[73] Hartwell D, Riis BJ, Christiansen C. Changes in vitamin D metabolism during natural and medical menopause. J Clin Endocrinol Metab 1990;71:127.

[74] Villareal DT, Civitelli R, Chines A, et al. Subclinical vitamin D deficiency in post- menopausal. Women with low vertebral bone mass. J Clin Endocrinol Metab 1992;72:628.

[75] Gallagher JC, Riggs BL, Eisman J, et al. Intestinal calcium absorption and serum vitamin D metabolites in normal subjects and osteoporotic patients: effect of age and dietary calcium. J Clin Invest 1979;64:729.

[76] Slovik DM, Adams JS, Neer RM, et al. Deficient production of 1,25-dihydroxyvitamin D in elderly osteoporotic patients. N Engl J Med 1981;305:372.

[77] Riggs BL, Hamstra A, DeLuca HF. Assessment of 25-hydroxyvitamin D 1α-hydroxylase reserve in postmenopausal osteoporosis by administration of parathyroid extract. J Clin Endocrinol Metab 1981;53:833.

[78] Kanis JA, Pitt FA. Epidemiology of osteoporosis. Bone 1992;13(Suppl):7.

[79] Armamonto-Villareal R, Villareal DT, Avioli LV, et al. Estrogen status and hereditary are major determinants of premenopausal bone mass. J Clin Invest 1992;90:2464.

[80] Cummings SR. Are patients with hip fractures more osteoporotic? Review of the evidence. Am J Med 1985;78:487.

[81] Johnston CC, Slemenda CW. Risk prediction of osteoporosis: a theoretic overview. Am J Med 1991;91(Suppl 5B):47.

[82] Kelsey JL, Browner WS, Seeley DG, et al. Risk factors for fractures of the distal forearm and proximal humerus. Am J Epdemiol 1992;135:477.

[83] Bell NH, Shary J, Stevens J, et al. Demonstration that bone mass is greater in black than in white children. J Bone Miner Res 1991;6:719.

[84] Gilsanz V, Roe TF, Mora S, et al. Changes in vertebral bone density in black girls and white girls during childhood and puberty. N Engl J Med 1991;325:1597.

[85] Sebastian A, Harris ST, Ottaway JH, et al. Improved mineral balance and skeletal metabolism in postmenopausal women treated with potassium carbonate. N Engl J Med 1994;330:1776–81.

[86] Daniell HW. Osteoporosis of the slender smoker: vertebral compression fractures and loss of metacarpal cortex in relation to postmenopausal cigarette smoking and lack of obesity. Arch Intern Med 1976;136:298.

[87] Seeman E, Melton III LJ, O'Fallon WM, et al. Risk factors for spinal osteoporosis in men. Am J Med 1983;75:977.

[88] Jensen J, Christiansen C, Rodbro P. Cigarette smoking, serum estrogens, and bone loss during hormone-replacement therapy early after menopause. N Engl J Med 1985;313:973.

[89] Aloia JF, Cohn SH, Vaswani A, et al. Risk factors for postmenopausal osteoporosis. Am J Med 1985;78:95.

[90] Spencer H, Rubio N, Rubio E, et al. Chronic alcoholism: frequently overlooked cause of osteoporosis in men. Am J Med 1986;80:393.

[91] Pocock NA, Eisman JA, Hopper JL, et al. Genetic determinants of bone mass in the adult. J Clin Invest 1987;80:706–10.

[92] Christian JC, Yu P-L, Slemenda CW, Johnston CCJ. Heretability of bone mass: a longitudinal study in aging male twins. Am J Hum Genet 1989;44:429–33.

[93] Cooper GS, Umbach DM. Are vitamin D receptor polymorphisms associated with bone mineral density? A meta-analysis. J Bone Miner Res 1996;11:1841–9.

[94] Frame B, Nixon RK. Bone-marrow mast cells in osteoporosis of aging. N Engl J Med 1968;279:626.

[95] Ramos-Remus C, Sibley J, Russell AS. Steroids in rheumatoid arthritis: the honeymoon revisited. J Rheumatol 1992;19:667.

[96] Nagant de Deuxchaisnes C, Devogelaer JP, Esselinckx W, et al. The effect of low dosage glucocorticoids on bone mass in rheumatoid arthritis: a cross-sectional and longitudinal study using single photon absorptiometry. In: Avioli LV, Gennari C, Imbimbo B, editors. Glucocorticoid effects and their biological consequences. New York: Plenum Press; 1982. p. 209.

[97] Baylink DJ. Glucocorticoid-induced osteoporosis [editorial]. N Engl J Med 1983;309:306.

[98] Bressot C, Meunier PJ, Chapuy MC, et al. Histomorphometric profile, pathophysiology, and reversibility of corticosteroid-induced osteoporosis. Metab Bone Dis Relat Res 1979;1:303.

[99] Hahn TJ, Halstead LR, Teitelbau SL, et al. Altered mineral metabolism in glucocorticoid-induced osteopenia: effect of 25-hydroxyvitamin D administration. J Clin Invest 1979;64:655.

[100] Villareal DT, Civitelli R, Genari C, et al. Is there an effective treatment for glucocorticoid-induced osteoporosis? Calcif Tissue Int 1991;49:141.

[101] American College of Rheumatology Task Force on Osteoporosis Guidelines. Recommendations for the prevention and treatment of glucocorticoid-induced osteoporosis. Arthritis Rheum 1996;39:1791–801.

[102] Buckley LM, Leib ES, Cartularo KS, et al. Calcium and vitamin D_3 supplementation prevents bone loss in the spine secondary to low-dose corticosteroids in patients with rheumatoid arthritis. Ann Int Med 1996;125:961–8.

[103] Cauley JA, Cummings SR, Seeley DG, et al. Effects of thiazide diuretic therapy on bone mass, fractures, and falls. Ann Intern Med 1993;118:666.

[104] Laan RFJM, van Riel PLCM, van de Putte LVBA, et al. Low dose prednisone induces rapid reversible axial bone loss in patients with rheumatoid arthritis. A randomized, controlled study. Ann Int Med 1993;119:963–8.

[105] Caldwell JR, Furst DE. The efficacy and safety of low-dose corticosteroids for rheumatoid arthritis. Semin Arthritis Rheum 1991;21:1.

[106] Joffe I, Epstein S. Osteoporosis associated with rheumatoid arthritis: pathogenesis and management. Semin Arthritis Rheum 1991;20:256.

[107] Riis B, Thomsen K, Christiansen C. Does calcium supplementation prevent post-menopausal bone loss? N Engl J Med 1987;316:173.

[108] Vedi S, Compston JE, Webb A, et al. Histomorphometric analysis of bone biopsies from the iliac crest of normal British subjects. Metab Bone Dis Relat Res 1982;4:231.

[109] Chavassieux PM, Arlot ME, Meunier PJ. Intermethod variation in bone histomorphometry: comparison between manual and computerized methods applied to iliac bone biopsies. Bone 1985;6:221.

[110] Reeve J, Arlot ME, Chavassieux PM, et al. The assessment of bone formation and bone resorption in osteoporosis: a comparison between tetracycline-based iliac histomorphometry and whole body [85]Sr kinetics. J Bone Miner Res 1987;2:479.

[111] Recker RR, Kimmel DB, Parfitt AM, et al. Static and tetracycline-based bone histomorphometric data from 34 normal postmenopausal females. J Bone Miner Res 1988;3:133.

[112] Taylor AK, Lueken SA, Libanati C, et al. Biochemical markers of bone turnover for the clinical assessment of bone metabolism. Clin Rheum Dis 1994;20:589.

[113] Charles P, Hasling C, Risteli L, et al. Assessment of bone formation by biochemical markers in metabolic bone disease: separation between osteoblastic activity at the cell and tissue level. Calcif Tiss Int 1992;51:406.

[114] Eriksen EF, Charles P, Melsen F, et al. Serum markers of type I collagen formation and degradation in metabolic bone disease: correlation to bone histomorphometry. J Bone Miner Res 1993;8:127.

[115] Hassager AC, Risteli J, Risteli L, et al. Diurnal variation in serum markers of type I collagen synthesis and degradation in healthy premenopausal women. J Bone Miner Res 1992;7:1307.

[116] Kushida K, Takahashi M, Kawana K, Inoue T. Comparison of markers for bone formation and

resorption in premenopausal and postmenopausal subjects, and osteoporosis patients. J Clin Endocrinol Metab 1995;80:2447–55.

[117] Delmas PD. Biochemical markers of bone turnover. J Bone Miner Res 1993;8(Suppl 2): S549–55.

[118] Simon LS, Krane SM, Wortman PD, et al. Serum levels of type I and type III procollagen fragments in Paget's disease of bone. J Clin Endocrinol Metab 1984;58:110–20.

[119] Robins SP, Black D, Paterson CR, et al. Evaluation of urinary hydroxypyridinium crosslink measurements as resorption markers in metabolic bone diseases. Eur J Clin Invest 1991;21:310.

[120] Delmas P, Geneyts E, Bertholin A, et al. Immunoassay of pyridinoline crosslink excretion in normal adults and in Paget's disease. J Bone Miner Res 1993;8:643–8.

[121] Kivirikko KI. Urinary excretion of hydroxyproline in health and disease. Int Rev Connect Tissue Res 1970;5:93.

[122] Weiss PH, Klein L. The quantitative relationship of urinary peptide hydroxyproline excretion to collagen degradation. J Clin Invest 1969;48:1.

[123] Parfitt AM, Simon L, Villanueva AR, et al. Procollagen type I carboxy-terminal extension peptide in serum as a marker of collagen synthesis in bone. Correlation with iliac bone formation rates and comparison with total alkaline phosphate. J Bone Miner Res 1987;2:427.

[124] Epstein S. Serum and urinary markers of bone remodeling. Endocr Rev 1988;9:437.

[125] Delmas PD. Clinical use of biochemical markers of bone remodeling in osteoporosis. Bone 1992;13:S17.

[126] Uebelhart D, Gineyts E, Chapuy M-C, et al. Urinary excretion of pyridinium crosslinks: a new marker of bone resorption in metabolic bone disease. Bone Miner 1990;8:87.

[127] Beardsworth LJ, Eyre DR, Dickson IR. Changes with age in the urinary excretion of Lysyl- and hydroxylysylpyridinoline, two new markers of bone collagen turnover. J Bone Miner Res 1990;5:671.

[128] Panigrahi K, Delmas PD, Singer F, et al. Characteristics of a two-site immunoradiometric assay for human skeletal alkaline phosphatase in serum. Clin Chem 1994;40:822–8.

[129] Black D, Marabani M, Sturrock RD, et al. Urinary excretion of the hydroxypyridinium cross links of collagen in patients with rheumatoid arthritis. Ann Rheum Dis 1989;48:641.

[130] Harvey RD, McHardy KC, Reid IW, et al. Measurement of bone collagen degradation in hyperthyroidism and during thyroxine replacement therapy using pyridium cross-links as specific urinary markers. J Clin Endocrinol Metab 1991;72:1189.

[131] Reiser K, McCormick RJ, Rucker RB. Enzymatic and nonenzymatic crosslinking of collagen and elastin. FASEB J 1992;6:2439.

[132] Greenwald RA. Monitoring collagen degradation in patients with arthritis. Arthritis Rheum 1996;39:1455–65.

[133] Cummings SR, Black D, Ensrud K, et al. Urine markers of bone resorption predict bone loss and fractures in older women: the study of osteoporotic fractures. J Bone Miner Res 1996; 11:S128.

[134] Ganero P, Hausherr E, Chapuy M-C, et al. Markers of bone resorption predict fractures in elderly women: the EPIDOS Prospective Study. J Bone Miner Res 1996;11:1531–8.

[135] Singh M, Riggs BL, Beabout JW, et al. Femoral trabecular-pattern index for evaluation of spinal osteoporosis. Ann Intern Med 1972;77:63.

[136] Meema HE, Meema S. Cortical bone mineral density versus cortical thickness in diagnosis of osteoporosis: a roentgenologic-densitometric study. J Am Geriatr Soc 1969;17:120.

[137] Hall FM, David MA, Baran DT. Bone mineral screening for osteoporosis. N Engl J Med 1987;316:212.

[138] Pouilles JM, Tremollieres F, Louvet JP, et al. Sensitivity of dual-photon absorptiometry in spinal osteoporosis. Calcif Tisse Int 1988;43:329.

[139] Bergot C, Laval-Jeantet A-M, Preteux F, et al. Measurement of anisotropic vertebral trabecular bone loss during aging by quantitative image analysis. Calcif Tissue Int 1988;43:143.

[140] Kelly TJ, Slovik DM, Schoenfeld DA, et al. Quantitative digital radiography versus dual photon absorptiometry of the lumbar spine. J Clin Endocrin Metab 1988;67:839

[141] Baran DR, Kelly AM, Karellas A, et al. Ultrasound attenuation of the os calcis in women with osteoporosis and hip fractures. Calcif Tissue Int 1988;43:138.

[142] Libanati CR, Schulz EE, Shook JE, et al. Hip mineral density in females with a recent hip fracture. J Clin Endocrinol Metab 1992;74:351.

[143] Johnston Jr CC, Melton III LJ, Lindsay R, Eddy DM. Clinical indications for bone mass measurements. A report from the Scientific Advisory Board of the National Osteoporosis Foundation. J Bone Miner Res 1989;4(Suppl):2.

[144] Slemenda CW, Hill SL, Longcope C, et al. Predictors of bone mass in perimenopausal women. Ann Intern Med 1990;112:96.

[145] Cosman F, Schnitzer MB, McCann PD, et al. Relationships between quantitative histological measurements and noninvasive assessments of bone mass. Bone 1992;13:237.

[146] Genant HK, Ettinger B, Cann CE, et al. Osteoporosis: assessment by quantitative computed tomography. Orthop Clin North Am 1985;16:557.

[147] Poss PD, Davis JW, Vogel JM, Wasnich RD. A critical review of bone mass and the risk of fractures in osteoporosis. Calcif Tissue Int 1990;46:149–61.

[148] Sartoris DJ, André M, Resnick C, et al. Trabecular bone density in the proximal femur: quantitative CT assessment. Radiology 1986;160:707.

[149] Gonnelli S, Cepollaro C, Agnusdei D, et al. Diagnostic value of ultrasound analysis and bone densitometry as predictors of vertebral deformity in postmenopausal women. Osteoporos Int 1995;5:413–8.

[150] Riggs BL, Wahner HW, Dunn WL, et al. Differential changes in bone mineral density of the appendicular and axial skeleton with aging. J Clin Invest 1981;67:328.

[151] Symmons DPM, Van Hemert AM, Vanderbroncke JP, et al. A longitudinal study of back pain and radiological changes in the lumber spine of middle aged women. II. Radiographic findings. Ann Rheum Dis 1991;50:162.

[152] Ryan PJ, Evans P, Gibson T, et al. Osteoporosis and chronic back pain: a study with single-photon emission computed tomography bone scintigraphy. J Bone Miner Res 1992;7:1455.

[153] Ryan PJ, Evans P, Gibson T, et al. Chronic low back pain: comparison of bone SPECT with radiography and CT. Radiology 1992;182:849.

[154] Christiansen C. Consensus development conference on osteoporosis. Am J Med 1991; 91(5B):1S.

[155] Prince RL, Smith M, Dick IM, et al. Prevention of postmenopausal osteoporosis. A comparative study of exercise, calcium supplementation, and hormone-replacement therapy. N Engl J Med 1991;325:1190.

[156] Dawson-Hughes BD, Dallal GE, Krall EA, et al. A controlled trial of the effect of calcium supplementation on bone density in postmenopausal women. N Engl J Med 1990; 323:878.

[157] Elders PJM, Netelenbos JC, Lips P, et al. Calcium supplementation reduces vertebral bone loss in perimenopausal women: a controlled trial in 248 women between 46 and 55 years of age. J Clin Endocrinol Metab 1991;73:533.

[158] Reid IR, Ames RW, Evans MC, et al. Effect of calcium supplementation on bone loss in postmenopausal women. N Engl J Med 1993;328:460.

[159] Christiansen C. Prevention and treatment of osteoporosis: a review of current modalities. Bone 1992;13:S35.

[160] Gallagher JC, Riggs BL, Eisman J, et al. Intestinal calcium absorption and serum vitamin D metabolites in normal subjects and osteoporotic patients. J Clin Invest 1979;64:729.

[161] Bullamore JR, Gallagher JC, Wilkinson R, et al. Effect of age on calcium absorption. Lancet 1970;2:535.

[162] Alevizaki CC, Ikkos DG, Singhelakis P. Progressive decrease of true intestinal calcium absorption with age in normal man. J Nucl Med 1973;14:760.

[163] Aloia JF, Vaswani A, Yeh JK, et al. Calcium supplementation with and without hormone replacement therapy to prevent postmenopausal bone loss. Ann Int Med 1994;120:97–103.

[164] Chapuy MC, Arlot ME, Duboeuf F, et al. Vitamin D_3 and calcium to prevent hip fractures in elderly women. N Engl J Med 1992;327:1637–42.

[165] Tilyard MW, Spears GFS, Thomson J, Dovey S. Treatment of postmenopausal osteoporosis with calcitriol or calcium. N Engl J Med 1992;326:357–62.

[166] Sambrook P, Birmingham J, Kelley P, et al. Prevention of corticosteroid osteoporosis: a comparison of calcium, calcitriol, and calcitonin. N Engl J Med 1993;328:1747–52.

[167] Richelson LS, Heinz WW, Melton LJ, Riggs BL. Relative contributions of aging and estrogen deficiency to postmenopausal bone loss. N Engl J Med 1984;311:1273–5.

[168] Prior JC, Vigna YM, Barr SI, et al. Cyclic medroxyprogesterone treatment increases bone density. Am J Med 1994;96:521.

[169] Felson DT, Zhang Y, Hannah MT, et al. The effect of postmenopausal estrogen therapy on bone density in elderly women. N Engl J Med 1993;329:1141–6.

[170] Lafferty FW, Fiske ME. Postmenopausal estrogen replacement: a long term cohort study. Am J Med 1994;97:66.

[171] Cauley JA, Seely DG, Ensrud K, et al. Estrogen replacement therapy and fractures in older women. Ann Int Med 1995;122:9–16.

[172] Grisso JA, Kelsey JL, Strom BL, et al. Risk factors for hip fracture in black women. N Engl J Med 1994;330:1555–9.

[173] Lindsay R, Hart DM, Forrest C, et al. Prevention of spinal osteoporosis in oophorectomised women. Lancet 1980;2:1151.

[174] Nachtigall LE, Nachtigall RH, Nachtigall RD, et al. Estrogen replacement therapy 1: a 10-year prospective study in the relationship to osteoporosis. Obstet Gynecol 1979;53:277.

[175] Munk-Jensen N, Nielsen SP, Eriksen PB. Reversal of postmenopausal vertebral bone loss by oestrogen and progestogen: a double blind placebo controlled study. BMJ 1988;296:1150.

[176] Ettinger B, Genant HK, Cann CE. Long-term estrogen replacement therapy prevents bone loss and fractures. Ann Intern Med 1985;102:319.

[177] Kiel DP, Felson DT, Anderson JJ, et al. Hip fracture and the use of estrogens in postmenopausal women. N Engl J Med 1987;317:1169.

[178] Naessen T, Persson I, Adami H-O, et al. Hormone replacement therapy and the risk for the first hip fracture. A prospective, population-based cohort study. Ann Intern Med 1990; 113:95.

[179] Paganini-Hill A, Ross RK, Gerkins VR, et al. Menopausal estrogen therapy and hip fractures. Ann Intern Med 1981;95:28.

[180] Weiss NS, Ure CL, Ballard JH, et al. Decreased risks of fractures of the hip and lower forearm with postmenopausal use of estrogen. N Engl J Med 1980;303:1195.

[181] Lufkin EG, Wahner HW, O'Fallon WM, et al. Treatment of postmenopausal osteoporosis with transdermal estrogen. Ann Intern Med 1992;117:1.

[182] Adami S, Suppi R, Bertoldo F, et al. Transdermal estradiol in the treatment of postmenopausal bone loss. Bone Min 1989;7:79.

[183] Lindsay R, Hart DM, Clark DM. The minimum effective dose of estrogen for prevention of postmenopausal bone loss. Obstet Gynecol 1984;63:759.

[184] Ettinger B, Genant HK, Cann CE. Postmenopausal bone loss is prevented by treatment with low-dosage estrogen with calcium. Ann Intern Med 1987;106:40.

[185] Whitehead MI, Townsend PT, Pryse-Davies J, et al. Effects of estrogens and progestins on the biochemistry and morphology of the postmenopausal endometrium. N Engl J Med 1981; 304:1599.

[186] Christiansen C, Riis BJ. 17β-estradiol and continuous norethisterone: a unique treatment for established osteoporosis in elderly women. J Clin Endocrinol Metab 1990;71:836.

[187] Grady D, Rubin SM, Petitti DB, et al. Hormone therapy to prevent disease and prolong life in postmenopausal women. Ann Intern Med 1992;117:1016.

[188] Steinberg KK, Thacker SB, Smith J, et al. A meta-analysis of the effect of estrogen replacement therapy on the risk of breast cancer. JAMA 1991;1:265.

[189] Colditz GA, Stampfer MJ, Willett WC, et al. Prospective study of estrogen replacement therapy and risk in breast cancer in postmenopausal women. JAMA 1990;264:2648.

[190] Berkvist L, Adami H-O, Persson I, et al. The risk of breast cancer after estrogen and estrogen-progestin replacement. N Engl J Med 1989;321:293.

[191] Henderson BE, Ross RK, Lobo RA, et al. Re-evaluating the role of progestogen therapy after the menopause. Fertil Steril 1988;49(Suppl 5):9S.

[192] Schneider DL, Barrett-Connor EL, Morton DJ. Thyroid hormone use and bone mineral density in elderly women. JAMA 1994;271:1245–9.

[193] Srivastava M, Deal C. Osteoporosis in elderly: prevention and treatment. Clin Geriatr Med 2002;18(3):529–55.

[194] Montemurro L, Schiraldi G, Fraiolo P, et al. Prevention of corticosteroid-induced osteoporosis with salmon calcitonin in sarcoid patients. Calcif Tissue Int 1991;49:71–6.

[195] Mazzuoli GF, Passeri M, Gennari C, et al. Effects of salmon calcitonin in postmenopausal osteoporosis: a controlled double-blind clinical study. Calcif Tissue Int 1986;38:3.

[196] Gennari C, Chierichetti SM, Bigazzi S, et al. Comparative effects on bone mineral content of calcium and calcium plus salmon calcitonin given in two different regimens in postmenopausal osteoporosis. Curr Ther Res 1985;38:455.

[197] MacIntyre I, Whitehead BI, Banks LM, et al. Calcitonin for prevention of postmenopausal bone loss. Lancet 1988;1:900.

[198] Overgaard K. Effect of intranasal salmon calcitonin therapy on bone mass and bone turn-over in early postmenopausal women: a dose response study. Calcific Tissue Int 1994;55:82–6.

[199] Overgaard K, Riis BJ, Christinasen C, Hansen MA. Effect of salcotonin given intranasally on early postmenopausal bone loss. Br J Med 1989;299:477–9.

[200] Overgaard K, Hansen MA, Jensen SB, et al. Effect of salcatonin given intranasally on bone mass and fracture rates in established osteoporosis. BMJ 1992;305:556.

[201] Overgaard K, Hansen MA, Christiansen C. Effect of intranasal calcitonin on bone mass and fracture rates in elderly women. A dose-response study [abstract]. J Bone Miner Res 1992;7(Suppl 1):S117.

[202] Gennari C, Agnusdei D, Montagnani M, et al. An effective regimen of intranasal calcitonin in early postmenopausal bone loss. Calcif Tissue Int 1992;50:381.

[203] Overgaard K, Riis BJ, Christiansen C, et al. Effect of salcatonin given intranasally on early postmenopausal bone loss. BMJ 1989;299:477.

[204] Reginster JY. Effect of calcitonin on bone mass and fracture rates. Am J Med 1991;91(Suppl 5B):19S.

[205] Reginster JY, Albert A, Lecart MP, et al. One-year controlled randomised trial of prevention of early postmenopausal bone loss by intranasal calcitonin. Lancet 1987;2:1481.

[206] Overgaard K, Hansen MA, Christiansen C. Effect of intranasal calcitonin on bone mass and bone turnover in early postmenopausal women [abstract]. J Bone Miner Res 1992;7(Suppl 1):S140.

[207] Civitelli R, Gonnelli S, Zachei F, et al. Bone turnover in postmenopausal osteoporosis. Effect of calcitonin therapy. J Clin Invest 1988;82:1268–74.

[208] Lyritis GP, Tsakalabos S, Magiasis B, et al. Analgesic effect of salmon calcitonin on osteo-porotic vertebral fractures. Double-blind, placebo-controlled study. Calcif Tissue Int 1991;49:369–72.

[209] Watts NB, Harris ST, Genant HK, et al. Intermittent cyclical etidronate treatment of post-menopausal osteoporosis. N Engl J Med 1990;323:73.

[210] Struys A, Snelden AA, Mulder H. Cyclic etidronate reverses bone loss of the spine and proximal femur in patients with established corticosteroid induced osteoporosis. Am J Med 1995;99:235–42.

[211] Harris ST, Watts NB, Jackson RD, et al. Four-year study of intermittent cyclic etidronate treatment of postmenopausal osteoporosis: three years of blinded therapy followed by one year of open therapy. Am J Med 1993;95:557.

[212] Storm T, Thamsborg G, Steiniche T, et al. Effect of intermittent cyclical etidronate therapy on bone mass and fracture rate in women with postmenopausal osteoporosis. N Engl J Med 1990;322:1265–71.

[213] Papapoulos SE, Landman SO, Bijvoet OLM, et al. The use of bisphosphonates in the treatment of osteoporosis. Bone 1992;13(Suppl 1):S41.

[214] Seedor G, Quartuccio HA, Thompson DD. The bisphosphonate alendronate (MK-217) inhibits bone loss due to ovariectomy in rats. J Bone Miner Res 1991;6:339.

[215] Liberman UA, Weiss SR, Broll J, et al. Effect of oral alendronate on bone mineral density and the incidence of fractures in postmenopausal osteoporosis. N Engl J Med 1995;333:1437–43.

[216] Licata AA. Bisphosphonate therapy. Am J Med Sci 1997;313:1.

[217] Cohen SB. An update on bisphosphonates. Curr Rheumatol Rep 2004;6:59–65.

[218] Black DM, Cummings SR, Karpf DB, et al. Randomized trial of effect of alendronate on risk of fracture in women with existing vertebral fractures. Lancet 1996;348:1535–41.

[219] Geusens P, Nijs J, Van der Perre G, et al. Longitudinal effect on tiludronate on bone mineral density, resonant frequency and strength in monkeys. J Bone Miner Res 1992;7:599.

[220] Reginster JY, Deroisy R, Denis D, et al. Prevention of postmenopausal bone loss by tiludronate. Lancet 1989;2:1469.

[221] Riggs BL, Baylink DJ, Kleerekoper M, et al. Incidence of hip fractures in osteoporotic women treated with sodium fluoride. J Bone Miner Res 1987;2:123.

[222] Riggs BL, Hodgson SF, O'Fallon WM, et al. Effect of fluoride treatment on the fracture rate in postmenopausal women with osteoporosis. N Engl J Med 1990;322:802.

[223] Pak CYC, Sakhaee K, Adams-Huet B, et al. Treatment of postmenopausal osteoporosis with slow-release sodium fluoride. Ann Int Med 1995;123:401–8.

[224] Reeve J, Meunier PJ, Parsons JA, et al. Anabolic effect of human parathyroid hormone fragment on trabecular bone in involutional osteoporosis: a multicenter trial. BMJ 1980; 280:1340.

[225] Reeve J, Bradbeer JN, Arlot M, et al. hPTH 1–34 treatment of osteoporosis with added hormone replacement therapy: biochemical, kinetic and histological responses. Osteoporos Int 1991;1:162.

[226] Slovik DM, Neer RM, Potts JT. Short-term effects of synthetic human parathyroid hormone-(1–34) administration on bone mineral metabolism in osteoporotic patients. J Clin Invest 1981;68:1261.

[227] Neer R, Slovik D, Daly M, et al. Treatment of postmenopausal osteoporosis with daily parathyroid hormone plus calcitriol. In: Chritstiansen C, Overgaard K, editors. Osteoporosis 1990: Proceedings of the Third International Symposium on Osteoporosis. Copenhagen: Osteopress Aps; 1990. p. 1314.

[228] Neer RM, Slovik DM, Doppelt S, et al. The use of parathyroid hormone plus 1,25-dihydroxyvitamin D to increase trabecular bone in osteoporotic men and postmenopausal women. In: Chritstiansen C, Overgaard K, editors. Osteoporosis 1990: Proceedings of the Third International Symposium on Osteoporosis. Copenhagen: Osteopress Aps; 1990. p. 829.

[229] Finkelstein JS, Klibanski A, Schaefer EH, et al. Parathyroid hormone for the prevention of bone loss induced by estrogen deficiency. N Engl J Med 1994;331:1618–23.

[230] Horwitz M, Stewart A, Greenspan SL. Sequential parathyroid hormone/alendronate therapy for osteoporosis—robbing Peter to pay Paul? J Clin Endocrinol Metab 2000;85:2129–34.

[231] Brixen KT, Christensen PM, Ejersted C, Langdahl BL. Teriparatide (biosynthetic human parathyroid hormone 1–34): a new paradigm in the treatment of osteoporosis. Basic Clin Pharmacol Toxicol 2004;94:260–70.

[232] Conn D. New ways with old bones. Osteoporosis researchers look for drugs to replace hormone replacement therapy. Lancet 2004;363:786–7.

[233] Chestnut III CH, Ivey JL, Gruber HE, et al. Stanazol in the postmenopausal osteoporosis: therapeutic efficacy and possible mechanisms of action. Metabolism 1983;32:571–80.

[234] Hassager C, Riis BJ, Podenphat J, Chrisitnasen C. Nadrolone decanoate treatment of postmenopausal osteoporosis for 2 years and effects of withdrawal. Maturitas 1989;11:305–17.

[235] Meunier PJ, Roux C, Seeman E, et al. The effects of strontium ranelate on the risk of vertebral fracture in women with postmenopausal osteoporosis. N Engl J Med 2004;350:459–68.

[236] Compston J. Prevention of vertebral fractures by strontium ranelate in postmenopausal women with osteoporosis. Osteoporosis International; published online October 12, 2004.

ELSEVIER
SAUNDERS

CLINICS IN
GERIATRIC
MEDICINE

Clin Geriatr Med 21 (2005) 631–647

Vasculitis in the Geriatric Population

Carol A. Langford, MD, MHS

*Center for Vasculitis Care and Research, Department of Rheumatic and Immunologic Diseases,
The Cleveland Clinic Foundation, 9500 Euclid Avenue, A50, Cleveland, OH 44195, USA*

Vasculitis is histologically defined by the presence of blood vessel inflammation. As a result of this vascular inflammation, stenoses may develop with subsequent tissue ischemia or there may be attenuation of the vessel wall leading to aneurysm formation or hemorrhage. Vasculitis can occur as a primary disease entity in which no currently identified cause has been identified or secondary to an underlying disease or exposure.

Patient age can play a very important role in many different facets of vasculitic disease. The most common form of systemic vasculitis seen in humans, giant cell arteritis (GCA), occurs almost exclusively in people over the age of 50. For this and many other forms of vasculitic disease that can develop in older patients the challenges of diagnosis and treatment can be further compounded by the presence of comorbid diseases and concomitant medications.

This article will seek to review the vasculitic diseases that may be most frequently encountered in patients over the age of 65 as well as management issues that warrant special consideration in geriatric vasculitis patients.

Vasculitic disease in patients over age 65

Primary vasculitic diseases

The first account of a primary systemic vasculitic disease was made in 1866 when Kussmaul and Maier [1] described a disease process characterized by nodular inflammation of the muscular arteries that they named periarteritis nodosa (later referred to as polyarteritis nodosa [PAN]). During the 1900s, the

---

E-mail address: langfoc@ccf.org

description of clinical entities associated with vasculitis emerged, and in 1952, Zeek [2] proposed the first classification system for the vasculitic diseases. Since that time, the nomenclature and classification of the vasculitides has continued to evolve. One means of categorizing the vasculitic diseases is based upon the predominant size of blood vessel involvement [3,4].

Large vessel vasculitis
Giant cell arteritis and polymyalgia rheumatica.   GCA, also called temporal arteritis, is a granulomatous arteritis of the aorta and its major branches that has a predilection to affect the extracranial branches of the carotid artery [5,6]. It is seen more frequently in women at a ratio of 2:1, and is the most common form of systemic vasculitis, with an incidence of 18.8 cases per 100,000 person-years in Olmstead County, Minnesota [7].

   The predilection for GCA to occur in older patients has been considered by many to be a defining parameter in its diagnosis. Takayasu's arteritis, another form of large vessel vasculitis, predominantly affects women of child-bearing age. However, the shared presence of granulomatous aortitis has raised the question as to whether these represent a similar underlying disease that can have a differing clinical spectrum.

   Patients with GCA will typically present with headache, jaw, or tongue claudication, scalp tenderness, constitutional features, or fever [8]. The most dreaded complication of GCA is vision loss due to optic nerve ischemia from arteritis involving vessels of the ocular circulation [9,10]. Limb claudication reflecting involvement of the primary branches of the aorta occurs in 15% of cases [11]. Findings on physical examination in GCA include nodularity, tenderness, or absent pulsations of the temporal arteries or other involved vessels.

   An elevated erythrocyte sedimentation rate (ESR) occurs in greater than 80% of patients, and when seen together with compatible clinical features, suggests the diagnosis of GCA. Temporal artery biopsy is confirmatory in 50% to 80% of cases with the demonstration of a panmural mononuclear cell infiltration that can be granulomatous with histiocytes and giant cells. To increase yield, the length of biopsy specimen should be at least 3 to 5 cm and sampled at multiple levels. In patients strongly suspected of having GCA, treatment should be instituted immediately to protect vision while a prompt temporal artery biopsy is being arranged [12].

   Glucocorticoids prevent visual complications in GCA and bring about a rapid improvement in clinical symptoms [9,13–15]. The optimal initial dosage has remained a point of differing opinion, but most investigators support that prednisone be initiated at a dose of 40 to 60 mg/d. In patients who present with acute visual loss, methylprednisolone 1 g/d for 3 days can be considered, with the goal being to protect the remaining vision [16]. Symptomatic improvement usually occurs within the first 1 to 2 weeks following the initiation of prednisone, accompanied by a reduction in ESR over the first month. Although there is no standardized prednisone tapering method, after 2 to 4 weeks when symptomatic improvement has occurred, prednisone can be reduced by 5-mg increments every 1 to 2 weeks until 20 mg is reached, at which time the decrements are made at 2- to 4-week intervals. After reaching a dosage of prednisone 10 mg/d, then the dosage would be reduced by 1-mg increments each month. Most patients require glucocorticoids for at least 2 years, with many receiving over 4 years of treatment [17–22]. The ability of methotrexate (MTX) to decrease relapses and lessen glucocorticoid treatment was examined in two randomized studies that reaching different conclusions [23,24]. To date, no cytotoxic or biologic agent has been reproducibly found to effectively reduce the use of prednisone and lower its risk of side effects, although novel therapeutic approaches remain under active investigation. Current evidence supports that low-dose aspirin may play a beneficial role in reducing cranial ischemic complications in GCA, and should be considered in all patients who do not have contraindications [25].

The clinical course of patients with GCA is assessed on the basis of symptoms and signs. ESR can be useful parameter to follow, but may remain elevated in some patients and is not consistently reliable in assessing disease activity or guiding therapy. Approximately 26% to 90% of patients experience one or more relapses requiring an increase or reinstitution of prednisone [17,18,20–22,24].

Acute mortality from GCA is uncommon, although thoracic aortic aneurysms may occur as a late complication of disease, and can be associated with rupture and death [26,27]. Morbidity may occur as a result of ocular or large vessel disease or from glucocorticoid-related toxicities.

Polymyalgia rheumatica (PMR) is characterized by aching and morning stiffness along the proximal muscles of the shoulder and hip girdle [28,29]. PMR can occur in 40% to 50% of patients with GCA or as an isolated entity in which 10% to 15% of patients may later go onto have GCA. This clinical association, together with evidence from the laboratory, has supported that PMR and GCA represent clinical subsets of a single disease process [30,31]. The diagnosis of isolated PMR is based upon consistent symptoms together with acute phase parameters that include an increased ESR and anemia. Further support for the diagnosis of PMR is provided by a rapid symptomatic response to prednisone 10 to 20 mg/d. Similar to GCA, prednisone is slowly tapered, based upon symptoms and acute phase parameters, and may require dosage increases for clinical relapses [32]. The use of MTX in PMR has been examined, and use of this agent must be weighed against its risks [33,34].

Medium vessel vasculitis
Polyarteritis nodosa. As understanding of the vasculitides has grown, the classification of PAN has undergone a number of changes. In the nomenclature system published in 1994 from the Chapel Hill Consensus Conference, PAN was defined by the presence necrotizing inflammation of medium-sized or small arteries without glomerulonephritis or vasculitis in arterioles, capillaries, or venules [3,35]. Using this definition, PAN is believed to be very uncommon, but it remains an important multisystem illness that can present acutely in older patients [36].

The most common clinical manifestations of PAN include hypertension, fever, musculoskeletal symptoms, and vasculitis involving the nerve, gastrointestinal tract, heart, and nonglomerular renal vessels. Laboratory findings reflect an acute inflammatory process with anemia, leukocytosis, thrombocytosis, and an increased ESR. Antineutrophil cytoplasmic antibodies (ANCA) are uncommon in patients with PAN [37].

The diagnosis of PAN is made on the basis of biopsy or arteriography. Biopsies of clinically involved areas such as the peripheral nerve or testicle reveal necrotizing inflammation involving the medium-sized or small arteries with abundant neutrophils, fibrinoid changes, and disruption of the internal elastic lamina. Arteriography is most often performed of the visceral and renal circulation, and demonstrates microaneurysms, stenoses, or a beaded pattern with areas of arterial narrowing and dilation.

Patients with immediately life-threatening disease affecting the gastrointestinal system, heart, or central nervous system (CNS) should be treated with daily cyclophosphamide (CYC) 2 mg/kg/d and glucocorticoids [38–40]. In patients where the disease manifestations do not pose an immediate threat to life or major organ function, glucocorticoids alone can be considered as initial therapy, with CYC being added in patients who continue to have evidence of active disease or who are unable to taper prednisone [39,41]. Relapses occur in <10% of patients with PAN [39].

A PAN-like vasculitis can also be seen in patients infected with hepatitis B, hepatitis C, or the HIV [42]. In these settings, antiviral therapy should be part of the treatment regimen, with the goal being to contain viral replication and favor seroconversion. To initially gain control of the vasculitis, patients may require glucocorticoids, alone or combined with CYC, depending on the disease severity. Some investigators also advocate the use of plasmapheresis [43–45]. Once clinical improvement is observed, immunosuppressive therapies should be rapidly withdrawn while antiviral treatment is continued, as the virus will persist and replicate in the setting of immunosuppression.

The estimated 5-year survival rate of PAN with treatment is 80%, with mortality being influenced by disease severity [39].

Small vessel vasculitic diseases

Vasculitis involving the small vessels clinically manifests in a variety of ways that can include cutaneous vasculitis, alveolar hemorrhage, and glomerulonephritis. These features can be seen in a spectrum of diseases that may have differing clinical presentations and severity.

Small vessel vasculitis is a prominent feature of three important forms of primary systemic vasculitis: Wegener's granulomatosis (WG), microscopic polyangiitis (MPA), and Churg-Strauss syndrome (CSS). Although these disease entities possess unique features, because they share similar involvement of the small vessels, glomerular histology, and the frequent association with ANCA, these diseases have been grouped together by some investigators for the purposes of therapeutic and epidemiologic studies.

The age of onset for the small vessel vasculitides has been an interesting area of epidemiologic investigation. Although some WG series have found a median age of diagnosis in the 40s [46,47], two studies from Europe demonstrated a much older age of disease presentation. In a study conducted in Sweden, Tidman and colleagues [48] found a frequency peak for ANCA-associated vasculitides in men ages 55 to 64. Watts and associates [49], in the United Kingdom, found the occurrence of primary systemic vasculitis to increase with age with a peak in the 65- to 74-year-old age group. These experiences underscore that the small vessel vasculitic diseases should remain a diagnostic consideration in all patients, regardless of age.

Wegener's granulomatosis. WG is characterized by a granulomatous inflammation involving the respiratory tract and necrotizing vasculitis affecting the small- to medium-sized vessels in which glomerulonephritis is common [46,47]. Over 90% of patients first seek medical attention for symptoms related to the upper or lower airways. Nasal and sinus mucosal inflammation may result in nasal crusting and epistaxis, with the potential for nasal septum perforation or collapse of the nasal bridge. A diverse range of pulmonary radiographic abnormalities can be seen including single or multiple nodules or infiltrates, cavities, and ground glass infiltrates. Glomerulonephritis can be rapidly progressive and asymptomatic, and is detected by the presence of an active urine sediment with microscopic hematuria and red blood cell casts. Although the sinuses, lungs, and kidneys are the most frequently affected locations, WG is a multisystem disease that can involve the eyes, skin, nerve, and heart with potentially serious consequences.

WG is highly ANCA associated [50,51]. Two types of ANCA have been identified in patients with a primary systemic small vessel vasculitis: ANCA that target the neutrophil serine protease, proteinase 3 (PR3) that causes a cytoplasmic immunofluorescence pattern (cANCA) on ethanol-fixed neutrophils [52] and ANCA directed against the neutrophil enzyme myeloperoxidase (MPO) that generate a perinuclear immunofluorescence pattern (pANCA) [53]. Approximately 75% to 90% of patients with active WG have PR3-ANCA, while 5% to 20% may have MPO-ANCA. With the exception of patients who present with sinus, lung, and renal disease, the predictive value of ANCA is usually insufficient to render a diagnosis of WG. ANCA levels are not static, and will vary during the course of a patient's illness. Although cohort studies observed that patients with active disease had higher levels of ANCA compared with those who were in remission [50,54], changes in sequential ANCA measurement in an individual patient have not been found to be uniformly reliable for assessing disease activity or predicting relapse, and should not be used to guide treatment [55,56]. The role of ANCA in disease pathogenesis remains an active area of investigation [57,58].

The diagnosis of WG is usually based on the presence of characteristic histologic findings in a clinically compatible setting. Nonrenal tissues demonstrate granulomatous inflammation, necrosis, often with aggregates of neutrophils, and necrotizing or granulomatous vasculitis. Surgically obtained biopsies of abnormal pulmonary parenchyma yield diagnostic changes in 91% of cases [59]. Biopsies of the upper airways are less invasive but demonstrate diagnostic features only 21% of the time [60]. The characteristic renal histology is that of a focal, segmental, necrotizing, crescentic glomerulonephritis with few to no immune complexes [61].

The outcome for patients with WG dramatically improved when Fauci and Wolff [62,63] introduced combined therapy with CYC 2 mg/kg/d and prednisone 1 mg/kg/d. This regimen has reproducibly been found to induce remission in 75% to 100% of patients with active WG [46,64,65]. After the first 4 weeks of treatment, if there is evidence of improvement, the prednisone is tapered and discontinued by 6 to 12 months. In the setting of fulminant disease, methylprednisolone 1 g/d may be given in combination with CYC 3 to 4 mg/kg/d for 3 days, after which time it is reduced to 2 mg/kg/d [63]. CYC is associated with substantial toxicity including bone marrow suppression, bladder injury, infertility, myeloproliferative disease, and transitional cell carcinoma of the bladder [66]. To reduce the risk of toxicity, staged therapeutic approaches are now used in which the duration of CYC exposure is limited to the 3- to 6-month period required to induce remission. Following that time, CYC is stopped and switched to azathioprine (AZA) 2 mg/kg/d [65] or MTX 20 to 25 mg/wk [64,67] to maintain remission. Maintenance therapy is given for 1 to 2 years, after which time if patients remain in remission, it is tapered and discontinued. In patients who have active but non–life-threatening disease who do not have renal or hepatic contraindications, MTX 20 to 25 mg/wk together with prednisone can be used to induce and maintain remission [68].

Despite the ability to successfully induce remission, relapse occurs in at least 50% of patients with WG. The ability of trimethoprim/sulfamethoxazole (T/S) to reduce relapse was examined in a randomized trial. Although an overall higher rate of relapse at 24 months was observed in patients who received placebo compared with T/S, T/S did not lessen relapses involving organ systems outside of the upper airways when examined by organ system [69]. As discussed later in this review, one of the most important roles for T/S in WG is in the prevention of *Pneumocystis carinii* pneumonia. In patients receiving MTX, T/S can safely be administered at prophylactic doses but should not be given twice daily as bone marrow suppression can occur [70].

Before the introduction of treatment, WG was uniformly fatal. Effective therapy has brought the potential for long-term survival, although substantial morbidity can still result from both the disease and its treatment.

Microscopic polyangiitis.   MPA is characterized by necrotizing vasculitis with few or no immune deposits affecting small vessels. It was nosologically separated from PAN in conjunction with the Chapel Hill consensus definitions, and there remain limited data on this entity as an independent process [3]. MPA has many similarities to WG, but is currently said to be differentiated by the absence of granulomatous inflammation.

The presentation of MPA can be acute and severe, with features including glomerulonephritis, pulmonary hemorrhage, mononeuritis multiplex, and fever [71,72]. MPA is diagnosed by histologic demonstration of necrotizing vasculitis of the small vessels or small- to medium-sized arteries in which granulomatous inflammation is absent. Biopsies of lung tissue typically reveal capillaritis, hemorrhage into the alveolar space, and the absence of immunofluorescence, as would be seen in antiglomerular basement membrane antibody disease (Goodpasture's syndrome). The renal histology is similar to that observed in WG in being a focal segmental necrotizing glomerulonephritis with few to no immune complexes. MPA is also highly ANCA-associated with 50% to 80% having MPO-ANCA while 10% to 50% may be PR3-ANCA positive.

Patients with MPA should initially be treated with CYC 2 mg/kg/d and prednisone 1 mg/kg/d, with transition to a less toxic maintenance agent after remission as discussed for WG [65,72,73]. Relapses occur in at least 34% of patients with MPA with the estimated 5-year survival rate being 74% [71].

Churg-Strauss syndrome. CSS is a rare disease characterized by asthma, peripheral and tissue eosinophilia, and necrotizing vasculitis affecting the small to medium sized vessels [74–77]. CSS has been thought of as having three phases: a prodromal phase, with allergic rhinitis and asthma, a phase characterized by peripheral eosinophilia and eosinophilic tissue infiltrates, and ultimately vasculitic disease, which can involve the nerve, lung, heart, gastrointestinal tract, and kidney. These phases may not be clinically identifiable in all patients, and they often do not occur in sequence.

Histologic features of CSS include eosinophilic tissue infiltrates, extravascular "allergic" granuloma, and small vessel necrotizing vasculitis [74]. The constellation of clinical manifestations in CSS is of great importance in the diagnosis, as evidence of vasculitis can be difficult to establish. ANCA are less commonly seen in CSS with 3% to 35% having PR3-ANCA and 2% to 50% having MPO-ANCA.

Prednisone 1 mg/kg/d is effective for many manifestations of CSS. Relapses of vasculitic disease occur in at least 26% of CSS patients, and asthma often persists after remission of the vasculitis, limiting the ability for prednisone to be completely tapered [75]. It is unclear whether an association exists between leukotriene receptor antagonists and CSS, and use of these agents should be avoided [78]. Combined therapy with glucocorticoids and CYC 2 mg/kg/d in CSS is reserved for patients with life-threatening vasculitis.

The outcome of patients with CSS is influenced by the presence of severe disease involving sites such as the heart, gastrointestinal tract, CNS, and kidney. Cardiac involvement is the main cause of patient mortality and is a poor prognostic sign.

Isolated cutaneous vasculitis. Cutaneous vasculitis is the most commonly encountered vasculitic manifestation. Cutaneous vasculitis typically manifests as palpable purpura, but may present as necrotic papules, or ulcerative lesions

[79,80]. Cutaneous vasculitis is histologically characterized by the presence of small vessel inflammation within the dermis, often with leukocytoclasis.

In over 70% of cases, cutaneous vasculitis occurs secondary to an underlying disease or exposure or as a heralding feature of a primary vasculitic disease [79–81]. An isolated idiopathic cutaneous vasculitis should only be diagnosed after other causes have been ruled out. Biopsy of a skin lesion can confirm the presence of vasculitis and provide clues to the underlying process through cultures and immunofluorescence studies.

The course of idiopathic cutaneous vasculitis can range from a single episode to multiple protracted recurrences, and progression to a systemic vasculitis occurs infrequently. There are no uniformly effective treatments for idiopathic cutaneous vasculitis, and the least toxic treatment that provides benefit should be employed. Glucocorticoids, nonsteroidal antiinflammatory agents, antihistamines, dapsone, and colchicine have been used. Because idiopathic cutaneous vasculitis is limited to the skin, the risks of cytotoxic agents must be weighed against the uncertain benefits, and should be reserved for very select cases in which patients have severe disease that is unresponsive to other measures or when glucocorticoids cannot be tapered.

Henoch-Schönlein purpura.   Henoch-Schönlein purpura (HSP) is a small vessel vasculitis characterized by the presence of IgA-dominant immune deposits [82]. Although HSP predominantly affects children with 75% of cases occurring before 8 years of age, adults can rarely be affected.

The clinical manifestations of HSP include palpable purpura, arthritis, glomerulonephritis, and gastrointestinal involvement. Less is known about HSP in adults, although several studies suggest a more severe clinical syndrome may occur, particularly with regard to glomerulonephritis [83–85].

The diagnosis of HSP is established by the characteristic pattern of clinical manifestations. Skin biopsy reveals leukocytoclastic vasculitis with IgA deposition in blood vessel walls.

HSP is a self-limited condition that rarely requires treatment. Glucocorticoids are of no proven benefit in skin or renal disease, and do not appear to lessen the likelihood of relapse. In patients with glomerulonephritis who have a rising creatinine, treatment with CYC and prednisone may be considered. Outcome data largely comes from pediatric series where recurrence occurs in up to 40% of cases. Disease-related mortality occurs in only 1% to 3% of patients.

Secondary vasculitides

Vasculitis occurring secondary to an underlying disease or exposure represents a significant proportion of the vasculitis that is encountered in clinical practice.

Secondary vasculitis most commonly occurs in association with medications, malignancies, infection, or connective tissue diseases [79–81]. Particularly in geriatric patients, the potential for a neoplastic disease or a medication reaction must be carefully examined in any patient who presents with a new cutaneous vasculitis.

Secondary vasculitis is often isolated to the skin, although systemic vasculitis can occur in conjunction with a connective tissue disease, cryoglobulinemic vasculitis, or rarely in conjunction with a medication. An increasing number of medications have been reported to cause vasculitis in association with a positive ANCA. The agents reported to cause ANCA-associated drug-induced vasculitis include propylthiouracil, hydralazine, penicillamine, minocycline, sulfasalzine, as well as others [86]. The clinical manifestations in affected patients range from cutaneous disease to glomerulonephritis and pulmonary hemorrhage. In suspected cases the drug should be withdrawn and immunosuppressive treatment initiated based upon the degree of severity of the vasculitis.

Cryoglobulinemic vasculitis

Cryoglobulins are cold-precipitable monoclonal or polyclonal immunoglobulins. Cryoglobulinemia can be associated with a small vessel vasculitis characterized by palpable purpura, arthritis, weakness, neuropathy, and a membranoproliferative glomerulonephritis [87–89]. Cryoglobulinemic vasculitis most commonly occurs in the setting of chronic hepatitis C viral infection (HCV), but can also be seen with plasma cell or lymphoid neoplasms, infection, inflammatory diseases, or rarely as an idiopathic process [87].

Laboratory features of cryoglobulinemic vasculitis include circulating cryoglobulins, a positive rheumatoid factor, hypocomplementemia, and an elevated ESR. Biopsies of the skin and kidney are not typically required for diagnosis but can be useful in demonstrating deposition of immunoglobulin or complement by immunofluoresence.

Management of cryoglobulinemic vasculitis is directed toward treatment of the underling disease. Antiviral therapy provides the best opportunity for improvement of cryoglobulinemic vasculitis occurring in association with HCV, but long-term resolution is limited to patients who have a sustained virologic response [89,90]. Immunosuppressive therapies and plasmapheresis have been used with brief improvement but are associated with toxicities that preclude them from being effective long-term treatment options.

Cryoglobulinemic vasculitis represents a chronic process in which mortality is usually related to the underlying disease rather than the vasculitis.

Management considerations in the geriatric vasculitis patient

Impact of comorbid diseases

Geriatric patients will frequently have other medical illnesses that can influence the signs and symptoms of a vasculitic disease. This is best exemplified by pulmonary vasculitis where the appearance of radiographic nodules or infiltrates in an older patient may appropriately raise concern for a neoplasm or infection. Concomitant factors such as tobacco use, chronic obstructive pulmonary disease, or other lung disorders may also influence clinical and radiographic presentations.

The presence of comorbid diseases can also impact vasculitis care following diagnosis. Worsening signs or symptoms of an underlying disease could have a similar appearance to vasculitis. In a patient with atherosclerotic coronary artery disease and a systemic vasculitis, new dyspnea and pulmonary infiltrates could be related to a variety of causes that include congestive heart failure, active vasculitis, a medication reaction, or infection.

Increased risk of medication toxicities

Treatment-related toxicities influence outcome in patients with vasculitis, and can present unique challenges in older individuals. Awareness, monitoring, and prevention of medication side effects play an important role in minimizing risk in geriatric patients.

Infection

Infection is a prominent cause of morbidity and mortality in vasculitis patients, and can develop in association with any type of immunosuppressive therapy. In one series of 43 prednisone-treated GCA patients, sepsis and other infectious complications were responsible for 6 of the 19 (32%) observed fatalities seen during the study period [91]. Infection risks are compounded when a cytotoxic agent is used in combination with glucocorticoids. Infections have been reported to occur in 10% to 70% of WG patients [46,64,65,92] and in a long-term survival study of WG patients from the American College of Rheumatology Classification Criteria cohort, Matteson and colleagues [93] found infection to be the number one cause of death responsible for 29% of patient fatalities.

P. carinii pneumonia is a serious opportunistic infection that has been found to occur in approximately 10% of WG patients receiving prednisone in combination with a cytotoxic agent [68,94]. Although large-scale studies in other vasculitic diseases are not available, the presence of published case reports suggests that vasculitis patients who receive similar treatment regimens are also at risk of Pneumocystis. Because of this association, it is recommended that all patients with a vasculitic disease who are receiving combined therapy with glucocorticoids and a cytotoxic agent be given Pneumocystis prophylaxis. Based upon the experience in HIV and leukemia, trimethoprim 160 mg/sulfamethoxazole 800 mg three times weekly or trimethoprim 80 mg/sulfamethoxazole 400 mg daily is recommended [95]. For patients with a severe sulfa allergy, atovaquone 1500 mg daily or inhaled pentamidine 300 mg every 4 weeks may be considered.

Influenza is a potentially life-threatening infection in all geriatric patients. There has been no clear evidence to suggest that influenza immunization has a deleterious impact on vasculitis or its treatment, and it is therefore recommended that all geriatric vasculitis patients continue to receive annual influenza vac-

cinations. Vasculitis patients should only receive inactivated influenza immuni-
zations, as live vaccinations are contraindicated in immunosuppressed hosts.

Glucocorticoids

Glucocorticoids comprise an essential therapeutic component for almost all
forms of primary systemic vasculitis that affect adults. In GCA, 35% to 65%
of treated patients have been found to experience glucocorticoid-related toxicity
[91,96]. Glucocorticoids possess a broad range of potential side effects, many of
which can occur at an increased frequency or have greater potential for clinical
impact in geriatric patients.

Osteoporosis. Glucocorticoids have been well established to reduce bone
density, and by so doing, place geriatric patients at greater risk of fractures
[91,96,97]. Although postmenopausal women are subject to the greatest risk
of bone loss, glucocorticoid-induced osteoporosis can also develop in men.
Glucocorticoid-treated patients should undergo a baseline dual energy x-ray
absorptiometer early in treatment, with regular monitoring thereafter. Preventive
measures to reduce the risk of bone loss and fractures should be initiated in all
glucocorticoid treated patients and include the use of exercise, calcium, and
bisphosphonates in eligible patients and evaluation of the home for fall risks.

Cataracts. Cataracts can occur in a high percentage of glucocorticoid treated
patients. In one series of patients with WG, 21% developed glucocorticoid-
related cataracts [46]. For patients who may already have established cataract
formation, progression may accelerate to the point of significantly impairing
vision. Ophthalmologic assessment at baseline and at regular intervals can be
useful in monitoring for cataract development.

Diabetes mellitus. Glucose intolerance can develop in glucocorticoid-treated
patients. In one study, patients with PMR had greater than two times the risk of
developing diabetes mellitus compared with age- and sex-matched individuals
from the same community [96]. Counseling regarding diet and monitoring of
the serum glucose form important parts in the care of geriatric vasculitis patients
who receive glucocorticoid treatment.

Hypertension. Hypertension is a critical cardiovascular risk factor for complications involving the heart, brain, and kidneys. The presence of renal vascular
disease affecting the large, medium, or small vessels and glucocorticoid treatment increases the potential for hypertension in vasculitis patients. Management
of hypertension in geriatric patients must take into account the presence of comorbid diseases, medication interactions, and the course of the vasculitic disease
and its management.

Myopathy. Myopathy can result from glucocorticoid therapy, and most commonly presents as weakness in the proximal muscles of the shoulder and hip

girdle, limiting the ability to rise from a chair or go up stairs. Glucocorticoid myopathy can be differentiated from muscle weakness due to other causes by location and the presence of normal muscle enzymes. Muscle weakness will characteristically improve as the glucocorticoid dosage is lowered, and may be helped by physical therapy. If myopathy is present, caution for falls should be raised and a careful assessment of the home should be undertaken to reduce the risk for potential injuries.

Cytotoxic therapies

For many vasculitic diseases, optimal treatment includes the use of cytotoxic agents such as CYC, MTX, or AZA. Although these therapies each have individual side effects, there are potential concerns that apply to many of these agents when prescribed in geriatric patients.

Cytopenias.   CYC, MTX, AZA, and many other cytotoxic agents are suppressive to the bone marrow. Geriatric patients receiving cytotoxic treatment may be particularly prone to the development of cytopenias, which can place them at risk of infection, bleeding, or anemia. In addition to caution regarding dosing, the most important measure that can be taken to minimize the occurrence of cytopenias is to perform frequent monitoring of the complete blood counts. Patients receiving CYC should have their blood counts monitored every 1 to 2 weeks. Blood counts should be performed in patients receiving MTX and AZA every 1 to 2 weeks during the first month and every 4 weeks thereafter.

Impact of renal function.   CYC and MTX are both renally eliminated making underlying kidney function an important parameter in dosing and protection. An association between age and decreasing glomerular filtration rate has been suggested by several studies. Accurate assessment of renal function may be confounded in older patients by the presence of comorbid diseases, medications, and low muscle mass. Depending upon the clinical setting, reduction of CYC dosage may be indicated in patients with renal insufficiency. MTX is contraindicated in patients with a creatinine clearance < 35 mL/min or serum creatinine of > 2.0 mg/dL, as ineffective elimination can lead to severe toxicity. AZA is not contraindicated in renal insufficiency, and can be considered in the treatment of vasculitic diseases where data has demonstrated its benefit.

Medication interactions

Medications that are being used to treat another underlying disease may have important interactions with agents that are used to treat vasculitis. Allopurinol inhibits the metabolism of AZA, leading to increased AZA levels when taken together [98,99]. For patients who must remain on allopurinol for the treatment of gout, the dosage of AZA should be reduced by one third to one quarter of the usual dosage to avoid toxicity.

As noted in the WG section, weekly MTX and T/S given at twice daily dosing represents another important interaction that is associated with bone marrow toxicity [70].

Summary

The vasculitic diseases represent a diverse range of clinical entities that are linked by the presence of blood vessel inflammation. For many forms of vasculitis, older patients comprise a significant proportion of the affected population. Recognition of the forms of vasculitis that may affect geriatric patients and an appreciation of how the disease and its treatment may uniquely impact this age group can play a meaningful role in improving patient outcome and quality of life.

References

[1] Kussmaul A, Maier K. Uber eine bischer nicht beschreibene eigenthumliche Arterienekrankkung (Periarteritis nodosa), die mit Morbus Brightii und rpaid fortschreitender allgemeiner Muskellahmung einhergeht. Dtsch Arch Klin 1866;1:484–517.

[2] Zeek PM. Periarteritis nodosa: critical review. Am J Clin Pathol 1952;22:777–90.

[3] Jennette JC, Falk RJ, Andrassy K, et al. Nomenclature of systemic vasculitides. Proposal of an international consensus conference. Arthritis Rheum 1994;37(2):187–92.

[4] Watts RA, Scott DG. Classification and epidemiology of the vasculitides. Baillieres Clin Rheumatol 1997;11(2):191–217.

[5] Weyand CM, Goronzy JJ. Giant-cell arteritis and polymyalgia rheumatica. Ann Intern Med 2003;139(6):505–15.

[6] Salvarani C, Cantini F, Boiardi L, et al. Polymyalgia rheumatica and giant-cell arteritis. N Engl J Med 2002;347(4):261–71.

[7] Salvarani C, Crowson CS, O'Fallon WM, et al. Reappraisal of the epidemiology of giant cell arteritis in Olmsted County, Minnesota, over a fifty-year period. Arthritis Rheum 2004;51(2): 264–8.

[8] Calamia KT, Hunder GG. Clinical manifestations of giant cell (temporal) arteritis. Clin Rheum Dis 1980;6:389–403.

[9] Aiello PD, Trautmann JC, McPhee TJ, et al. Visual prognosis in giant cell arteritis. Ophthalmology 1993;100(4):550–5.

[10] Hayreh SS, Podhajsky PA, Zimmerman B. Ocular manifestations of giant cell arteritis. Am J Ophthalmol 1998;125(4):509–20.

[11] Brack A, Martinez-Taboada V, Stanson A, et al. Disease pattern in cranial and large-vessel giant cell arteritis. Arthritis Rheum 1999;42(2):311–7.

[12] Achkar AA, Lie JT, Hunder GG, et al. How does previous corticosteroid treatment affect the biopsy findings in giant cell (temporal) arteritis? Ann Intern Med 1994;120(12):987–92.

[13] Birkhead NC, Wagener HP, Shick RM. Treatment of temporal arteritis with adrenal corticosteroids. JAMA 1957;163:821–7.

[14] Myles AB, Perera T, Ridley MG. Prevention of blindness in giant cell arteritis by corticosteroid treatment. Br J Rheumatol 1992;31:103–5.

[15] Ross Russell RW. Giant cell arteritis. QJM 1959;112:471–89.

[16] Liu GT, Glaser JS, Schatz NJ, et al. Visual morbidity in giant cell arteritis. Clinical characteristics and prognosis for vision. Ophthalmology 1994;101(11):1779–85.

[17] Fauchald P, Rygvold O, Oystase B. Temporal arteritis and polymyalgia rheumatica. Clinical and biopsy findings. Ann Intern Med 1972;77:845–52.

[18] Huston KA, Hunder GG, Lie JT, et al. Temporal arteritis: a 25-year epidemiologic, clinical, and pathologic study. Ann Intern Med 1978;88:162–7.

[19] Sorensen S, Lorenzen I. Giant-cell arteritis, temporal arteritis and polymyalgia rheumatica. A retrospective study of 63 patients. Acta Med Scand 1977;201(3):207–13.

[20] Bengtsson BA, Malmvall BE. Prognosis of giant cell arteritis including temporal arteritis and polymyalgia rheumatica. A follow-up study on ninety patients treated with corticosteroids. Acta Med Scand 1981;209(5):337–45.

[21] Lundberg I, Hedfors E. Restricted dose and duration of corticosteroid treatment in patients with polymyalgia rheumatica and temporal arteritis. J Rheumatol 1990;17:1340–5.

[22] Fernandez-Herlihy L. Duration of corticosteroid therapy in giant cell arteritis. J Rheumatol 1980; 7(3):361–4.

[23] Jover JA, Hernandez-Garcia C, Morado IC, et al. Combined treatment of giant-cell arteritis with methotrexate and prednisone. a randomized, double-blind, placebo-controlled trial. Ann Intern Med 2001;134(2):106–14.

[24] Hoffman GS, Cid MC, Hellmann DB, et al. A multicenter, randomized, double-blind, placebo-controlled trial of adjuvant methotrexate treatment for giant cell arteritis. Arthritis Rheum 2002;46(5):1309–18.

[25] Nesher G, Berkun Y, Mates M, et al. Low-dose aspirin and prevention of cranial ischemic complications in giant cell arteritis. Arthritis Rheum 2004;50(4):1332–7.

[26] Evans JM, Bowles CA, Bjornsson J, et al. Thoracic aortic aneurysm and rupture in giant cell arteritis. A descriptive study of 41 cases. Arthritis Rheum 1994;37(10):1539–47.

[27] Evans JM, O'Fallon WM, Hunder GG. Increased incidence of aortic aneurysm and dissection in giant cell (temporal) arteritis. A population-based study. Ann Intern Med 1995;122(7):502–7.

[28] Salvarani C, Cantini F, Boiardi L, et al. Polymyalgia rheumatica. Best Pract Res Clin Rheumatol 2004;18(5):705–22.

[29] Chuang TY, Hunder GG, Ilstrup DM, et al. Polymyalgia rheumatica: a 10-year epidemiologic and clinical study. Ann Intern Med 1982;97(5):672–80.

[30] Weyand CM, Tetzlaff N, Bjornsson J, et al. Disease patterns and tissue cytokine profiles in giant cell arteritis. Arthritis Rheum 1997;40(1):19–26.

[31] Weyand CM, Hicok KC, Hunder GG, et al. Tissue cytokine patterns in patients with polymyalgia rheumatica and giant cell arteritis. Ann Intern Med 1994;121(7):484–91.

[32] Weyand CM, Fulbright JW, Evans JM, et al. Corticosteroid requirements in polymyalgia rheumatica. Arch Intern Med 1999;159(6):577–84.

[33] Caporali R, Cimmino MA, Ferraccioli G, et al. Prednisone plus methotrexate for polymyalgia rheumatica: a randomized, double-blind, placebo-controlled trial. Ann Intern Med 2004;141(7): 493–500.

[34] Stone JH. Methotrexate in polymyalgia rheumatica: kernel of truth or curse of Tantalus? Ann Intern Med 2004;141(7):568–9.

[35] Guillevin L, Lhote F, Guillevin L, et al. Distinguishing polyarteritis nodosa from microscopic polyangiitis and implications for treatment. Curr Opin Rheumatol 1995;7(1):20–4.

[36] Watts RA, Jolliffe VA, Carruthers DM, et al. Effect of classification on the incidence of polyarteritis nodosa and microscopic polyangiitis. Arthritis Rheum 1996;39(7):1208–12.

[37] Guillevin L, Visser H, Noel LH, et al. Antineutrophil cytoplasm antibodies in systemic polyarteritis nodosa with and without hepatitis B virus infection and Churg-Strauss syndrome— 62 patients. J Rheumatol 1993;20(8):1345–9.

[38] Fauci AS, Doppman JL, Wolff SM. Cyclophosphamide-induced remissions in advanced polyarteritis nodosa. Am J Med 1978;64:890–4.

[39] Gayraud M, Guillevin L, le Toumelin P, et al. Long-term followup of polyarteritis nodosa, microscopic polyangiitis, and Churg-Strauss syndrome: analysis of four prospective trials including 278 patients. Arthritis Rheum 2001;44(3):666–75.

[40] Guillevin L, Lhote F. Treatment of polyarteritis nodosa and microscopic polyangiitis. Arthritis Rheum 1998;41(12):2100–5.

[41] Guillevin L, Lhote F, Gayraud M, et al. Prognostic factors in polyarteritis nodosa and Churg-Strauss syndrome. A prospective study in 342 patients. Medicine (Baltimore) 1996;75(1):17–28.

[42] Guillevin L, Lhote F, Gherardi R. The spectrum and treatment of virus-associated vasculitides. Curr Opin Rheumatol 1997;9(1):31–6.

[43] Guillevin L, Lhote F, Cohen P, et al. Polyarteritis nodosa related to hepatitis B virus. A prospective study with long-term observation of 41 patients. Medicine (Baltimore) 1995;74(5): 238–53.

[44] Guillevin L, Lhote F, Sauvaget F, et al. Treatment of polyarteritis nodosa related to hepatitis B virus with interferon-alpha and plasma exchanges. Ann Rheum Dis 1994;53(5):334–7.

[45] Guillevin L, Lhote F, Leon A, et al. Treatment of polyarteritis nodosa related to hepatitis B virus with short term steroid therapy associated with antiviral agents and plasma exchanges. A prospective trial in 33 patients. J Rheumatol 1993;20:289–98.

[46] Hoffman GS, Kerr GS, Leavitt RY, et al. Wegener granulomatosis: an analysis of 158 patients. Ann Intern Med 1992;116(6):488–98.

[47] Reinhold-Keller E, Beuge N, Latza U, et al. An interdisciplinary approach to the care of patients with Wegener's granulomatosis: long-term outcome in 155 patients. Arthritis Rheum 2000; 43(5):1021–32.

[48] Tidman M, Olander R, Svalander C, et al. Patients hospitalized because of small vessel vasculitides with renal involvement in the period 1975–95: organ involvement, anti-neutrophil cytoplasmic antibodies patterns, seasonal attack rates and fluctuation of annual frequencies. J Intern Med 1998;244(2):133–41.

[49] Watts RA, Lane SE, Bentham G, et al. Epidemiology of systemic vasculitis: a ten-year study in the United Kingdom. Arthritis Rheum 2000;43(2):414–9.

[50] van der Woude FJ, Rasmussen N, Lobatto S, et al. Autoantibodies against neutrophils and monocytes: tool for diagnosis and marker of disease activity in Wegener's granulomatosis. Lancet 1985;1(8426):425–9.

[51] Hoffman GS, Specks U. Antineutrophil cytoplasmic antibodies. Arthritis Rheum 1998;41(9): 1521–37.

[52] Niles JL, McCluskey RT, Ahmad MF, et al. Wegener's granulomatosis autoantigen is a novel neutrophil serine proteinase. Blood 1989;74(6):1888–93.

[53] Falk RJ, Jennette JC. Anti-neutrophil cytoplasmic autoantibodies with specificity for myeloperoxidase in patients with systemic vasculitis and idiopathic necrotizing and crescentic glomerulonephritis. N Engl J Med 1988;318(25):1651–7.

[54] Nölle B, Specks U, Lüdemann J, et al. Anticytoplasmic autoantibodies: their immunodiagnostic value in Wegener's granulomatosis. Ann Intern Med 1989;111:28–40.

[55] Boomsma MM, Stegeman CA, van der Leij MJ, et al. Prediction of relapses in Wegener's granulomatosis by measurement of antineutrophil cytoplasmic antibody levels: a prospective study. Arthritis Rheum 2000;43(9):2025–33.

[56] Kerr GS, Fleisher TA, Hallahan CW, et al. Limited prognostic value of changes in antineutrophil cytoplasmic antibody titer in patients with Wegener's granulomatosis. Arthritis Rheum 1993; 36(3):365–71.

[57] Falk RJ, Jennette JC. ANCA are pathogenic—oh yes they are! J Am Soc Nephrol 2002;13(7): 1977–9.

[58] Russell KA, Specks U. Are antineutrophil cytoplasmic antibodies pathogenic? Experimental approaches to understand the antineutrophil cytoplasmic antibody phenomenon. Rheum Dis Clin North Am 2001;27(4):815–32.

[59] Travis WD, Hoffman GS, Leavitt RY, et al. Surgical pathology of the lung in Wegener's granulomatosis. Review of 87 open lung biopsies from 67 patients. Am J Surg Pathol 1991; 15:315–33.

[60] Devaney KO, Travis WD, Hoffman GS, et al. Interpretation of head and neck biopsies in Wegener's granulomatosis. A pathologic study of 126 biopsies in 70 patients. Am J Surg Pathol 1990;14:555–64.

[61] Jennette JC, Falk RJ. The pathology of vasculitis involving the kidney. Am J Kidney Dis 1994; 24(1):130–41.

[62] Fauci A, Wolff S. Wegener's granulomatosis: studies in eighteen patients and a review of the literature. Medicine 1973;52:535–61.

[63] Fauci A, Haynes B, Katz P, et al. Wegener's granulomatosis: Prospective clinical and therapeutic experience with 85 patients for 21 years. Ann Intern Med 1983;98:76–85.

[64] Langford CA, Talar-Williams C, Barron KS, et al. Use of a cyclophosphamide-induction methotrexate-maintenance regimen for the treatment of Wegener's granulomatosis: extended follow-up and rate of relapse. Am J Med 2003;114(6):463–9.

[65] Jayne D, Rasmussen N, Andrassy K, et al. A randomized trial of maintenance therapy for vasculitis associated with antineutrophil cytoplasmic autoantibodies. N Engl J Med 2003; 349(1):36–44.

[66] Talar-Williams C, Hijazi YM, Walther MM, et al. Cyclophosphamide-induced cystitis and bladder cancer in patients with Wegener granulomatosis. Ann Intern Med 1996;124(5):477–84.

[67] Reinhold-Keller E, Fink CO, Herlyn K, et al. High rate of renal relapse in 71 patients with Wegener's granulomatosis under maintenance of remission with low-dose methotrexate. Arthritis Rheum 2002;47(3):326–32.

[68] Sneller MC, Hoffman GS, Talar-Williams C, et al. An analysis of forty-two Wegener's granulomatosis patients treated with methotrexate and prednisone. Arthritis Rheum 1995;38(5): 608–13.

[69] Stegeman CA, Cohen Tervaert JW, de Jong PE, et al. Trimethoprim-sulfamethoxazole (co-trimoxazole) for the prevention of relapses of Wegener's granulomatosis. N Engl J Med 1996; 335(1):16–20.

[70] Govert JA, Patton S, Fine RL. Pancytopenia from using trimethoprim and methotrexate. Ann Intern Med 1992;117(10):877–8.

[71] Guillevin L, Durand-Gasselin B, Cevallos R, et al. Microscopic polyangiitis: clinical and laboratory findings in eighty-five patients. Arthritis Rheum 1999;42(3):421–30.

[72] Savage CO, Winearls CG, Evans DJ, et al. Microscopic polyarteritis: presentation, pathology and prognosis. Q J Med 1985;56(220):467–83.

[73] Nachman PH, Hogan SL, Jennette JC, et al. Treatment response and relapse in antineutrophil cytoplasmic autoantibody-associated microscopic polyangiitis and glomerulonephritis. J Am Soc Nephrol 1996;7(1):33–9.

[74] Churg J, Strauss L. Allergic granulomatosis, allergic angiitis and periarteritis nodosa. Am J Pathol 1951;27:277–301.

[75] Guillevin L, Cohen P, Gayraud M, et al. Churg-Strauss syndrome. Clinical study and long-term follow-up of 96 patients. Medicine (Baltimore) 1999;78(1):26–37.

[76] Lanham JG, Elkon KB, Pusey CD, et al. Systemic vasculitis with asthma and eosinophilia: a clinical approach to the Churg-Strauss syndrome. Medicine (Baltimore) 1984;63(2):65–81.

[77] Chumbley LC, Harrison Jr EG, DeRemee RA. Allergic granulomatosis and angiitis (Churg-Strauss syndrome). Report and analysis of 30 cases. Mayo Clin Proc 1977;52(8):477–84.

[78] Weller PF, Plaut M, Taggart V, et al. The relationship of asthma therapy and Churg-Strauss syndrome: NIH workshop summary report. J Allergy Clin Immunol 2001;108(2):175–83.

[79] Stone JH, Nousari HC. Essential cutaneous vasculitis: what every rheumatologist should know about vasculitis of the skin. Curr Opin Rheumatol 2001;13(1):23–34.

[80] Lotti T, Ghersetich I, Comacchi C, et al. Cutaneous small-vessel vasculitis. J Am Acad Dermatol 1998;39(5 Pt 1):667–87 [quiz 88–90].

[81] Gibson LE. Cutaneous vasculitis: appraoch to diagnosis and systemic associations. Mayo Clin Proc 1990;65:221–9.

[82] Saulsbury FT. Henoch-Schonlein purpura in children. Report of 100 patients and review of the literature. Medicine (Baltimore) 1999;78(6):395–409.

[83] Fogazzi GB, Pasquali S, Moriggi M, et al. Long-term outcome of Schonlein-Henoch nephritis in the adult. Clin Nephrol 1989;31(2):60–6.

[84] Ballard HS, Eisenger RP, Gallo G. Renal manifestations of Henoch-Schonlein syndrome in adults. Am J Med 1970;49:328–35.

[85] Blanco R, Martinez-Taboada VM, Rodriguez-Valverde V, et al. Henoch-Schonlein purpura in

adulthood and childhood: two different expressions of the same syndrome. Arthritis Rheum 1997;40(5):859–64.

[86] Choi HK, Merkel PA, Walker AM, et al. Drug-associated antineutrophil cytoplasmic antibody-positive vasculitis: prevalence among patients with high titers of antimyeloperoxidase antibodies. Arthritis Rheum 2000;43(2):405–13.
[87] Lamprecht P, Gause A, Gross WL. Cryoglobulinemic vasculitis. Arthritis Rheum 1999;42(12): 2507–16.
[88] Agnello V, Romain PL. Mixed cryoglobulinemia secondary to hepatitis C virus infection. Rheum Dis Clin North Am 1996;22(1):1–21.
[89] Vassilopoulos D, Calabrese LH. Hepatitis C virus infection and vasculitis: implications of antiviral and immunosuppressive therapies. Arthritis Rheum 2002;46(3):585–97.
[90] Dammacco F, Sansonno D, Han JH, et al. Natural interferon-alpha versus its combination with 6-methyl-prednisolone in the therapy of type II mixed cryoglobulinemia: a long-term, randomized, controlled study. Blood 1994;84(10):3336–43.
[91] Nesher G, Sonnenblick M, Friedlander Y. Analysis of steroid related complications and mortality in temporal arteritis: a 15-year survey of 43 patients. J Rheumatol 1994;21(7):1283–6.
[92] Guillevin L, Cordier JF, Lhote F, et al. A prospective, multicenter, randomized trial comparing steroids and pulse cyclophosphamide versus steroids and oral cyclophosphamide in the treatment of generalized Wegener's granulomatosis. Arthritis Rheum 1997;40(12):2187–98.
[93] Matteson EL, Gold KN, Bloch DA, et al. Long-term survival of patients with Wegener's granulomatosis from the American College of Rheumatology Wegener's Granulomatosis Classification Criteria Cohort. Am J Med 1996;101(2):129–34.
[94] Ognibene FP, Shelhamer JH, Hoffman GS, et al. Pneumocystis carinii pneumonia: a major complication of immunosuppressive therapy in patients with Wegener's granulomatosis. Am J Respir Crit Care Med 1995;151(3 Pt 1):795–9.
[95] Masur H. Prevention and treatment of pneumocystis pneumonia. N Engl J Med 1992;327(26): 1853–60.
[96] Gabriel SE, Sunku J, Salvarani C, et al. Adverse outcomes of antiinflammatory therapy among patients with polymyalgia rheumatica. Arthritis Rheum 1997;40(10):1873–8.
[97] Pearce G, Ryan PF, Delmas PD, et al. The deleterious effects of low-dose corticosteroids on bone density in patients with polymyalgia rheumatica. Br J Rheumatol 1998;37(3):292–9.
[98] el-Gamel A, Evans C, Keevil B, et al. Effect of allopurinol on the metabolism of azathioprine in heart transplant patients. Transplant Proc 1998;30(4):1127–9.
[99] Prager D, Rosman M, Bertino JR. Letter: azathioprine and allopurinol. Ann Intern Med 1974; 80(3):427.

ELSEVIER
SAUNDERS

CLINICS IN
GERIATRIC
MEDICINE

Clin Geriatr Med 21 (2005) 649–669

Disease-Modifying Antirheumatic Drug use in the Elderly Rheumatoid Arthritis Patient

Veena K. Ranganath, MD[a,b], Daniel E. Furst, MD[a,*]

[a]*Division of Rheumatology, Department of Medicine,*
David Geffen School of Medicine at University of California, Los Angeles,
1000 Veteran Avenue, Room 32-59, Los Angeles, CA 90025-1670, USA
[b]*VA Greater Los Angeles Healthcare System, West Los Angeles, 11301 Wilshire Boulevard,*
Los Angeles, CA 90073, USA

Rheumatoid arthritis (RA) is an autoimmune disease of unknown etiology. RA causes an inflammatory destructive arthritis with a prevalence of 1% worldwide. It can be rapidly destructive, with 60% of patients having erosions of joints seen on radiographs within 2 years of disease onset [1,2]. RA patients suffer from a loss of functional ability leading to an inability to work, causing an economic burden to society [1]. As early as 1953, patients with RA were shown to have an approximate 10-year premature mortality [3]. RA patients who had higher functional disability, longer walk time, or increased number of involved joints had a two- to sixfold higher relative risk for death within 5 to 15 years compared with those with lower functional disability, shorter walk time, or decreased number of involved joints, as answered by patient questionnaires [4]. Unfortunately, there is no cure for RA, and the mainstay of therapy is treatment with disease-modifying antirheumatic drugs (DMARDs).

Schnell [5], in 1941, was the first to describe an elderly patient with RA in his paper entitled, "The clinical features of rheumatic infection in the old." The fastest growing population currently in the United States is comprised of people over the age of 65 [6], and approximately one third of all RA patients now fall in this category. Thus, there is increasing interest in evaluating the diagnostic, therapeutic, and prognostic implications of RA in the elderly. Although there continues to be debate about whether, and to what degree, RA differs in the

---
* Corresponding author.
E-mail address: defurst@mednet.ucla.edu (D.E. Furst).

0749-0690/05/$ – see front matter © 2005 Elsevier Inc. All rights reserved.
doi:10.1016/j.cger.2005.02.010

elderly versus the young [7], there is information pointing to some differences in response to DMARDs in the older RA patients.

In addition to an increased number of comorbidities (with more than 80% of elderly patients using at least one prescribed medication) [8], there is also an increased incidence of polypharmacy, noncompliance, risk for dosage errors and difficulties with access to medications (secondary to inability to pay) [9]. This review will not attempt to deal with these factors.

Instead, this article will briefly review the clinical pharmacology of humans as they age, and detail the effects of aging on the specific pharmacokinetics and responses to commonly used DMARDs such as methotrexate, sulfasala- zine, leflunomide, hydroxychloroquine, and cytokine therapies. We will not re- view less commonly used DMARDs in the elderly RA patient, including gold, d-penicillamine, cyclosporine, cyclophosphomide, or azathioprine. However, it is important to understand that the goals for the elderly RA patient are the same as in the younger RA patient: to decrease inflammation and prevent destruction of the joint in a safe, effective manner.

The question of who is considered to be an elderly RA patient is not clear. For the purpose of this review, we will use the arbitrary age cutoff of 65 years of age, and we will specify if articles presented use a different definition.

Physiologic changes in older patients

Pharmacokinetics

Pharmacokinetics describes the action of the body on the drug over time. This is governed by absorption, distribution, metabolism, and elimination. Phar- macokinetics are known to change with age, with the most important factors being decreases in elimination via renal excretion and type 1 hepatic metabolism [8,10,11]. Even though the elderly consume more than one third of all prescribed medications and more than half of over-the-counter medications in the United States, only a small percentage of these patients are entered into clinical trials [8]. Thus, responses of the older patients who are prescribed multiple medications for numerous comorbidities cannot be inferred with confidence from the results of published clinical trials. Many DMARDs have not been specifically examined in this area, so little is known regarding DMARD pharmacokinetics per se in the elderly RA patient.

Absorption

The older patient has decreased saliva production, decreased gastric acid, increased gastric emptying time, and decreased gastrointestinal motility. This may affect the rate of absorption. Nonetheless, most drugs are absorbed by pas- sive diffusion from the gastrointestinal tract so overall absorption is not usually affected by age-related changes. Some exceptions may occur; for example, indomethacin has both decreased clearance (by 43%) and absorbion (by 23%) in the elderly patient [12]. There were 16 patients above the age of 65 (range 69–86 years) and 10 patients younger than 65 (range 26–53 years) in this study, and it was recommended that the dose be decreased by 25%.

Distribution

Compared with younger persons, elderly patients tend to have decreased cardiac output, decreased renal blood flow, decreased hepatic blood flow, decreased total body water, increased body fat, and decreased serum albumin levels. Lean body mass is decreased in the older patient by 12% to 19%, fat stores are increased by 14% to 35%, and albumin is decreased by 10% to 20% [8,11, 13–15]. These changes can affect the distribution of drugs, especially when elderly patients are taking multiple medications, thus causing transient toxic or subtherapeutic levels.

For example, the known decrease in body water and increase in body fat with age would cause a decrease in the volume of distribution (Vd) of hydrophilic compounds such as alcohol and increase in Vd of lipophilic compounds such as diazepam. Age-dependent decreases in albumin concentration are small. However, tolbutamine, coumarins, meperidine, naproxen, salicylates, phenytoin, valproic acid, acetazolamide, diazepam, and ceftriaxone are noted to have decreased plasma protein binding in the elderly [11].

Metabolism

The older patient has decreased hepatic blood flow by 40%, decreased liver size by 25% to 35%, and decreased production of proteins, lipids, and glucose. With some drugs such as coumarin, some benzodiazepines, theophylline, imipramine, propranolol, levodopa, and indomethacin, there is a 20% to 40% decrease in metabolic clearance [11]. The model used for evaluating hepatic clearance in the elderly uses phenazone metabolism as a marker; phenazone metabolism decreases 6% for every 10 years of age [16,17]. There is some evidence to support a decline in phase I drug metabolism (hydroxylation, oxidation, hydrolysis, and demethylation), but not much in support of age-related changes in phase II drug metabolism (such as glucuronidation and sulfation).

Furthermore, nutritional status can play a major role in drug metabolism. Frail elderly patients with poor nutritional intake have generally decreased drug metabolism compared with elderly patients with good nutritional intake [11,18].

Elimination

In the elderly patient, an important pharmacokinetic change is a decrease in renal drug excretion. With age, renal plasma flow, renal tubular clearance, and creatinine clearance decrease. After the age of 30, the glomerular filtration rate declines by 1 mL/min/y. By the age of 90, glomerular filtration rate (GFR) may be reduced by 25% to 50% in comparison to a 20-year-old [10,11]. Muscle mass decreases with age, so the serum creatinine levels (which can reflect tissue breakdown from muscle) can be lower than expected for a given level of renal function. Creatinine may remain the same as GFR decreases because muscle mass is decreasing.

Pharmacodynamics

Pharmacodynamics describes the action of a drug on the body. Drug pharmacodynamics may be altered in the elderly if there are changes in the number of receptors in the target organ, in how the cells respond by signal transduction, or other conterregulatory processes. The beta-adrenergic system and homeostatic mechanisms have been studied in the elderly. Decreased responses are seen in salbutamol and propranolol in elderly patients, thought to be secondary to a decrease in postreceptor binding events occurring in the cell [8,19]. Overall, data are slim in elucidating changes of pharmacodynamics in the elderly compared with pharmacokinetics in this group.

Summary

There are many important pharmacokinetic and pharmacodynamic changes that occur in the elderly patient. The mainstay of therapy in RA is the use of DMARDs. When evaluating an elderly RA patient it is essential to understand age-related changes as described above to help prevent unnecessary adverse events (AEs). The remainder of the review will discuss commonly used DMARDs in more detail in the context of the above information, and as applicable to the elderly RA patient.

Commonly used disease-modifying antirheumatic drugs in RA

Methotrexate

History

Farber et al, in 1948, developed methotrexate's parent compound, aminopterin, to treat childhood leukemia. Methotrexate (MTX) was first found to be effective in two psoriatric arthritis and six RA patients in 1951 by Gubner and colleagues [20,21]. It wasn't until the 1980s that this chemotherapeutic agent was used in pilot studies. Four randomized controlled clinical trials were conducted in the mid-1980s and played a pivotal role in MTX's Food and Drug Administration's (FDA) approval for use in RA patients [22–25]. Since the 1990s, MTX has been gradually accepted as a first-line agent for RA.

Mechanism of action

The mechanism of action of MTX is still unclear, although many mechanisms have been proposed (Box 1). MTX is an antimetabolite that competitively inhibits dihydrofolate reductase, causing interference with synthesis of purines and pyrimidines necessary for DNA synthesis and cell division. MTX may inhibit angiogenesis, affecting both fibroblasts and lymphocytes in RA patients [26,27].

Box 1. Proposed mechanisms of action of MTX

- Inhibits metabolism of adenosine (a potent inhibitor of neutrophil chemotaxis)
- Induces apoptosis of activated T cells
- Decreases IL-6 and IL-1B (proinflammatory cytokines)
- Decreases IgG production

Clinical pharmacology

The chemical structure of MTX is the result of substituting an amine residue and a methyl group in folic acid. Oral MTX has a bioavailability of 70% to 75% compared with intravenous administration, although marked variability has been demonstrated. There is no credible data that food affects bioavailability, so MTX may be taken with or without food. After parenteral therapy, peak plasma concentrations are reached in 1 to 2 hours and elimination half-life is 8 to 24 hours [28–31]. Approximately 30% to 60% of MTX is protein bound, and a small proportion (10%) is monohydroxylated to 7-OH-MTX in the liver, which enters cells and then is polyglutamated to MTX glutamates of varying lengths. MTX glutamates have a long half-life of approximately 1 week, and may be important to understanding the kinetics of MTX in RA [30]. Renal clearance accounts for 50% to 80% of MTX elimination, and 10% to 30% is eliminated through the bile.

Cotrimoxazole and MTX can interact to promote hematologic abnormalities with severe life-threatening pancytopenias. This occurs due to cotrimoxazole's folic acid antagonist activity [32]. In double-blind studies, folic acid or leucovorin can decrease MTX's toxicity, although they may also decrease its efficacy (unpublished data).

Nonsteroidal anti-inflammtory drugs (NSAIDs) and MTX pharmacokinetic interactions are a topic of debate. NSAIDs (eg, Sulindac; indomethacin) and MTX interactions were said to result in an increase in serum MTX concentrations by inhibiting renal clearance of MTX, although some feel that MTX excretion may be compensated by increases in biliary clearance [30–32]. Clinical interactions are not often significant. However, because elderly patients have an age-related decrease in renal function, this group of patients should be watched particularly carefully when MTX and NSAIDs are used together.

Studies have evaluated MTX pharmacokinetics in elderly RA patients. One study evaluated MTX pharmacokinetics after an intramuscular dose in 38 older RA patients (65–83 years of age) compared with 24 younger RA patients (21–45 years of age) [33]. Patients received anywhere between 7.5 and 15 mg of MTX intramuscularly every week. Plasma and ultrafiltrate samples were assayed by a fluorescence polarization immunoassay for MTX concentration. The Vd and the unbound fraction of MTX were not different between the two groups. However, the elimination half life of the free and total MTX was greater in the elderly RA group at 14.5 and 14.3 compared with 9.4 and 9.4 in the younger patients, respectively. The free and total clearance of MTX was 169 and 95.9 mL/min in the elderly patients compared with 225 and 126 in the younger RA patients, respectively, with P-values of <0.001. However, MTX clearance was more highly correlated with creatinine clearance than with age. It was concluded that MTX clearance decreases with decreasing creatinine clearance, and that dosing regimen should be adjusted in elderly patients with renal insufficiency.

Efficacy

After Gubner [20,21], in 1951, showed that six patients with RA and two patients with PsA responded to treatment with MTX, there was still reluctance to embrace a new therapy with gold and corticosteroids then being the mainstay of therapy. It took approximately 30 to 40 years until the first short-term, randomized double-blind placebo-controlled trials evaluated low-dose MTX for efficacy in RA. Most studies have shown that 50% or more of RA patients using MTX continue on it for 5 years or more [34]. Patients receiving MTX remain on it longer than any other DMARD, with a median duration of treatment of 4.3 years compared with 2.0 years with hydroxychloroquine [35]. Patients discontinue therapy secondary to toxicity rather than lack of efficacy [34,36]. In addition, some studies have shown that MTX has a more rapid efficacy of onset than other DMARDs [29].

Several studies have shown that MTX slows progression of radiographic damage, and a few patients seem to show healing of erosions [31]. In comparison to oral gold, penicillamine, and azathioprine, the rate of radiographic progression is slower with MTX [37].

Meta-analysis of available trials has demonstrated that MTX is one of the most effective medications for the treatment of RA [38,39]. Data from 11 MTX clinical trials with 496 RA patients were evaluated, where patients were grouped above and below the age of 60 [40], and approximately 69% of patients were below the age of 60. The results of the study showed that age did not affect MTX efficacy on tender/swollen joint count, erythrocyte sedimentation rate, and pain. Wolfe [41], in 1991, also did not show a difference in efficacy in a cohort of 235 RA patients with a cutoff of 65 years of age and a mean of 1.9 years follow-up. These studies suggest that MTX is just as effective in the elderly RA patient as in young RA patients [38] (Table 1).

Although 10% to 30% of patients taking MTX discontinue this drug secondary to toxicity, most AEs when using MTX are mild and do not lead to termination of the drug [29–31]. The most common pulmonary side effect is acute interstitial pneumonitis which, nevertheless, occurs in <1% of patients. Patients can present with dypsnea, hypoxia, fevers, nonproductive cough, and infiltrates on chest X-ray [42].

A small retrospective study evaluated the safety of low dose MTX (7.5 mg/wk) in older RA patients, where 4 of 33 (12%) patients discontinued MTX. Two patients had elevated liver enzymes and two patients suffered gastrointestinal irritation (no further information was provided) [43]. Felson et al [38], in 1995,

Table 1
Toxicity

Side effects of methotrexate	
Gastrointestinal (20–70% of all AEs)	nausea, vomiting, abdominal pain, stomatitis (causes 10% of all discontinuation of MTX), elevation of hepatic enzymes two to three times normal (causes 5% of all discontinuation of MTX)
Pulmonary	acute interstitial pneumonitis, interstitial fibrosis, pleuritis, pulmonary nodules
Skin	photosensitivity, increase in size of RA nodules, alopecia
CNS	headaches
Hematology	megaloblastic anemia, leukopenia, thrombocytopenia, pancytopenia
Genitourinary	teratogenesis, decreased sperm count
Oncology	Epstein-Barr-related lymphoma
Renal	decreased creatinine clearance

Abbreviations: AEs, adverse events; CNS, central nervous system; MTX, methotrexate; RA, rheumatoid arthritis.

performed a meta-analysis of 11 clinical trials with a total of 496 patients, and 341 patients were below the age of 60, 65 patients were between the ages of 60 to 64, 57 patients were between the ages of 65 to 69, and 33 patients were above the age of 70. In this selected group of RA patients, renal function rather than age determined toxicity of MTX. Bologna et al [44] studied 53 patients who were older than 65 years and 416 patients who were younger than 65 years of age for influence of age on MTX efficacy and toxicity. Clinical markers, biologic markers, number of patients achieving remission, and AEs were similar in the young and old RA groups. On the other hand, older RA patients trended toward a lower MTX maintenance dose with a *P*-value of 0.07. Both studies were limited by their size and by the nature of the patients studied. Nonetheless, the PDR recommends that older patients on MTX should be monitored for renal function every 1 to 2 months.

In a review by Nyfors in 1980 [45,46], there was some, although sparse, data that hepatic toxicity was more common in the elderly patients. However, age-related changes in renal function were not accounted for in these articles.

Engelbrecht et al [47] described six case reports with acute MTX pneumonitis after low-dose MTX, and the patients' ages ranged between 58 to 75 years of age. However, there is no evidence at present that there is any clear-cut age-related increase of MTX pneumonitis in the elderly.

Sulfasalazine

History

In 1938, Professor Nana Svartz created sulfasalazine (SSZ), specifically for the treatment of "rheumatic polyarthritis." In 1948, Svartz [28] treated 400 patients with SSZ, demonstrating a 67% response. Unfortunately, around the same time period Sinclair and Duthie [48] published a study with SSZ in comparison with gold that was not favorable, with only one patient still on SSZ

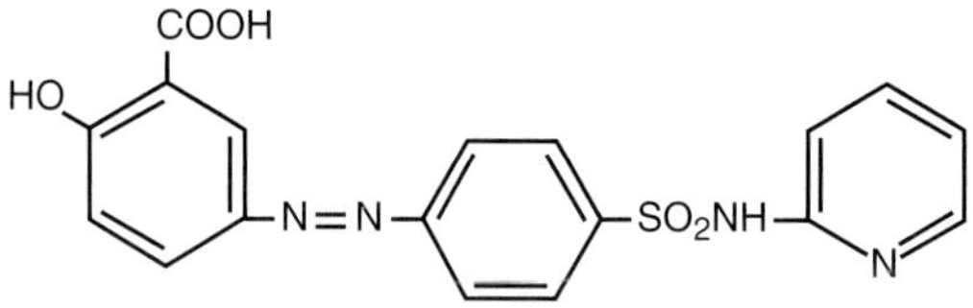

Fig. 1. Structure of sulfasalazine (SSZ) (the strucutre is not really relevant to the elderly).

at the time of assessment. It was not until the early 1980s, with McConkey's [49] publication of her experience with SSZ in RA, and two additional articles confirming SSZ's efficacy compared with intramuscular gold and penicillamine, that SSZ began to be used more widely [29].

Mechanism of action

SSZ is a combination of sulfapyridine and 5-ASA linked by a diazo bond, which is broken enzymatically in the large intestine by colonic bacteria (Fig. 1). Sulfapyridine and possibly SSZ, are the active agents in RA, and the 5-ASA portion is the active agent in inflammatory bowel disease. The mechanisms of action of SSZ and its metabolites are not fully understood, although Box 2 outlines many of their potential mechanisms of action.

Approximately 30% of SSZ is absorbed, mainly in the small intestine, and it undergoes enterohepatic circulation, providing an SSZ bioavailability of 10%. The other 70% of SSZ reaches the colon intact where the azo bond is reduced by bacteria, releasing sulfapyridine and 5-ASA. Sulfapyridine is rapidly absorbed, with only 7% excreted in the feces; virtually no 5-ASA is absorbed. Sulfapyridine is detected in the serum in 4 to 6 hours, and steady state is achieved in 4 to 5 days. Sulfapyridine is metabolized in the liver where it is acetylated and hydroxylated. The metabolites are then excreted in the urine.

Box 2. SSZ mechanism of action: (this is not necessarily relevant to the elderly)

- Neutrophil—inhibits function and recruitment
- Natural killer cell—accelerates ability to induce apoptosis
- T Cells—inhibits IL-2 induction and proliferation
- B Cells—decreases immunoglobulin
- Cytokines—decreases reduce levels of IL-6, TNF-α, IL-1, and IL-12
- Transcriptional factors—inhibits NFkB
- Folate-dependent enzymes—inhibits purine synthesis and increases adenosine levels
- Fibroblasts—inhibits endothelial cell proliferation and development into new blood vessels

The rate of hepatic sulfapyridine acetylation is genetically determined, and is categorized as slow or fast acetylators. Slower acetylators may have a longer sulfapyridine half-life, and this can explain part of SSZ's toxicity as some studies (not all) evaluating slow acetylators demonstrated that these patients had more side effects than fast acetylators [50–52].

The pharmacokinetics of SSZ have been described in elderly RA patients. Twelve patients were elderly (ages 71–83) and eight patients were young RA patients (ages 35–46) [52]. There were equal numbers of slow and fast acetylators in each group. Serum and urine specimens were obtained from patients over a 96-hour time period at regular intervals. The elimination half-life of SSZ was longer in the elderly RA patients. However, acetylator phenotype, not age, played a role in determining the serum concentration of sulfapyridine.

To date, interaction studies of SSZ with antibiotics or cholestyramine have not shown clinically significant effects. On the other hand, digoxin serum levels may be decreased by 25% when using SSZ [32].

Efficacy

There have been six controlled studies and a meta-analysis, all showing the benefit of SSZ over placebo in RA [53–58]. The onset of response to SSZ is more rapid than hydroxychloroquine (HCQ) or gold therapy, with some patients responding in 4 to 6 weeks. As with MTX, SSZ slows the progression of erosions [53,54,59].

SSZ has been compared with many DMARDs. According to published articles, SSZ is more effective than HCQ, oral gold, and azathioprine in treating RA. SSZ is as effective as leflunomide, intramuscular gold, and penicillamine, with less toxicity than the latter two [42]. In a 1999, double-blind multicenter randomized study by Smolen et al, American College of Rheumatology (ACR) response scores were compared between SSZ and leflunomide [57]. Patients using SSZ achieved an ACR_{20} of 56% and an ACR_{50} 30% compared with an ACR_{20} 55% and ACR_{50} 33% for the leflunomide-treated group. Comparisons of MTX with SSZ have been less clear. One study showed that both MTX and SSZ have similar efficacy at 52 weeks, although maximum doses of SSZ (2–3 g/d) were compared with relatively low doses of MTX (7.5–15 mg/wk) [60].

Table 2
SSZ toxicities

Gastrointestinal	nausea (cause of 10–15% discontinuation of SSZ), anorexia, vomiting, diarrhea
CNS	headache, fever, and lightheadedness
Dermatologic	photosensitivity
Genitourinary	oligospermia
Rare SE	elevated transaminines, alopecia, peripheral neuropathy
Serious SE	leucopenia (1.4% of patients with SSZ treatment), thrombocytopenia, and agranulocytosis

Abbreviations. SE, side effects; SSZ, sulfasalazine

SSZ has a withdrawal rate related to AEs of 17% to 30%. Most side effects occur within the first few months of therapy, and can be decreased by starting a lower dose and gradually increasing to the dose of 2–3 g daily (Table 2). Although it does reduce sperm count, SSZ is safe to use in pregnancy [29–31,42].

Elderly patients were found to have a higher dropout rate due to the side effects of nausea and vomiting than younger patients [59]. In addition, folate deficiency is thought to be more prevalent in the elderly [61–64], a population with poor nutritional status, exposing them to the possibility of hematologic toxicities. However, when Wilkieson et al [65], in 1993, performed a combined analysis of five prospective SSZ studies with a total of 352 patients (wherein patients were categorized into young, middle aged, and elderly); no age-related differences in either toxicity or efficacy were seen.

Leflunomide

History

Bartlett and Schleyerbach [63], in 1985, originally developed leflunomide for use in RA, showing its activity in adjuvant arthritis models of RA. Later, many animal models and organ graft models showed efficacy by decreasing inflammation and rejection. The first use of leflunomide in RA was reported in 1991. It was approved by the FDA in September, 1998, and since that time more than 400,000 patients have been treated with leflunomide worldwide [30,66,67].

Mechanism of action

Leflunomide is an N-(4-trifluoromethylphenyl)-5-methylisoxazole-4-carbox-amine ($C_{12}H_9F_3N_2O_2$), an isoxazole derivative. After absorption of leflunomide, a prodrug, it is rapidly converted in the submucosal wall of the intestine, plasma, and liver into its active metabolite A77 1726 (M1 derivative) (Box 3).

Box 3. Mechanism of action of Leflunomide: (this is not really relevant to the elderly)

- Inhibits pyramidine synthesis
- Inhibits T-cell proliferation
- Inhibits diapedesis and chemotaxis
- Inhibits cell–cell contact
- Inhibits intracellular signaling
- Inhibits leukocyte adhesion
- Inhibits tyrosine kinases
- Inhibits NFkB gene expression
- Inhibits IL-1beta expression
- Inhibits metalloproteinase—production
- Inhibits synthesis of dUMP

M1 inhibits dihydroorotate dehydrogenase (DHODH), a mitochondrial enzyme, which is important in de novo pyrimidine synthesis. Leflunomide also inhibits tyrosine kinases and NFkB gene expression in a human T-cell line and affects T-cell proliferation [68]. Leflunomide inhibits synthesis of dUMP from deoxythymidylate (dTMP), which occurs later in the G1 phase of the cell cycle. These mechanisms of action are different from MTX, making it easier to understand why leflunomide and MTX can work additively [69].

Clinical pharmacology

Approximately 50% of leflunomide is absorbed in the gastrointestinal tract and the remaining portion is excreted in the feces. As stated above, leflunomide is metabolized to A77 1726 (M1 derivative), which is highly protein bound (>99%), and has a low Vd. Metabolites of M1 found in the urine are glucuronide conjugates, and oxanilic acid derivatives are found as long as 36 days after discontinuation of medication. Approximately two thirds of M1 is excreted in the feces and one third in the urine. Leflunomide steady state is reached in 7 weeks at 20 mg/d. Its half-life is 15–18 days, a rather long half-life, due to enterohepatic circulation and biliary recycling. This was the rationale behind the loading dose of 100 mg/d of leflunomide for 3 days, followed by the maintenance dose of 20 mg/d.

M1 readily binds to activated charcoal or cholestyramine. Patients who suffer an AE can take 8 g of cholestyramine three times a day for 2 days, which results in a 65% reduction of plasma drug levels, and may ameliorate the AE. To avoid leflunomide-induced embryo toxicity, women who have been taking leflunomide but wish to become pregnant should take cholestyramine for 11 days for complete drug washout. It can take up to 2 years to completely washout drug without taking cholestyramine [67].

Not many drug interactions have been noted, even though M1 does inhibit isoenzyme 2C9 of the cytochrome P450 system. Warfarin, tolbutamide, phenytoin, and many NSAIDs are metabolized by this pathway; however, the unbound drug fraction of these drugs is below the IC_{50} for this enzyme, making clinically important drug interactions unlikely [42].

Specific pharmacodynamic or pharmacokinetic studies have not been done in the elderly.

Efficacy

The efficacy of leflunomide as monotherapy has been evaluated in four multicenter double-blind randomized controlled trials, showing that it is better than placebo, approximately equal to SSZ, and MTX [57,70–73].

An open-label 52-week study of active RA patients showed no significant pharmacokinetic interactions between MTX and leflunomide [74]. Leflunomide (10 mg/d after loading) plus MTX together resulted in an additional 51.5% benefit compared with MTX alone. However, 23% of patients had a small increase in liver enzyme; three times the upper limit of normal elevation or more occurring only in 1.5% to 3.8% of patients, and most of these elevations returning to normal with observation alone. Liver biopsies done in three patients showed mild hepatic fibrosis in two of the patients. Some authors have stated, although without supporting data, that not loading patients with leflunomide should be considered in patients who are elderly.

Toxicity

The side effect and safety profile of leflunomide is similar to SSZ and MTX, as shown by reviewing 1339 patients in clinical trials; although it is important to note that the side effects last longer due to the long half-life of leflunomide [42]. The most common leflunomide-associated gastrointestinal side effects are diarrhea (17%), nausea (9%), abdominal pain (5%), and increased hepatic enzymes (5–10%) [42,67]. Diarrhea lasted longer than 1 month in 35% of patients. Elevation of hepatic enzymes greater than three times normal was seen in 1.5% to 4.4% of patients in clinical trials [67]. In a review of managed care cohorts by the FDA in 2003, the estimated risk of hospitalization due to leflunomide-related hepatitis was 1/5000. Other side effects occur including hypertension (increased in 10%, with new onset <2%), alopecia (10%), rash (10%), headache (7%), anorexia (7%) parasthesias (2%), and rare Stevens-Johnson syndrome, epidermal necrolysis, pancytopenia, agranulocytosis, and thrombocytopenia.

No studies have specifically evaluated leflunomide's toxicities in the elderly RA patient. However, a recent article reported 19 cases of pancytopenia associated with leflunomide use in Australia. Median age was 65.5 years (range 18–79 years), and 14 patients were on MTX as well. There were 16 of 19 patients who were older than 60 years of age. Five patients died of secondary to pancytopenia and 3 of 5 were older than 60 years of age. The authors felt that the risk for pancytopenia increased with concomitant use of MTX and in older patients [75].

Antimalarials

History

Payne [72], in 1894, was the first to use antimalarial therapy in rheumatology for the treatment of discoid lupus erythematosus. The first report of efficacy in RA with use of antimalarial therapy was in 1951. However, enthusiasm for antimalarial drugs waned when patients developed ocular toxicities in the late 1970s. Appreciation for this safe DMARD did not recur until the rarity of ocular toxicities was recognized (when appropriate doses were used). Presently, two antimalarial medications are in use in the treatment of RA: HCQ and chloroquine (CQ).

Mechanism of action

The exact mechanism of action of antimalarial drugs is unknown. In in vitro experiments, CQ and HCQ (both alkaline compounds) accumulate in lysosomes (stabilizing the lysosomal membranes) causing alkalinization of vesicles and inhibiting proteases. This, in turn, inhibits T cell–macrophage interaction and impairs autoantigen presentation on MHC. In older studies, sometimes using very high drug concentrations, antimalarials inhibit chemotaxis, phagocytosis, and superoxide anion production.

Clinical pharmacology

Approximately 75% of an oral dose of HCQ or CQ is rapidly absorbed. HCQ has a long terminal elimination half-life of up to 7 to 40 days due to tissue uptake and trapping [76]. Thus, antimalarials have a large Vd. The liver metabolizes 30% to 60% of HCQ, with metabolites having even longer half-lives. Other tissue affinities, from lowest to highest, are fat red blood cells, muscle, brain, liver, spleen, and leukocytes. HCQ has the highest affinity for melanized tissue of the skin and retinal pigment [77].

HCQ metabolites are 50% bound to albumin, and HCQ is excreted via the kidneys (45%), intestine (5%), skin (7.3%), and feces (24%). Chloroquine binds more avidly to corneal tissue than does hydroxychloroquine. Because 45% of HCQ is renally excreted, it was suggested by the author of a 1983 paper that patients with renal insufficiency may have increased risk of retinal damage [78]. In addition, it was suggested that patients who are older, with declining renal function, should be monitored more closely. It is recommended that HCQ dosing not exceed 6.5 mg/kg/d and CQ dosing not to exceed 4 mg/kg/d. In addition, onset of action is slow and may take 6 months or even up to 9 months of therapy.

CQ decreases MTX levels secondary to increased gastric emptying, and may account for a decrease in hepatic toxicity when used in combination [79]. D-penicillamine concentrations increase by 34% in patients treated with CQ [80]. Antimalarials increase free digoxin levels by displacing digoxin from binding sites and by decreasing renal clearance as seen in two patients [81]. In addition, HCQ can increase the bioavailability of metoprolol. Cimetidine doubles the elimination half-life of HCQ in healthy volunteers [32].

There are no studies that have specifically examined the pharmacodynamics or pharmacokinetics in the elderly population.

Efficacy

Antimalarials have a relatively mild DMARD effect and slow onset of action compared with many other DMARDs. In placebo controlled studies by Davis et al in 1991 and Clark et al in 1993, HCQ was more effective than placebo but no inhibition of radiographic progression was found [82,83]. HCQ has been found to have less toxicity and efficacy than CQ by Avina-Zubieta et al [84]. Two meta-analyses demonstrated that antimalarial therapies were as effective as azathioprine and more effective than oral gold [38,85].

Toxicity

Antimalarials are generally well tolerated and have minimal serious side effects. The most concerning adverse reaction occurs very rarely, namely maculopathic retinopathy. Rarely, the retinal lesion progresses even after medication is withdrawn, and may result in blindness [31]. A confounding factor appears to be that age-related macular degeneration is similar to HCQ-related retinopathy.

Other side effects include gastrointestinal symptoms of nausea, abdominal discomfort, and diarrhea. Patients can develop rash and depigmentation. Tinnitus and headaches also can occur. Other rare but serious complications of anti-malarial medications include cardiomyopathy, heart block, and dyskinesias. This medication is considered to be safe in pregnancy, although it can cross the placenta.

Cytokine therapies

History

Biologic agents are the newest class of DMARDs and were specifically designed to target cytokines thought to play a major role in inflammation. There was a great deal of interest in tumor necrosis factor (TNF) inhibition, which was felt to play a large role in the pathogenesis of RA. Three different TNF inhibitors have been marketed: etanercept (ETN), infliximab (IFX), and adalimumab (ADA).

Mechanism of Action

TNF-α is a homotrimer produced intracellularly as a transmembrane protein, cleaved off by TNF-α converting enzyme (TACE). TNF-α has many functions including promoting synthesis of: adhesion molecules, proinflammatory cytokines, chemokines, matrix metalloproteinases, RANK ligand expression, promotion of angiogenesis, activation of cells (T cells, B cell, macrophages), and antiviral and antitumor effects [86]. Due to its pleiotrophic effects, TNF-α has been an attractive therapeutic candidate and is felt to play a central role in the pathogenesis of RA. Thus, inhibition of TNF-α blocks the effects of pro-inflammatory cytokines or enhances the anti-inflammatory cytokines. ETN is a receptor, while IFX and ADA are antibodies. ETN is produced in Chinese hamster ovary cell cultures and binds both TNF-α and lymphotoxin-α. IFX binds only to TNF-α, and has been shown to promote apoptosis of TNF receptor expressing cells in vitro. ADA is presumed to be more similar to IFX than ETN, although not much has been published with respect to ADA's specific mechanisms of action.

Another biologic agent that has been marketed for the treatment of RA is rhIL-1ra. IL-1 inhibition also blocks many of the same pathways as TNF-α. It was the first proinflammatory cytokine to be well characterized, and anakinra (ANK), an IL-1 inhibitor, has also been approved for use in RA. However, as will be described below, ANK has modest clinical effects in RA.

Clinical pharmacology

ETN is subcutaneously injected with a terminal half-life of between 4 to 12 days. IFX is administered intravenously and has a terminal half-life of 8 to 9.5 days. IFX generally is used in combination with some other DMARD because these DMARDs may block the development of human antichimeric antibodies (HACA). ADA is also subcutaneously injected and has a half life of 10 to 20 days. The pharmacokinetics of IFX or ADA have not been studied in the elderly patient. According to the package insert for ETN in 2001, the pharmacokinetics of ETN do not change with age.

Efficacy

The efficacy of ETN was demonstrated in four different clinical trials including a total of 2000 patients, with ongoing safety trials [87]. Greater efficacy has been shown with the use of the combination of ETN and MTX compared with either one alone [88]. FDA approval of IFX in combination with MTX to decrease HACA was based on 771 RA patients in five clinical trials. ADA was recently FDA approved in 2003 based on 2468 RA patients in 17 different clinical trials. Neutralizing human antihuman antibodies (HAHA) are occasionally seen in ADA treated patients and they decrease with the addition of MTX. TNF inhibitors have been shown to slow radiographic progression [87]. ANK was approved by the FDA based on five randomized placebo-controlled clinical trials with a total of 2932 RA patients. Dose-related increases of ANK have not been shown to increase efficacy in RA [86].

In 2002, Fleischmann et al [89] retrospectively analyzed 1128 patients treated with ETN in clinical trials to evaluate the safety and efficacy in elderly patients. Approximately 17% (197) of patients were above the age of 65, and their clinical response was not different than that in younger patients. ACR 20 responses were 66% for older RA patients and 69% for younger RA patients (after 1 year of treatment with ETN). However, this may not be a typical elderly population for few had comorbid conditions or polypharmacy.

Toxicity

The most common side effect of subcutaneous injections with biologic agents was injection side reactions (ISRs) ranging in incidence from 18.5% to 71%. These reactions cause discontinuation of therapy only rarely (ANK 7%, ETN <2%, ADA 0.3%) [67]. There is a 50% reduction of ISRs with the combination of ETN and MTX (unpublished data). Infusion reactions with IFX occur in up to 22% of patients within 1 to 2 hours after treatment (uriticaria, pruritus, rash, headache, flushing, fever, chills, nausea, tachycardia, shortness of breath), but cause discontinuation in only 2% of patients. Symptoms in those patients who discontinued IFX sometimes included feelings of chest tightness, bronchospasm, hypotension, diaphoresis, anaphylaxis or "impeding doom."

Infection is a concern with immunomodulatory biologic agents. In controlled clinical trials, one third of RA patients suffered from minor infections including upper respiratory infections, bronchitis, sinusitis, pharyngitis, and urinary tract infections [66,67]. These did not occur more frequently than in the placebo groups, however. In postmarketing surveillance registries, these infections occurred about twice as frequently as before the use of biologics. Serious infections were not common (eg, pneumonia, sepsis, cellulites, or joint infections). Tuberculosis (TB) and opportunistic infections have been a concern, with the knowledge that TNF-α is important in granuloma formation. The risk of reactivation of latent tuberculosis is increased when using TNF-blocking agents. Although numerical trends seem to implicate a reactivation among IFX users, these numbers are fraught with methodologic problems, and the best approach is to assume that this danger is present for all TNF-blocking agents. After screening for TB, appropriate prophylaxis should be initiated.

Use of TNF inhibitors with ANK is not advisable, with recent papers showing increased rate of serious infections when ANK and ETN were combined (with no increased benefit). Demyelinating disorders, hematologic effects (pancytopenia, aplastic anemia), and drug-induced lupus are rare, but have been described with TNF inhibitors [66,67,86]. TNF inhibitor therapy should be used with caution in patients with NYHA class II, III, or IV heart failure, due to increased CHF events, particularly at higher doses.

RA patients have a 2 to 23-fold increase in the rate of lymphoma and non-Hodgkin's lymphoma possibly dependent on disease activity. In a 2003 compilation of controlled clinical trials by the FDA, 6 of 6303 RA patients treated with TNF inhibitors were found to have lymphomas, compared with none in the placebo group. In follow-up of the same patients, a total of 23 lymphomas were observed, with an increased relative risk of 3.47 to 6.35. As these risks clearly overlap with the background risk of lymphomas in the RA population, it is still not clear if TNF-blocking agent-treated patients are exposed to an excessive lymphoma risk. ANK is not generally associated with lymphomas.

Fleischmann et al [89], in 2002, demonstrated that neither elderly nor younger RA patients tolerated ETN differently; injection site reactions, headache, and rhinitis were the only statistically different AEs, and were noted more in the younger RA patients.

Summary

During the 10-year period since the last review was done by Gardner and Furst [29], studies have furthered our knowledge regarding the pharmacokinetics of methotrexate in the elderly RA patient, and leflunomide and cytokine therapy have now become a part of our armamentarium. There has been some progress in understanding the elderly RA patient. Specifically, pharmacokinetics are different in the elderly and can affect AEs, especially as renal function and metabolism change in the elderly. There is insufficient good data for much confidence in DMARD effects in the elderly, and there is a need for concentration on sufficient numbers and good methodology. It is quite apparent that more work needs to be done in other areas as well. There are many areas where a lack of knowledge is obvious—what is the effect of polypharmacy and comorbidities on kinetics or dynamics in the older RA patient? Importantly, what is the effect of the previous confounders and age, per se, on cellular pharmacodynamics, an area that may be very critical in the elderly? Also, what about formal drug interaction studies? In addition, emerging therapies (CTLA-IgG, rituximab, and so on) are on the horizon for RA, further increasing the need and importance of doing additional specific studies in the one third of RA patients who are elderly.

Acknowledgments

The authors acknowledge Dr. Harold Paulus and Dr. Janet Elashoff for their valuable contribution and assistance in preparing this article.

References

[1] Fuchs HA, Kaye JJ, Callahan LF, et al. Evidence of significant radiographic damage in rheumatoid arthritis within the first 2 years of disease. J Rheumatol 1989;16(5):585–91.

[2] van der Heijde DM, van Leeuwen MA, van Riel PL, et al. Radiographic progression on radiographs of hands and feet during the first 3 years of rheumatoid arthritis measured according to Sharp's method (van der Heijde modification). J Rheumatol 1995;22(9):1792–6.

[3] Cobb S, Anderson F, Bauer W. Length of life and cause of death in rheumatoid arthritis. N Engl J Med 1953;249(14):553–6.

[4] Pincus T, Brooks RH, Callahan LF. Prediction of long-term mortality in patients with rheumatoid arthritis according to simple questionnaire and joint count measures. Ann Intern Med 1994; 120(1):26–34.

[5] Schnell A. The clinical features of rheumatic infection in the old. Acta Med Scand 1941; 106:345–51.

[6] Schmucker DL, Vesell ES. Are the elderly underrepresented in clinical drug trials? J Clin Pharmacol 1999;39(11):1103–8.

[7] Kavanaugh AF. Rheumatoid arthritis in the elderly: is it a different disease? Am J Med 1997; 103(6A):40S–8S.

[8] Beyth RJ, Shorr RI. Principles of drug therapy in older patients: rational drug prescribing. Clin Geriatr Med 2002;18(3):577–92.

[9] Chutka DS, Takahashi PY, Hoel RW. Inappropriate medications for elderly patients. Mayo Clin Proc 2004;79(1):122–39.

[10] Turnheim K. Drug dosage in the elderly. Is it rational? Drugs Aging 1998;13(5):357–79.

[11] Turnheim K. When drug therapy gets old: pharmacokinetics and pharmacodynamics in the elderly. Exp Gerontol 2003;38(8):843–53.

[12] Oberbauer R, Krivanek P, Turnheim K. Pharmacokinetics of indomethacin in the elderly. Clin Pharmacokinet 1993;24(5):428–34.

[13] Lonergan ET. Medications. In: Lonergan ET, editor. Geriatrics. New York: Appleton and Lange; 1996. p. 38–46.

[14] Morgan J, Furst DE. Implications of drug therapy in the elderly. Clin Rheum Dis 1986; 12(1):227–44.

[15] Percy LA, Fang MA. Geropharmacology for the rheumatologist. Rheum Dis Clin North Am 2000;26(3):433–4vi.

[16] Greenblatt DJ, Divoll M, Abernethy DR, et al. Antipyrine kinetics in the elderly: prediction of age-related changes in benzodiazepine oxidizing capacity. J Pharmacol Exp Ther 1982; 220(1):120–6.

[17] Sotaniemi EA, Arranto AJ, Pelkonen O, et al. Age and cytochrome P450-linked drug metabolism in humans: an analysis of 226 subjects with equal histopathologic conditions. Clin Pharmacol Ther 1997;61(3):331–9.

[18] Montamat SC, Cusack BJ, Vestal RE. Management of drug therapy in the elderly. N Engl J Med 1989;321(5):303–9.

[19] Noble RE. Drug therapy in the elderly. Metabolism 2003;52(10 Suppl 2):27–30.

[20] Gubner R. Therapeutic supression of tissue reactivity: I. Comparison of the effects of cortisone and aminopterin. Am J Med Sci 1951;221:169–75.

[21] Gubner R, August S, Ginsberg V. Therapeutic supression of tissue reactivity. II. Effect of amniopterin in rheumatoid arthritis and psoriasis. Am J Med Sci 1951;221:176–82.

[22] Andersen PA, West SG, O'Dell JR, et al. Weekly pulse methotrexate in rheumatoid arthritis. Clinical and immunologic effects in a randomized, double-blind study. Ann Intern Med 1985; 103(4):489–96.

[23] Thompson RN, Watts C, Edelman J, et al. A controlled two-centre trial of parenteral methotrexate therapy for refractory rheumatoid arthritis. J Rheumatol 1984;11(6):760–3.

[24] Weinblatt ME, Coblyn JS, Fox DA, et al. Efficacy of low-dose methotrexate in rheumatoid arthritis. N Engl J Med 1985;312(13):818–22.

[25] Williams HJ, Willkens RF, Samuelson Jr CO, et al. Comparison of low-dose oral pulse methotrexate and placebo in the treatment of rheumatoid arthritis. A controlled clinical trial. Arthritis Rheum 1985;28(7):721–30.

[26] Billington DC. Angiogenesis and its inhibition: potential new therapies in oncology and non-neoplastic diseases. Drug Des Discov 1991;8(1):3–35.

[27] Hirata S, Matsubara T, Saura R, et al. Inhibition of in vitro vascular endothelial cell proliferation and in vivo neovascularization by low-dose methotrexate. Arthritis Rheum 1989;32(9):1065–73.

[28] Svartz N. The treatment of rheumatic polyarthritis with acid azo compound. Rheumatism 1948: 56–60.

[29] Case JP. Old and new drugs used in rheumatoid arthritis: a historical perspective. Part 1: the older drugs. Am J Ther 2001;8(2):123–43.

[30] Drosos A. Methotrexate intolerance in elderly patients with rheumatoid arthritis: what are the alternatives? Drugs Aging 2003;20(10):723–36.

[31] Gardner G, Furst DE. Disease-modifying antirheumatic drugs. Potential effects in older patients. Drugs Aging 1995;7(6):420–37.

[32] Haagsma CJ. Clinically important drug interactions with disease-modifying antirheumatic drugs. Drugs Aging 1998;13(4):281–9.

[33] Bressolle F, Bologna C, Kinowski JM, et al. Total and free methotrexate pharmacokinetics in elderly patients with rheumatoid arthritis. A comparison with young patients. J Rheumatol 1997;24(10):1903–9.

[34] Bannwarth B, Labat L, Moride Y, et al. Methotrexate in rheumatoid arthritis. An update. Drugs 1994;47(1):25–50.

[35] Wolfe F, Hawley DJ, Cathey MA. Termination of slow acting antirheumatic therapy in rheumatoid arthritis: a 14-year prospective evaluation of 1017 consecutive starts. J Rheumatol 1990; 17(8):994–1002.

[36] Alarcon GS, Tracy IC, Blackburn Jr WD. Methotrexate in rheumatoid arthritis. Toxic effects as the major factor in limiting long-term treatment. Arthritis Rheum 1989;32(6):671–6.

[37] Alarcon GS, Lopez-Mendez A, Walter J, et al. Radiographic evidence of disease progression in methotrexate treated and nonmethotrexate disease modifying antirheumatic drug treated rheumatoid arthritis patients: a meta-analysis. J Rheumatol 1992;19(12):1868–73.

[38] Felson DT, Anderson JJ, Meenan RF. Use of short-term efficacy/toxicity tradeoffs to select second-line drugs in rheumatoid arthritis. A metaanalysis of published clinical trials. Arthritis Rheum 1992;35(10):1117–25.

[39] Furst DE. Rational use of disease-modifying antirheumatic drugs. Drugs 1990;39(1):19–37.

[40] The effect of age and renal function on the efficacy and toxicity of methotrexate in rheumatoid arthritis. Rheumatoid Arthritis Clinical Trial Archive Group. J Rheumatol 1995;22(2): 218–23.

[41] Wolfe F, Cathey MA. The effect of age on methotrexate efficacy and toxicity. J Rheumatol 1991;18(7):973–7.

[42] Hochberg MC, Silman AJ, Smoten JS, et al. Rheumatology. 3rd edition. New York: Mosby; 2003.

[43] Hirshberg B, Muszkat M, Schlesinger O, et al. Safety of low dose methotrexate in elderly patients with rheumatoid arthritis. Postgrad Med J 2000;76(902):787–9.

[44] Bologna C, Viu P, Jorgensen C, et al. Effect of age on the efficacy and tolerance of methotrexate in rheumatoid arthritis. Br J Rheumatol 1996;35(5):453–7.

[45] Nyfors A. Liver biopsies from psoriatics related to methotrexate therapy. 3. Findings in post-methotrexate liver biopsies from 160 psoriatics. Acta Pathol Microbiol Scand [A] 1977;85(4): 511–8.

[46] Roenigk Jr HH, Bergfeld WF, St Jacques R, et al. Hepatotoxicity of methotrexate in the treatment of psoriasis. Arch Dermatol 1971;103(3):250–61.

[47] Engelbrecht JA, Calhoon SL, Scherrer JJ. Methotrexate pneumonitis after low-dose therapy for rheumatoid arthritis. Arthritis Rheum 1983;26(10):1275–8.

[48] Sinclair RJG, Duthie JJR. Salazopyrin in the treatment of rheumatoid arthritis. Ann Rheum Dis 1948;8:226–31.

[49] McConkey B, Amos RS, Durham S, et al. Sulphasalazine in rheumatoid arthritis. BMJ 1980; 280(6212):442–4.

[50] Kitas GD, Farr M, Waterhouse L, et al. Influence of acetylator status on sulphasalazine efficacy and toxicity in patients with rheumatoid arthritis. Scand J Rheumatol 1992;21(5):220–5.

[51] Pullar T, Hunter JA, Capell HA. Effect of acetylator phenotype on efficacy and toxicity of sulphasalazine in rheumatoid arthritis. Ann Rheum Dis 1985;44(12):831–7.

[52] Taggart AJ, McDermott B, Delargy M, et al. The pharmacokinetics of sulphasalazine in young and elderly patients with rheumatoid arthritis. Scand J Rheumatol Suppl 1987;64:29–36.

[53] Sulfasalazine in early rheumatoid arthritis. The Australian Multicentre Clinical Trial Group. J Rheumatol 1992;19(11):1672–7.

[54] Hannonen P, Mottonen T, Hakola M, et al. Sulfasalazine in early rheumatoid arthritis. A 48-week double-blind, prospective, placebo-controlled study. Arthritis Rheum 1993;36(11):1501–9.

[55] Nuver-Zwart IH, van Riel PL, van de Putte LB, et al. A double blind comparative study of sulphasalazine and hydroxychloroquine in rheumatoid arthritis: evidence of an earlier effect of sulphasalazine. Ann Rheum Dis 1989;48(5):389–95.

[56] Pinals RS, Kaplan SB, Lawson JG, et al. Sulfasalazine in rheumatoid arthritis. A double-blind, placebo-controlled trial. Arthritis Rheum 1986;29(12):1427–34.

[57] Smolen JS, Kalden JR, Scott DL, et al. Efficacy and safety of leflunomide compared with placebo and sulphasalazine in active rheumatoid arthritis: a double-blind, randomised, multicentre trial. European Leflunomide Study Group. Lancet 1999;353(9149):259–66.

[58] Williams HJ, Ward JR, Dahl SL, et al. A controlled trial comparing sulfasalazine, gold sodium thiomalate, and placebo in rheumatoid arthritis. Arthritis Rheum 1988;31(6):702–13.

[59] Pullar T, Hunter JA, Capell HA. Sulphasalazine in rheumatoid arthritis: a double blind comparison of sulphasalazine with placebo and sodium aurothiomalate. Br Med J (Clin Res Ed) 1983;287(6399):1102–4.

[60] Haagsma CJ, van Riel PL, de Jong AJ, et al. Combination of sulphasalazine and methotrexate versus the single components in early rheumatoid arthritis: a randomized, controlled, double-blind, 52 week clinical trial. Br J Rheumatol 1997;36(10):1082–8.

[61] Figlin E, Chetrit A, Shahar A, et al. High prevalences of vitamin B12 and folic acid deficiency in elderly subjects in Israel. Br J Haematol 2003;123(4):696–701.

[62] Hurdle AD, Williams TC. Folic-acid deficiency in elderly patients admitted to hospital. BMJ 1966;5507:202–5.

[63] Bartlett RR, Schleyerbach R. Immunopharmacological profile of a novel isoxazol derivative, HWA 486, with potential antirheumatic activity–I. Disease modifying action on adjuvant arthritis of the rat. Int J Immunopharmacol 1985;7:7–18.

[64] Tucker KL, Mahnken B, Wilson PW, et al. Folic acid fortification of the food supply. Potential benefits and risks for the elderly population. JAMA 1996;276(23):1879–85.

[65] Wilkieson CA, Madhok R, Hunter JA, et al. Toleration, side-effects and efficacy of sul-phasalazine in rheumatoid arthritis patients of different ages. Q J Med 1993;86(8):501–5.

[66] Case JP. Old and new drugs used in rheumatoid arthritis: a historical perspective. Part 2: the newer drugs and drug strategies. Am J Ther 2001;8(3):163–79.

[67] Cush JJ. Safety overview of new disease-modifying antirheumatic drugs. Rheum Dis Clin North Am 2004;30(2):237–55.

[68] Manna SK, Aggarwal BB. Immunosuppressive leflunomide metabolite (A77 1726) blocks TNF-dependent nuclear factor-kappa B activation and gene expression. J Immunol 1999;162(4): 2095–102.

[69] Fox RI. Mechanism of action of leflunomide in rheumatoid arthritis. J Rheumatol Suppl 1998; 53:20–6.

[70] Cohen S, Cannon GW, Schiff M, et al. Two-year, blinded, randomized, controlled trial of treatment of active rheumatoid arthritis with leflunomide compared with methotrexate. Utilization of Leflunomide in the Treatment of Rheumatoid Arthritis Trial Investigator Group. Arthritis Rheum 2001;44(9):1984–92.

[71] Mladenovic V, Domljan Z, Rozman B, et al. Safety and effectiveness of leflunomide in the treat-ment of patients with active rheumatoid arthritis. Results of a randomized, placebo-controlled, phase II study. Arthritis Rheum 1995;38(11):1595–603.

[72] Payne JF. A postgraduate lecture on lupus erythematosus. Clin J 1984;4:223–9.

[73] Strand V, Cohen S, Schiff M, et al. Treatment of active rheumatoid arthritis with leflunomide compared with placebo and methotrexate. Leflunomide Rheumatoid Arthritis Investigators Group. Arch Intern Med 1999;159(21):2542–50.

[74] Weinblatt ME, Kremer JM, Coblyn JS, et al. Pharmacokinetics, safety, and efficacy of com-bination treatment with methotrexate and leflunomide in patients with active rheumatoid arthritis. Arthritis Rheum 1999;42(7):1322–8.

[75] Chan J, Sanders DC, Du L, et al. Leflunomide-associated pancytopenia with or without metho-trexate. Ann Pharmacother 2004;38(7–8):1206–11.

[76] Furst DE. Pharmacokinetics of hydroxychloroquine and chloroquine during treatment of rheumatic diseases. Lupus 1996;5(Suppl 1):S11–5.

[77] Sturrock Rd. Disease-modifying antirheumatic drugs 1: antimalarials, gold and penicillamine. In: Hochberg MC, Silman AJ, Smolen JS, Weinblatt ME, Weismann MH, editors. Rheuma-tology. St. Louis (MO): Mosby; 2004. p. 399–403.

[78] Ferris III FL. Senile macular degeneration: review of epidemiologic features. Am J Epidemiol 1983;118(2):132–51.

[79] Seideman P, Albertioni F, Beck O, Peterson C, et al. Chloroquine reduces the bioavailability of methotrexate in patients with rheumatoid arthritis. A possible mechanism of reduced hepa-totoxicity. Arthritis Rheum 1994;37(6):830–3.

[80] Seideman P, Lindstrom B. Pharmacokinetic interactions of penicillamine in rheumatoid arthritis. J Rheumatol 1989;16(4):473–4.

[81] Leden I. Digoxin-hydroxychloroquine interaction? Acta Med Scand 1982;211(5):411–2.

[82] Clark P, Casas E, Tugwell P, et al. Hydroxychloroquine compared with placebo in rheumatoid arthritis. A randomized controlled trial. Ann Intern Med 1993;119(11):1067–71.

[83] Davis MJ, Dawes PT, Fowler PD, et al. Should disease-modifying agents be used in mild rheumatoid arthritis? Br J Rheumatol 1991;30(6):451–4.

[84] Avina-Zubieta JA, Galindo-Rodriguez G, Newman S, et al. Long-term effectiveness of antimalarial drugs in rheumatic diseases. Ann Rheum Dis 1998;57(10):582–7.

[85] Felson DT, Anderson JJ, Meenan RF. The comparative efficacy and toxicity of second-line drugs in rheumatoid arthritis. Results of two metaanalyses. Arthritis Rheum 1990;33(10):1449–61.

[86] Cush JJ. Cytokine therapies. In: Hochberg MC, Silman AJ, Smolen JS, Weinblatt ME, Weisman MH, editors. Rheumatology. St. Louis (MO): Mosby; 2003. p. 461–84.

[87] Klarenskog L, Moreland LM, Cohen SB, et al. Global sefety and efficacy of up to five years of etanercept (Enbrel) therapy. Arthritis Rheum 2001;44:S77.

[88] Weinblatt ME, Kremer JM, Bankhurst AD, et al. A trial of etanercept, a recombinant tumor

necrosis factor receptor:Fc fusion protein, in patients with rheumatoid arthritis receiving methotrexate. N Engl J Med 1999;340(4):253–9.

[89] Fleischmann RM, Baumgartner SW, Tindall EA, et al. Response to etanercept (Enbrel) in elderly patients with rheumatoid arthritis: a retrospective analysis of clinical trial results. J Rheumatol 2003;30(4):691–6.

ELSEVIER
SAUNDERS

Clin Geriatr Med 21 (2005) 671–675

CLINICS IN
GERIATRIC
MEDICINE

Index

Note: Page numbers of article titles are in **boldface** type.

Changing Your Address?

Make sure your subscription changes too! When you notify us of your new address, you can help make our job easier by including an exact copy of your Clinics label number with your old address (see illustration below.) This number identifies you to our computer system and will speed the processing of your address change. Please be sure this label number accompanies your old address and your corrected address—you can send an old Clinics label with your number on it or just copy it exactly and send it to the address listed below.

We appreciate your help in our attempt to give you continuous coverage. Thank you.

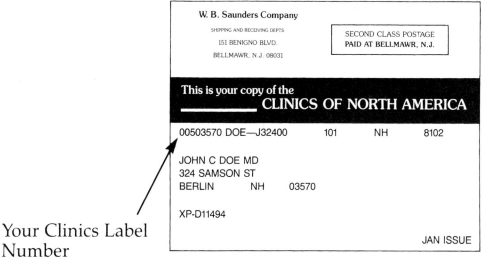

Your Clinics Label Number
Copy it exactly or send your label along with your address to:
W.B. Saunders Company, Customer Service
Orlando, FL 32887-4800
Call Toll Free 1-800-654-2452

Please allow four to six weeks for delivery of new subscriptions and for processing address changes.